PUBLIC HEALTH IN THE 21ST CENTURY

HEALTH EFFECTS OF MENTHOL CIGARETTES

AN EVALUATION OF EXISTING DATA AND RESEARCH

PUBLIC HEALTH IN THE 21ST CENTURY

Additional books in this series can be found on Nova's website under the Series tab.

Additional e-books in this series can be found on Nova's website under the e-book tab.

PUBLIC HEALTH IN THE 21ST CENTURY

HEALTH EFFECTS OF MENTHOL CIGARETTES

AN EVALUATION OF EXISTING DATA AND RESEARCH

MARK C. ELDRIDGE
AND
EDWARD FORESTER
EDITORS

New York

For permission to use material from this book please contact us:
Telephone 631-231-7269; Fax 631-231-8175
Web Site: http://www.novapublishers.com

Library of Congress Cataloging-in-Publication Data

ISBN: 978-1-62948-291-0

Published by Nova Science Publishers, Inc. † New York

Contents

Preface vii

Chapter 1 Preliminary Scientific Evaluation of the Possible Public Health Effects of Menthol Versus Nonmenthol Cigarettes **1**
Food and Drug Administration

Chapter 2 Reference Addendum: Preliminary Scientific Evaluation of the Possible Public Health Effects of Menthol versus Nonmenthol Cigarettes **165**
Food and Drug Administration

Index **225**

Preface

Menthol is widely used in consumer and medicinal products and has long been used in cigarettes, often as a flavor-characterizing additive. In medical products, menthol is regulated as a drug with restrictions on allowable doses and use. There are no product standards for menthol when used in cigarettes. In this report, The FDA has undertaken a thorough review of the available science concerning menthol cigarettes. To accomplish this task, FDA weighed the collective body of evidence for the impact of the use of menthol in cigarettes on public health. In reviewing the science of menthol smoking, FDA divided the scientific evidence into the following broad categories: smoke chemistry and nonclinical toxicology; physiology; biomarkers; patterns of use; marketing and consumer perception of risk; initiation and progression to regular use; dependence; cessation; and disease risk.

Chapter 1 – Menthol is widely used in consumer and medicinal products and has long been used in cigarettes, often as a flavor-characterizing additive. In medical products, menthol is regulated as a drug with restrictions on allowable doses and use. There are no product standards for menthol when used in cigarettes.

Approximately one-fourth of all cigarettes sold in the United States are menthol (Giovino, 2004). The vast majority (88%) of adult smokers in the United States start to smoke before age 18 (U.S. Department of Health and Human Services, 2012). Thus, youth and young adulthood appear to be a critical age-span for initiation of cigarette smoking, and research suggests that menthol cigarettes may have an impact on initiation rates that differ from nonmenthol cigarettes. Further, the impact of menthol cigarettes on dependence, cessation, and health risks has been the topic of scientific inquiry and intense debate.

The Federal Food, Drug, and Cosmetic Act (FD&C Act) (Section 907 (e)) requires FDA's Tobacco Products Scientific Advisory Committee (TPSAC) to submit a report and recommendation to the Secretary of Health and Human Services (HHS) on the impact of the use of menthol in cigarettes on public health – including use among children, women, African Americans, Hispanics, and other racial or ethnic minorities – by March 23, 2011. In March 2010, TPSAC began its process of reviewing the available evidence as well as soliciting and receiving valuable input from researchers, tobacco industry representatives, consultants to the tobacco industry, representatives of the public health sector, and others. On July 21, 2011, TPSAC voted on its final report and recommendations on menthol, which concluded "removal of menthol cigarettes from the marketplace would benefit public health in the United States." TPSAC noted that a variety of options were available for FDA to consider, and they made no specific suggestions for follow-up by FDA should the agency decide it should pursue this recommendation. In addition, the non-voting industry representatives of TPSAC submitted a separate document reflecting the industry perspective. That document acknowledged the inherent risks of all tobacco products, including those that have menthol as a characterizing flavor, and raised the possibility of countervailing effects, including potential risks of contraband menthol products, should a ban be imposed.

Independently, FDA has undertaken a thorough review of the available science concerning menthol cigarettes. To accomplish this task, FDA weighed the collective body of evidence for the impact of the use of menthol in cigarettes on public health. One of the first considerations in weighing the value of a particular study was the relevance of the information to the consumption of menthol cigarettes in the United States. Findings that were replicated in different studies, especially different types of studies, were given greater weight. FDA also considered the source of information, the type of study, and the quality of study methods and data. In drawing conclusions, more consideration was given to peer-reviewed studies, studies in humans, and studies that were appropriately powered and designed. In this process, FDA evaluated the peer- reviewed literature, industry submissions and other materials provided to TPSAC, and performed or commissioned additional analyses in an attempt to fill in and inform some of the gaps in the literature.

Chapter 2 – The "Preliminary Scientific Evaluation of the Possible Public Health Effects of Menthol versus Nonmenthol Cigarettes" was submitted for Peer Review in August 2011. Since that time, several peer-reviewed articles have been published that relate to this topic. This reference addendum provides a summary of updated research relevant to the full scientific review. On March 27, 2013, a systematic literature search was conducted in the PubMed database using the search term "menthol" and including articles published between July 1, 2011 and March 27, 2013.

As with the full scientific review, only original peer-reviewed publications were used. Basic information on menthol has been included here only as background; as with the full scientific review, this addendum is not intended to be a comprehensive review of menthol itself but rather menthol as related to its use in menthol cigarettes. General methodology caveats (e.g., self-report) and descriptions (e.g., TRPM8 channels, large national surveys) were discussed in the full scientific review, and will not be duplicated here.

In: Health Effects of Menthol Cigarettes
Editors: Mark C. Eldridge and Edward Forester
ISBN: 978-1-62948-291-0

Chapter 1

Preliminary Scientific Evaluation of the Possible Public Health Effects of Menthol Versus Nonmenthol Cigarettes*

Food and Drug Administration

I. Executive Summary

Menthol is widely used in consumer and medicinal products and has long been used in cigarettes, often as a flavor-characterizing additive. In medical products, menthol is regulated as a drug with restrictions on allowable doses and use. There are no product standards for menthol when used in cigarettes.

Approximately one-fourth of all cigarettes sold in the United States are menthol (Giovino, 2004). The vast majority (88%) of adult smokers in the United States start to smoke before age 18 (U.S. Department of Health and Human Services, 2012). Thus, youth and young adulthood appear to be a critical age-span for initiation of cigarette smoking, and research suggests that menthol cigarettes may have an impact on initiation rates that differ from nonmenthol cigarettes. Further, the impact of menthol cigarettes on dependence, cessation, and health risks has been the topic of scientific inquiry and intense debate.

The Federal Food, Drug, and Cosmetic Act (FD&C Act) (Section 907 (e)) requires FDA's Tobacco Products Scientific Advisory Committee (TPSAC) to submit a report and recommendation to the Secretary of Health and Human Services (HHS) on the impact of the use of menthol in cigarettes on public health – including use among children, women, African Americans, Hispanics, and other racial or ethnic minorities – by March 23, 2011. In March 2010, TPSAC began its process of reviewing the available evidence as well as soliciting and receiving valuable input from researchers, tobacco industry representatives,

* This is an edited, reformatted and augmented version of a Food and Drug Administration publication, dated August 2011.

consultants to the tobacco industry, representatives of the public health sector, and others. On July 21, 2011, TPSAC voted on its final report and recommendations on menthol, which concluded "removal of menthol cigarettes from the marketplace would benefit public health in the United States." TPSAC noted that a variety of options were available for FDA to consider, and they made no specific suggestions for follow-up by FDA should the agency decide it should pursue this recommendation. In addition, the non-voting industry representatives of TPSAC submitted a separate document reflecting the industry perspective. That document acknowledged the inherent risks of all tobacco products, including those that have menthol as a characterizing flavor, and raised the possibility of countervailing effects, including potential risks of contraband menthol products, should a ban be imposed.

Independently, FDA has undertaken a thorough review of the available science concerning menthol cigarettes. To accomplish this task, FDA weighed the collective body of evidence for the impact of the use of menthol in cigarettes on public health. One of the first considerations in weighing the value of a particular study was the relevance of the information to the consumption of menthol cigarettes in the United States. Findings that were replicated in different studies, especially different types of studies, were given greater weight. FDA also considered the source of information, the type of study, and the quality of study methods and data. In drawing conclusions, more consideration was given to peer-reviewed studies, studies in humans, and studies that were appropriately powered and designed. In this process, FDA evaluated the peer- reviewed literature, industry submissions and other materials provided to TPSAC, and performed or commissioned additional analyses in an attempt to fill in and inform some of the gaps in the literature.

In making its assessment, FDA used a "weight of scientific evidence" approach. Studies were evaluated to determine the strength of both negative and positive associations of menthol in cigarettes with the impact under consideration. Scientific determinations fell into one of five categories, where x is the impact under consideration:

- The weight of evidence supports the conclusion that menthol in cigarettes is associated with x
- The weight of evidence supports the conclusion that menthol in cigarettes is likely associated with x
- The weight of evidence supports the conclusion that menthol in cigarettes is likely not associated with x
- The weight of evidence supports the conclusion that menthol in cigarettes is not associated with x
- The evidence is not sufficient to support a conclusion of an association of menthol in cigarettes with x

The purpose of this evaluation was to determine whether there are independent associations between menthol in cigarettes and various outcomes of interest. In doing so, FDA evaluated the weight of evidence, taking into account potential threats to validity, such as bias or confounding, and whether the findings were generalizable to the U.S. population The evaluations were not an attempt to establish causality. In reviewing the science of menthol smoking, FDA divided the scientific evidence into the following broad categories:

Smoke Chemistry and Nonclinical Toxicology: This review assessed information on *in vitro* and *in vivo* studies, as well as studies that examined menthol alone or tobacco smoke from menthol cigarettes. Two particular areas of interest were the comparison of menthol to nonmenthol cigarettes and whether the addition of menthol impacted the presence and levels of harmful and potential harmful constituents in the smoke. The studies examined did not show increased toxicity in menthol cigarettes compared to the already-toxic nonmenthol cigarettes. From the available studies, the weight of evidence supports the conclusion that, from a nonclinical toxicity standpoint, menthol in cigarettes is not associated with increased or decreased smoke toxicity.

Physiology: FDA considered information on menthol's effect on cooling, desensitization, anesthesia, and potential effect on nicotine and tobacco specific nitrosamines (TSNAs). FDA reviewed both *in vitro* and *in vivo* studies in human and animal models. In addition, analysts reviewed studies looking at the effect of menthol on smoking topography. There are some *in vivo* and *in vitro* studies that show menthol has cooling, desensitizating, and proanalgesic effects. Menthol acts primarily through receptors on sensory nerves. From the available studies, the weight of evidence supports the conclusion that menthol in cigarettes is likely associated with altered physiological responses to tobacco smoke.

Biomarkers: FDA analyzed studies measuring biomarkers of exposure in smokers of menthol and nonmenthol cigarettes. Biomarkers included levels of smoke constituents or their metabolites in exhaled air, saliva, blood, and urine such as expired carbon monoxide (CO) and plasma carboxyhemoglobin (COHb) for levels of CO exposure; cotinine (main nicotine metabolite) and other nicotine equivalents in plasma and urine for exposure to nicotine. Some studies show that smoking menthol cigarettes modulates the exposure or metabolism of nicotine and tobacco-specific nitrosamines (TSNAs), while other studies fail to show a significant association. From the available studies, the weight of evidence supports the conclusion that menthol in cigarettes is likely not associated with increased or decreased levels of biomarkers of exposure.

Patterns of Use: FDA reviewed scientific literature focusing on the general trends and patterns in menthol smoking. Articles reporting data on national estimates or very large representative populations were given highest priority in order to draw estimations of patterns of use that would be applicable and generalizable for the U.S. population overall. Data support that a majority of African American smokers smoke menthol cigarettes, but other minority groups are also more likely to smoke menthol cigarettes as compared to Whites. Further, younger populations have the highest rate of smoking menthol cigarettes, and female smokers are more likely to smoke menthol cigarettes than male smokers. Also, the use of menthol cigarettes is associated with lower socioeconomic status (SES). From the available studies, the weight of evidence supports the conclusion that menthol in cigarettes is associated with particular patterns of smoking.

Marketing and Consumer Perception of risk: FDA reviewed studies of brand preference, advertising receptivity, marketing strategies, and consumer perception of risk in an effort to determine what role, if any, marketing and consumer perception of risk play in the use of menthol cigarettes. Of particular interest was whether there is a stronger relationship between marketing and/or consumer perceptions and the use of menthol among subpopulations (e.g., youth, African Americans, Hispanics, women). The available data show that advertising is a strong driver of brand preference among adolescents and that it is likely that the standard marketing mix approach of price, promotion, product, and place has been used to drive menthol cigarette preference among the urban African American community. From the available studies, the weight of evidence supports the conclusion that, like nonmenthol cigarettes, the marketing of menthol cigarettes is associated with brand preference. The marketing of menthol cigarettes is associated with menthol brand preference among adolescents and the African American community. Given the limited data reviewed and mixed results reported, the weight of evidence is not sufficient to support a conclusion that consumer perceptions are associated with the use of menthol cigarettes.

Initiation and Progression to Regular Use: FDA assessed data on the possible impact of menthol cigarettes on initiation and progress to regular use of cigarette smoking with a particular focus on smoking behavior by youth and young adults. Included in the analysis were studies looking at differences in prevalence rates, age of first cigarette, and progression to regular smoking. Data show that newer smokers prefer menthol at levels substantially above that of the general population, with an inverse correlation between age and menthol preference that reaches a plateau in adulthood. From the available studies, the weight of evidence supports the conclusion that menthol in cigarettes is likely associated with increased initiation and progression to regular of cigarette smoking.

Dependence: FDA reviewed studies utilizing a variety of measures of nicotine dependence and/or craving. This included studies measuring: time to first cigarette (TTFC), cigarettes per day (cpd), the Fagerström Test for Nicotine Dependence (FTND), and craving.

Night waking to smoke was also included since it is emerging as a reliable indicator of strength of dependence. Data are included on other scales of nicotine dependence and craving if there were direct menthol versus nonmenthol assessments. There were consistent findings that menthol smokers are more likely to smoke their first cigarette within five minutes of waking. From the available studies, the weight of evidence supports the conclusion that menthol in cigarettes is likely associated with increased dependence.

Cessation: FDA analyzed studies addressing questions of whether menthol smokers were differentially successful in smoking cessation. These included cross-sectional studies, community-based or population-based prospective cohort studies, and clinical trial cessation studies. None of the studies were specifically designed to prospectively evaluate the effect of menthol on cessation. Several of the studies that failed to find an association between menthol smoking and cessation may have "over-adjusted" their analyses by controlling for the level of dependence. In the reviewed studies, menthol smokers, especially African American menthol smokers, were less likely to successfully stop smoking than their nonmenthol smoking counterparts. This is consistent with the observation that menthol smokers appear to be more nicotine dependent than nonmenthol smokers which can be an important factor in smoking cessation success. From the available studies, the weight of evidence supports the conclusion that menthol in cigarettes is likely associated with reduced success in smoking cessation, especially among African American menthol smokers.

Disease Risk: FDA analyzed studies that addressed the impact of smoking menthol cigarettes on disease risk as compared to those risks posed by smoking nonmenthol cigarettes. Studies investigating impact on lung cancer, non-lung smoking-related cancers (esophageal cancer, oropharyngeal cancer), cardiovascular disease, and respiratory outcomes in addition to one study that evaluated health wellness and health conditions such as body mass index (BMI) and emergency room visits were reviewed. No studies found an increased risk of cancer or non-cancer diseases in menthol smokers compared to nonmenthol smokers. From the available studies, the weight of evidence supports the conclusion that menthol in cigarettes is not associated with an increase in disease risk to the user compared to non-menthol cigarette smokers.

Summary of Evidence. The impact of cigarette smoking upon public health is indisputable. More than 400,000 deaths per year in the United States are caused by tobacco use. Consistent patterns have emerged as a result of FDA's evaluation of the scientific evidence relevant to the impact of menthol tobacco products on public health. While there is little evidence to suggest that menthol cigarettes are more or less toxic or contribute to more disease risk to the user than nonmenthol cigarettes, adequate data suggest that menthol use is likely associated with increased smoking initiation by youth and young adults. Further, the data indicate that menthol in cigarettes is likely associated with greater addiction. Menthol smokers show greater signs of nicotine dependence and are less likely to successfully quit smoking. These findings, combined with the evidence indicating that menthol's cooling and anesthetic properties can reduce the harshness of cigarette smoke and the evidence indicating that menthol cigarettes are marketed as a smoother alternative to nonmenthol cigarettes, make it likely that menthol cigarettes pose a public health risk above that seen with nonmenthol cigarettes.

This document is a scientific assessment of public health issues related to the use of menthol in cigarettes. This document does not constitute a decision about what regulatory action, if any, FDA might take with respect to menthol in cigarettes. If FDA determines, after reviewing all of the available information from this assessment and the anticipated public comments, from the TPSAC report and associated public comments, and from the tobacco industry perspective document, that restrictions on the sale and/or distribution of menthol cigarettes or product standards should be established, the Agency would do so pursuant to rulemaking procedures that include public notice and an opportunity for public comment. There is no required deadline or timeline for FDA to make a determination about what regulatory action, if any, is appropriate.

References

Giovino, GA, Sidney, S, Gfroerer, JC, O'Malley, PM Allen, JA. et al. (2004) Epidemiology of menthol cigarette use. Nicotine and Tobacco Research 6 Suppl 1:S67-S81. [No funding source(s) provided. Authors affiliated with the Roswell Park Cancer Institute, Kaiser Permanente Medical Care Program, Substance Abuse and Mental Health Services Administration, University of Michigan, American Legacy Foundation, Centers for Diease Control and Prevention]

U.S. Department of Health and Human Services (2012). Preventing tobacco use among youth and young adults – A report of the Surgeon General. Rockville, MD.

II. Science Reviews

The following is a list of abbreviations commonly used in this report:

1-OHP: 1-hydroxypyrene
3-HPMA: 3-hydroxypropyl mercapturic acid
3OH: 3-hydroxy
4-ABP: 4-ABP
AOR: Adjusted odds ratio
BMI: Body Mass Index
CARDIA: Coronary Artery Risk Development in Young Adults
CDC: Centers for Disease Control and Prevention
CI: Confidence interval
CO: Carbon monoxide
COHb: carboxyhemoglobin
COMMIT: Community Intervention Trial for Smoking Cessation
COPD: Chronic obstructive pulmonary disease
CPD: Cigarettes per day
CPS-TUS: Tobacco Use Supplement to the Current Population Survey
DHBMA: 1, 2-dihydroxybutyl mercapturic acid
FDA: Food and Drug Administration
FEV1: Forced expiratory volume in one second
FTC: Federal Trade Commission
FTND: Fagerstrom Test for Nicotine Dependence
FVC: Forced vital capacity
HDL: high-density lipoprotein
HHS: Health and Human Services
HR:Hazard Ratio
LDL: low-density lipoprotein
MCh: methacholine
MHBMA: monohydroxy-3-butenyl mercapturic acids
MTF: Monitoring the Future Survey
NDI: National Death Index
NE: Nicotine equivalents
NHANES: National Health and Nutrition Examination Survey
NHIS: National Health Information Survey
NHIS-CCS: National Health Interview Survey – Cancer Control Supplement
NHIS-LMF: National Health Interview Survey Linked Mortality File
NNAL: 4-(Methylnitrosamino)-1-(3-pyridyl)-1-butanol
NSDUH: National Survey on Drug Use and Health
NTP: National Toxicology Program
NYTS: National Youth Tobacco Survey
OR: Odds ratio
RTI: Research Triangle Institute
SES: Socio-economic status
TDC: Tar delivery category
TES: Total Exposure Study
TPSAC: Tobacco Products Scientific Advisory Committee
TSNA: Tobacco specific nitroamine
TTFC: Time to first cigarette upon waking

A. Smoke Chemistry and Nonclinical Toxicology

Scientific studies have investigated the smoke chemistry and nonclinical toxicology of nonmenthol cigarettes, but very few studies have directly compared the exposure of nonmenthol cigarettes to menthol cigarettes. Nonmenthol cigarettes produce an array of harmful chemicals during combustion and result in significant and substantial toxicological effects. Studies that evaluate whether menthol cigarettes produce greater quantities of harmful chemicals or result in more pronounced toxicological outcomes are limited. FDA reviewed scientific papers in order to examine differences in the smoke chemistry and nonclinical toxicology.

Smoke Chemistry

The comparison of menthol to nonmenthol cigarettes is of interest to determine if the addition of menthol impacts the presence or measured levels of and occurrence of harmful smoke constituents. Schmeltz and Schlotzhauer (1968) evaluated the pyrolysis of menthol and reported the formation of phenols and polyaromatic hydrocarbons. But their study examined the pyrolysis of menthol alone and not as part of the process of burning tobacco. So while it is informative, it must be interpreted with this consideration.

In two papers from 2004, Baker et al. reported only minimal differences in harmful smoke constituents. They reported their results normalized to the levels of total particulate matter in smoke which provides relative increases or decreases between constituents, but does not necessarily reflect overall changes to the amount of harmful smoke constituents delivered per cigarette.

They reported an increase in aldehydes in the smoke from the menthol cigarettes, likely due to the combustion of simple and complex sugars, as well as increased lead. Some constituents were lower compared to the nonmenthol cigarette, such as benzo[a]pyrene. From the limited data and differences in how these data can be interpreted, there is a lack of evidence showing that menthol in cigarettes yields substantial changes in smoke chemistry.

Menthol as a Singular Compound – Toxicology, Pharmacology and Therapeutic Applications

A review of the National Toxicology Program (NTP) database (Ashby and Tennant, 1991) shows that menthol has neither a structural alert for DNA reactivity or mutagenic activity. Menthol is listed in the database as Level F on their carcinogenicity scale, which indicates that adequate tests have been conducted and the compound is concluded to be non-carcinogenic.

The racemic mixture of menthol was tested in an Ames, sister chromatid exchange and chromosomal aberration assays. In these studies, menthol alone had no effect under the conditions of these assays (Ishidate et al., 1984; Ivett et al., 1989; and Murthy et al., 1991).

Rabinoff et al. (2007) reviewed industry documents looking for information on the pharmacological activity of tobacco additives. Possible effects listed for menthol include anesthetic action, complex interaction with nicotine, and increase in P1-N2 amplitudes, an objective electrophysiological measure of brain activity.

Harris (2006) presented a review of the therapeutic applications of menthol alone, based on the interaction at the thermoreceptor. Some therapeutic actions discussed include local anesthesia, nasal decongestant and cough relief.

Antiproliferative Effects of Menthol as a Singular Compound

There were several papers that examined the effects of menthol on *in vitro* cell proliferation and have shown that in several cancer cell lines, menthol had a significant growth inhibition effect (Bernhardt et al., 2008; Li et al., 2009; Lu et al., 2006; Lu et al., 2007; Sidell et al., 1991; Tatman and Mo 2002; Yamamura et al., 2008; and Zhang and Barritt 2004).

Ruch and Sigler (1994) examined a mechanism for terpene-induced growth inhibition of rat liver epithelial cells and found that while some terpenes (such as limonene and pinene) appeared to inhibit 3-hydroxy-3-methylglutaryl CoA reductase and mevalonic acid synthesis, menthol did not act through this mechanism. It is important to note that any anti-proliferative effects of menthol have been shown with menthol alone, and not with menthol in combination with tobacco or in a smoke condensate.

In fact, as has already been stated, menthol smoke condensate from burned tobacco is genotoxic. Additionally, one should not assume that a compound that had anti-proliferative effects in a tumor cell line or even in a transfected animal model would definitively have oncolytic effects in humans.

In vitro studies have examined the pharmacological activity of menthol to help elucidate the mechanism by which it had antiproliferative effects (Kim et al., 2009; Li et al., 2009; Yamamura et al., 2008; and Zhang and Barritt 2004). These studies all show that menthol acts at the transient receptor potential melastatin 8 (TRPM8) thermoreceptor. Activation of this receptor appears to increase intracellular Ca^{2+} levels by increasing the influx of extracellular Ca^{2+} through this channel. These studies also showed the antiproliferative effects of menthol in tumor cell lines.

Lu et al. (2006) showed increased Ca^{2+} levels in human leukemia cells treated with menthol and showed that the decreased cell growth seen could be blocked by the calcium chelator, BAPTA. This is further evidence of the link between the antiproliferative effects of menthol and the increase in intracellular Ca^{2+} that it has been shown to cause cell death.

Sidell et al. (1991) also showed menthol down-regulated the IL-6 receptors in a human myeloma cell line.

In Vitro Toxicity of Menthol Tobacco Exposure

Several reports reviewed here have examined smoke condensate from menthol cigarettes and found no increase in mutagenicity, clastogenicity or cytotoxicity when compared to a comparable nonmenthol cigarette. This was done with mainstream and sidestream smoke, with the same results. Some studies also included cigarettes that heat, but do not burn the tobacco as test cigarettes.

These heated cigarettes included menthol and nonmenthol versions. All the cigarettes in which the tobacco was burned were positive in these assays, and cigarettes with added ingredients such as menthol were not significantly different from the control (Baker et al., 2004; Doolittle et al., 1990a and 1990b; Ivett et al., 1989; and Roemer et al., 2002). The cigarettes that heat tobacco but do not burn it were negative in these assays with and without menthol added (Doolittle et al., 1990a and 1990b; Lee et al., 1990).

Other *in vitro* assays showed menthol to be toxic at concentrations greater than 0.1 mM (Bernson and Pettersson 1983). This application produced lesions in biological membranes in the isolated mitochondria assay and increased the permeability over the inner mitochondrial membrane. While interesting, the relevance of these studies to menthol exposure via menthol cigarettes is not strong, as menthol overdose is not likely via this exposure.

In Vivo Toxicity of Menthol Tobacco Exposure

Several studies reported on *in vivo* inhalation toxicity studies with test cigarettes that had menthol added as a flavoring ingredient (Baker et al., 2004; Gaworski et al., 1997). These studies all show no discernable differences in the toxicity of the test cigarettes when compared to the nonmenthol cigarettes.

In vivo carcinogenesis studies also have shown no significant effects of menthol compared to nonmenthol. These studies included the SENCAR mouse skin painting assays with smoke condensate from menthol and nonmenthol cigarettes (Gaworski et al., 1999), DMBA-induced rat mammary carcinogenesis model with menthol in the feed (Russin et al., 1989) and azoxymethane-induced neoplasia of the large intestine and duodenum with menthol in the feed (Wattenberg, 1991).

BALB/c mice injected with WEHI-3 leukemia cells also showed effects of menthol exposure, having slowed leukemia-induced spleen growth,and limited differentiation of the precursors of macrophages and granulocytes (Lu et al., 2007).

Industry Reviews of Menthol

Two tobacco industry reviews (Lorillard (Heck 2010); Altria (Werley et al., 2007)) of the available literature on menthol and the possible effects of menthol cigarettes provided no additional information and no information that provided new insight into the potential toxicology of exposure to menthol from a menthol cigarette.

Conclusion

While menthol toxicity does occur, the reviewed studies show that this occurs at high levels of menthol as a singular compound and has not been shown with menthol exposure from cigarettes. The nonclinical toxicology data, *in vitro* or *in vivo* indicate that menthol exposure from a menthol cigarette does not cause the menthol cigarettes to be substantially more toxic than nonmenthol cigarettes already are.

Menthol in smoke condensate is no more genotoxic than condensate from the control cigarettes. Menthol has not been shown to be carcinogenic or to increase the number of tumors or alter the time to tumor emergence from known carcinogens.

In the few *in vivo* inhalation studies comparing menthol cigarette smoke to a control cigarette's smoke, researchers found no increased toxicity due to the added menthol. From the available studies, the weight of evidence supports the conclusion that, from a nonclinical toxicity standpoint, menthol in cigarettes is not associated with increased or decreased smoke toxicity.

Smoke Chemistry and Nonclinical Toxicology: Table of Referenced Sources

Author Name(s)	Article Title	Year Pub.	Funded By	Type of Study	Subject Description (Including Special population(s))	Sample Size (N)	Authors' Results/Conclusion(s) related to Menthol* (excerpted directly from article)
Ashby J, Tennant RW.	Definitive relationships among chemical structure, carcinogenicity and mutagenicity for 301 chemicals tested by the U.S. NTP.	1991	Funded though the National Institute of Environmental Health Sciences	Bioassay	Rodents	Not Applicable	Concepts of genotoxic and non-genotoxic rodent carcinogenicity are worthy of continued attention; it's meaningless to discuss the sensitivity/specificity without defining the broad chemical classes under discussion-> important to any model for screening environmental chemicals for potential carcinogens.
Baker RR, Massey, ED, Smith, G.	An overview of the effects of tobacco ingredients on smoke chemistry and toxicity.	2004	No funding source(s) provided. Authors affiliated with British American Tobacco Company	Evaluation of series of studies; pyrolysis studies	Not Applicable	Not Applicable	All of these studies have indicated that commonly used tobacco ingredients do not change the toxicity of smoke as measured in specified assays. Also, the ingredients have no effect on the levels of most smoke constituents that may be relevant to smoking-related diseases.
Baker RR, Pereira da Silva JA, Smith G.	The effect of tobacco ingredients on smoke chemistry. Part I: flavourings and additives.	2004	No funding source(s) provided. Authors affiliated with British American Tobacco Company	Experimental	The levels of the "Hoffmann analytes" in the smoke from the test cigarettes containing the ingredient mixture were compared to those from control cigarettes without the ingredients.	Not Applicable	It was found that, in most cases, the mixtures of flavouring ingredients (generally added in parts per million levels) had no statistically significant effect on the analyte smoke yields relative to the control cigarette.
Bernhardt G, Biersack B, Bollwein S, Schobert R, Zoldakova M.	Terpene conjugates of diaminedichlorido platinum(II) complexes: antiproliferative effects in HL-60 leukemia, 518A2 melanoma, and HT-29 colon cancer cells.	2008	No funding source(s) provided. Authors affiliated with two German universities	28 dichloridoplatin um (II) complexes	Not Applicable	Not Applicable	In the melanoma cells, the propane-1,2-cliyl-spacered conjugates of (-)-menthol (1a2,), (+)-neomenthol (1b2), (-)-carvomenthol (1h2,), and (-)-isolongifolol (1n2) displayed growth inhibition at IC50<4 uM which is ten times smaller than that of cisplatin.
Bernson VS,	The toxicity of	1983	Swedish Work	Animal Studies	Short Term Bioassays	Not	Menthol was found to be toxic on *in vitro*

Author Name(s)	Article Title	Year	Funded By	Type of Study	Subject Description	Sample	Authors' Results/Conclusion(s) related to
Pettersson B.	menthol in short-term bioassays.		Environment Fund (79/91:3) and the Swedish Tobacco Company		(trachea from chicken embryos, Ascites sarcoma BP 8 cells, isolated hamster brown adipocytes and rat liver mitochondria)	Applicable	biological model systems in concentrations >0.1mM. One effect of menthol was a lesion of biological membranes as demonstrated by experiments on isolated mitochondria.
Doolittle DJ, Lee CK, Ivett JL, Mirsalis JC, Riccio E, Rudd CJ, Burger GT, Hayes AW.	Comparative studies on the genotoxic activity of mainstream smoke condensate from cigarettes which burn or only heat tobacco.	1990	No funding source(s) provided. Authors affiliated with R.J. Reynolds Tobacco Company	Short term genotoxicity assays	Mice and hamsters	Not Specified	These results demonstrate that the mainstream CSCs [cigarette smoke concentrate] from the TEST and TEST-menthol cigarettes are neither genotoxic nor cytotoxic under conditions where CSCs from 1R4f, ULT, and ULT-menthol cigarettes are genotoxic and/or cytotoxic in a concentration-dependent manner.
Doolittle DJ, Lee CK, Ivett JL, Mirsalis JC, Riccio E, Rudd CJ, Burger GT, Hayes AW.	Genetic toxicology studies comparing the activity of sidestream smoke from cigarettes which burn or only heat tobacco.	1990	No funding source(s) provided. Authors affiliated with R.J. Reynolds Tobacco Company	Genotoxicity assays	Not Applicable	Not Applicable	Results demonstrate that side stream smoke from cigarettes that heat but do not burn tobacco (TEST and TEST-menthol) was neither genotoxic or cytotoxic under conditions where sidestream smoke from cigarettes which burn tobacco (1R4F, ULT, ULT-menthol) was genotoxic and/or cytotoxic in a concentration- dependent manner.
Gaworski CL, Dozier MM, Gerhart JM, Rajendran N, Brennecke LH, Aranyi C, Heck JD.	13-week inhalation toxicity study of menthol cigarette smoke.	1997	No funding source(s) provided. Authors affiliated with Lorillard Tobacco Company	Smoke inhalation study	Groups of male and female rats (21 per sex for reference and 15 per sex for menthol) were exposed at target smoke concentrations of 200, 600 and 1200mg TPM/m 3 for 1 hr/day, 5days/wk, for 13 wk.	N=72	Addition of menthol to cigarettes does not significantly alter the pattern, incidence, severity or reversibility of any of the effects attributable to smoke exposure in rats.
Gaworski CL, Heck JD, Bennett MB, Wenk ML.	Toxicologic evaluation of flavor ingredients added to cigarette tobacco: skin painting bioassay of cigarette	1999	No funding source(s) provided. Authors affiliated with Lorillard Tobacco Company	Skin painting biassays; experimental design	Female SENCAR mice	N=30-50	Study did not indicate any substantive effect of flavoring ingredients.

Smoke Chemistry and Nonclinical Toxicology: Table of Referenced Sources (Continued)

Author Name(s)	Article Title	Year Pub.	Funded By	Type of Study	Subject Description (Including Special population(s))	Sample	Authors' Results/Conclusion(s) related to Menthol* (excerpted directly from article)
	smoke condensate in SENCAR mice.						
Harris, B.	Menthol: A review of its thermo receptor interactions and their therapeutic applications.	2006	No funding source(s) provided. Author affiliated with Essential Oil Resource Consultants	Literature Review	Not Applicable	Not Applicable	This review has confirmed the therapeutic benefits of menthol containing oils in: topical applications for cooling, warming, relief of pain and itch; inhaled preparation and chest rub for relief of cough; and oral preparations such as lozenges for relief of cough.
Heck JD.	A review and assessment of menthol employed as a cigarette flavoring ingredient.	2010	No funding source(s) provided. Author affiliated with Lorillard Tobacco Company	Literature Review	Not Applicable	Not Applicable	...a broad convergence of findings supports a judgment that menthol employed as a cigarette tobacco flavoring ingredient does not meaningfully affect the inherent toxicity of cigarette smoke or the human risks that attend smoking.
Ishidate, Jr, M, Sofuni T, Yoshikawa K, Hayashi M, Nohmi T, Sawada M, and Matsuoka A	Primary mutagenicity screening of food additives currently used in Japan.	1984	The Food Chemistry Division, Environmental Health Bureau, Ministry of Health and Welfare of Japan	*In Vitro*	Chinese hamster fibroblast cells	Not Specified	[No narrative. Listed in Table 1]
Ivett JL, Brown BM, Rodgers C, Anderson BE, Resnick MA, Zeiger E.	Chromosomal aberrations and sister chromatid exchange tests in Chinese hamster ovary cells *in vitro*. IV. Results with 15 chemicals.	1989	National Institute of Environmental Health Sciences. Grant Number NO1-ES-3–5030	*In Vitro*	Chinese hamster ovary cells	Not Specified	There was no increase in the trial with activation, and the chemical was judged negative in the SCE assay. The aberration assays were both negative.
Kim SH, Nam JH, Park EJ, Kim BJ, Kim SJ, So I, Jeon JH.	Menthol regulates TRPM8- independent processes in PC-3 prostate cancer cells.	2009	Funded by a grant of the Korea Health 21R and D project, Ministry of Health, Welfare and Family Affairs, Republic of Korea	Experimental	Prostate cancer cells	Not Specified	There is an apparent lack of causality between TRPM8 activation and menthol-induced cell death and that menthol can regulate TRPM8-independent Ca(2+)-transport and cellular processes.

Author Name(s)	Article Title	Year Pub.	Funded By	Type of Study	Subject Description (Including Special population(s))	Sample	Authors' Results/Conclusion(s) related to Menthol* (excerpted directly from article)
			(A060058), and by the Seoul National University Hospital Research Fund (03-2005-026-0), and the BK21 project from Ministry of Education, Science and Technology				
Lee CK, Doolittle DJ, Burger GT, Hayes AW.	Comparative genotoxicity testing of mainstream whole smoke from cigarettes which burn or heat tobacco.	1990	No funding source(s) provided. Authors affiliated with R.J. Reynolds Tobacco Company	Comparative	Not Applicable	Not Applicable	Mainstream whole smoke from the heat tobacco (TEST) cigarettes, with either regular or menthol flavor, was neither cytotoxic nor mutagenic in any of these assays.
Li Q, Wang X, Yang Z, Wang B, Li S.	Menthol induces cell death via the TRPM8 channel in the human bladder cancer cell line T24.	2009	National Natural Science Foundation of China (No. 30872572/C160603)	Experimental	Cells of the human bladder cancer cell line T24.	Not Specified	Menthol can induce mitochondrial membrane depolarization via the TRPM8 channel in cells of the human bladder cancer cell line T24, resulting in cell death. It would be helpful to explore the precise mechanism of action of menthol in bladder cancer with a view to its possible use as intravesical chemotherapy.
Lu HF, Liu JY, Hsueh SC, Yang YY, Yang JS, Tan TW, Kok LF, Lu CC, Lan SH, Wu SY, Liao SS, Ip SW, Chung JG.	(-)-Menthol inhibits WEHI-3 leukemia cells *in vitro* and *in vivo*.	2007	grant CMU94-103 from the China Medical University, Taichung, Taiwan, and by grant 95-31 from the Cheng Hsin Rehabilitation Medical Center, Paipei, Taiwan	Experimental	*In vivo* Mice cells	Not Specified	(-)- menthol was found to induce cell death and inhibited leukemia-related spleen growth.
Lu HF, Hsueh SC, Yu FS, Yang JS, Tang NY, Chen SC, Chung JG.	The role of Ca2+ in (-)-menthol-induced human promyelocytic leukemia HL-60 cell death.	2006	Grant 93-32 from the Cheng Hsin Rehabilitation Medical Center (Taipei, Taiwan, R.O.C.)	Experimental	Human promyelocytic leukemia HL-60 cell line	Not Specified	Ca2+ production is associated with the induction of (-)-Menthol-induced cell death.

Smoke Chemistry and Nonclinical Toxicology: Table of Referenced Sources (Continued)

Author Name(s)	Article Title	Year Pub.	Funded By	Type of Study	Subject Description (Including Special population(s))	Sample	Authors' Results/Conclusion(s) related to Menthol* (excerpted directly from article)
Murthy PBK, Ahmed MM, Regu K.	Lack of genotoxicity of menthol in chromosome aberration and sister chromatid exchange assays using human lynphocytes *in vitro*.	1991	Department Science and Technology, Government of India (SP/YS/L35/85)	Experimental	Heparinized peripheral blood samples obtained from male and female adult non-smokers.	N=24 (12 male, 12 female)	These results suggest that menthol does not have a chromosomal-damaging effect in human lymphocytes.
Rabinoff M, Caskey N, Rissling A, Park C.	Pharmacological and chemical effects of cigarette additives.	2007	National Institute of Mental Health (NRSA training grant MH 14585)	Review	Tobacco industry documents and other sources	5 Primary Sources	Findings indicated that more than 100 of 599 documented cigarette additives have pharmacological actions that camouflage the odor of environmental tobacco smoke emitted from cigarettes, enhance or maintain nicotine delivery, could increase the addictiveness of cigarettes, and mask symptoms and illnesses associated with smoking behaviors.
Roemer E, Tewes FJ, Meisgen TJ, Veltel DJ, Carmines EL.	Evaluation of the potential effects of ingredients added to cigarettes. Part 3: *In vitro* genotoxcity and cytotoxicity.	2002	No funding source(s) provided. Author affiliated with R.J. Reynolds Tobacco Company	*In vitro*	Ingredients commonly used in cigarette manufacturing	N=333	Within the sensitivity and specificity of the test systems, the *in vitro* mutagenicity and cytotoxicity of the cigarette smoke were not increased by the addition of the ingredients.
Ruch RJ, Sigler K.	Growth inhibition of rat liver epithelial tumor cells by monoterpenes does not involve	1994	Grant from the American Institute for Cancer Research to RJ Reynolds Tobacco Company	*In Vitro*	Rat liver epithelial cells	Not Applicable	Monoterpene-induced growth inhibition of rat liver epithelial cells was dissimilar to lovastatin and did not appear to involve altered Ras plasma membrane association.
	Ras plasma membrane association.						
Russin WA, Hoesly JD, Elson CE, Tanner MA, Gould MN.	Inhibition of rat mammary carcinogenesis by monoterpenoids.	1989	Grant from the National Cancer Institute CA38128	Experimental	Terpenes	Not Specified	Dietary additions of each of the monocyclic terpenes, d-limonene or (-)-menthol resulted in a significant inhibition of mammary carcinogenesis. Furthermore, menthol was found to be a more

Author Name(s)	Article Title	Year Pub.	Funded By	Type of Study	Subject Description (Including Special population(s))	Sample	Authors' Results/Conclusion(s) related to Menthol* (excerpted directly from article)
							potent chemopreventive agent than limonene during the DMBA initiation of rat mammary tumors.
Schmeltz I, Schlotzhauer WS.	Benzo(a)pyrene, phenols and other products from pyrolysis of the cigarette additive, (d,1)-menthol.	1968	No funding source(s) provided. Authors affiliated with the U.S. Dept of Agriculture	Experimental	Menthol	Not Specified	The contribution of menthol to the chemical and biological effects of cigarette smoke must be weighed in relation to the amount used as an additive, and the amount that undergoes pyrolytic conversion.
Sidell N, Taga T, Hirano T, Kishimoto T, Saxon A.	Retinoic acid-induced growth inhibition of a human myeloma cell line via down- regulation of IL-6 receptors.	1991	United States Public Health Service Grants A115251. A115332, CA30515. CA43503 and CA12800 from the National Institutes of Health and Grant-in-Aid for Specially Promoted Research from the Ministry of Education. Science and Culture. Japan	Experimental	Human B cell lines	Not Specified	Menthol, a structurally unrelated compountdo RA, also suppressed IL-6R expression and, correspondingly, inhibited cell growth.
Tatman D, Mo H.	Volatile isoprenoid constituents of fruits, vegetables and herbs cumulatively suppress the proliferation of murine B16 melanoma and	2002	Public Health Service grant CA 73418	Experimental	Fruits, vegetables, herbs	Not Applicable	The cancer-protective property of fruits, vegetables, and related products is partly conferred by the cumulative impact of volatile isoprenoid constituents.
	human HL-60 leukemia cells.						
Wattenberg LW.	Inhibition of azoxymethane-induced neoplasia of the large bowel by 3-hydroxy- 3,7,11-trimethyl1,6,10-	1991	Funded by grant SIG 5A from the American Cancer Society	Experimental	Male F344 rats	Not Applicable	The chemical structure of nerolidol suggests the possibility that the compound might have an impact on protein prenylation or some other aspect of the mevalonate pathway, but this remains to be established.

Smoke Chemistry and Nonclinical Toxicology: Table of Referenced Sources (Continued)

Author Name(s)	Article Title	Year Pub.	Funded By	Type of Study	Subject Description (Including Special population(s))	Sample	Authors' Results/Conclusion(s) related to Menthol* (excerpted directly from article)
	dodecatriene (nerolidol).						
Werley MS, Coggins CR, Lee PN.	Possible effects on smokers of cigarette mentholation: a review of the evidence relating to key research questions.	2007	No funding source(s) provided. Authors affiliated with Philip Morris USA	Review	Not Applicable	Not Applicable	Smoking mentholated cigarettes did not affect the rate of decline in lung function in Year 1 or between Year 1 and Year 5 (p=0.229 and 0.64, respectively, data not shown).
Yamamura H, Ugawa S, Ueda T, Morita A, Shimada S.	TRPM8 activation suppresses cellular viability in human melanoma.	2008	Grants-in-Aid for Young Scientists from the Ministry of Education, Culture, Sports, Science and Technology (to H. Yamamura) and for Scientific Research and Exploratory Research from the Japan Society for the Promotion of Sciences (to S. Shimada).	In situ hybridization	Human melanoma	Not Specified	The viability of melanoma cells was dose-dependently depressed in the presence of menthol. These results reveal that a functional TRPM8 protein is expressed in human melanoma cells to involve the mechanism underlying tumor progression via the Ca(2+) handling pathway, providing us with a novel target of drug development for malignant melanoma.
Zhang L, Barritt GJ.	Evidence that TRPM8 is an androgen- dependent Ca2+ channel required for the survival of prostate cancer cells	2004	No funding source(s) provided. Authors affiliated with Flinders University	Experimental	Prostate cancer cell lines	Not Specified	TRPM8 is an important determinator of Ca2+ homeostasis in prostate epithelial cells and may be a potential target for the action of drugs in the management of prostate cancer.

* Note: these statements are taken directly from articles and may not include all relevant results/conclusions. [Bracketed notes added by FDA]

References

Ashby J, Tennant RW. (1991) Definitive relationships among chemical structure, carcinogenicity and mutagenicity for 301 chemicals tested by the U.S. NTP. Mutatation Research: Reviews in Genetic Toxicology 257(3):229–306. [Funded though the National Institute of Environmental Health Sciences]

Baker RR, Massey, ED, Smith, G (2004a) An overview of the effects of tobacco ingredients on smoke chemistry and toxicity. Food and Chemical Toxicology 42S: S53- S83. [No funding source(s) provided. Authors affiliated with British American Tobacco Company]

Baker RR, Pereira da Silva JA, Smith G (2004b) The effect of tobacco ingredients on smoke chemistry. Part I: flavourings and additives. Food and Chemical Toxicology 42(suppl):S3–S37. [No funding source(s) provided. Authors affiliated with British American Tobacco Company]

Bernhardt G, Biersack B, Bollwein, S, Schobert R, Zoldakova, M (2008) Terpene conjugates of diaminedichloridoplatinum(II) complexes: antiproliferative effects in HL-60 leukemia, 518A2 melanoma, and HT-29 colon cancer cells. Chemistry and Biodiversity 5(8):1645–1659. [No funding source(s) provided. Authors affiliated with two German universities]

Bernson VS, Pettersson B (1983) The toxicity of menthol in short-term bioassays. Chemico-Biological Interactions 46(2):233–246. [Funded by grants from the Swedish Work Environment Fund (79/91:3) and the Swedish Tobacco Company]

Doolittle DJ, Lee CK, Ivett JL, Mirsalis JC, Riccio E, Rudd CJ, Burger GT, Hayes AW (1990a) Comparative studies on the genotoxic activity of mainstream smoke condensate from cigarettes which burn or only heat tobacco. Environmental and Molecular Mutagenesis 15(2):93–105. [No funding source(s) provided. Authors affiliated with R.J. Reynolds Tobacco Company]

Doolittle DJ, Lee CK, Ivett JL, Mirsalis JC, Riccio E, Rudd CJ, Burger GT, Hayes AW (1990b) Genetic toxicology studies comparing the activity of sidestream smoke from cigarettes which burn or only heat tobacco. Mutation Research 240(2):59–72. [No funding source(s) provided. Authors affiliated with R.J. Reynolds Tobacco Company]

Gaworksi CL, Dozier MM, Gerhart JM, Rajendrans N, Brennecke LH, Aranyi C, Heck JD (1997) 13-week inhalation toxicity study of menthol cigarette smoke. Food and Chemical Toxicology 35(7):683–692. [No funding source(s) provided. Authors associated with Lorillard Tobacco Company]

Gaworski CL, Heck JD, Bennet MB, Wenk ML (1999) Toxicologic evaluation of flavor ingredients added to cigarette tobacco: skin painting bioassay of cigarette smoke condensate in SENCAR mice. Toxicology 139(1–2):1–17. [No funding source(s) provided. Authors affiliated with Lorillard Tobacco Company]

Harris B (2006) Menthol: a review of its thermoreceptor interactions and their therapeutic applications. International Journal of Aromatherapy 16(3–4):117–131. [No funding source(s) provided. Author affiliated with Essential Oil Resource Consultants]

Heck JD (2010) A review and assessment of menthol employed as a cigarette flavoring ingredient. Food and Chemical Toxicology 48(suppl):S1–S38. [No funding source(s) provided. Author affiliated with Lorillard Tobacco Company]

Ishidate, Jr, M, Sofuni T, Yoshikawa K, Hayashi M, Nohmi T, Sawada M, and Matsuoka A (1984) Primary mutagenicity screening of food additives currently used in Japan. Food and Chemical Toxicology 22(8):623–636. [Funding provided by the Food Chemistry Division, Environmental Health Bureau, Ministry of Health and Welfare of Japan.

Ivett JL, Brown BM, Rodgers C, Anderson BE, Resnick MA, Zeiger E (1989) Chromosomal aberrations and sister chromatid exchange tests in Chinese hamster ovary cells *in vitro*. IV. Results with 15 chemicals. Environmental and Molecular Mutagenesis 14:165–187. [Funded by contract number N01-ES-3-5030 with the National Institute of Environmental Health Sciences]

Kim SH, Nam JH, Park EJ, Kim BJ, Kim SJ, So I, Jeon JH (2009) Menthol regulates TRPM8-independent processes in PC-3 prostate cancer cells. Biochimica et Biophysica Acta 1792(1):33–38. [Funded by a grant of the Korea Health 21R and D project, Ministry of Health, Welfare and Family Affairs, Republic of Korea (A060058), and by the Seoul National University Hospital Research Fund (03-2005-026-0), and the BK21 project from Ministry of Education, Science and Technology]

Lee CK, Doolittle DL, Burger GT, Hayes AW (1990) Comparative genotoxicity testing of mainstream whole smoke from cigarettes which burn or heat tobacco. Mutation Research 242(1):37–45. [No funding source(s) provided. Authors affiliated with R.J. Reynolds Tobacco Company]

Li Q, Wang X, Yang Z, Wang B, Li S (2009) Menthol induces cell death via the TRPM8 channel in the human bladder cancer cell line T24. Oncology 77:335–341. [Funded by the National Natural Science Foundation of China (No. 30872572/C160603).

Lu HF, Liu JY, Hsueh SC, Yang YY, Yang JS, Tan TW, Kok LF, Lu CC, Lan SH, Wu SY, Liao SS, Ip SW, Chung JG (2007) (-)-Menthol inhibits WEHI-3 leukemia cells *in vitro* and *in vivo*. *In Vivo* 21(2):285–289. [Funded by grant CMU94-103 from the China Medical University, Taichung, Taiwan, and by grant 95-31 from the Cheng Hsin Rehabilitation Medical Center, Paipei, Taiwan]

Lu HF, Hsueh SC, Yu FS, Yang JS, Tang NY, Chen SC, Chung JG (2006) The role of Ca2+ in (-)-menthol-induced human promyelocytic leukemia HL-60 cell death. *In Vivo* 20(1):69–75. [Funded by grant 93-32 from the Cheng Hsin Rehabilitation Medical Center, Taipei, Taiwan]

Murthy PBK, Ahmend MM, Regu K (1991) Lack of genotoxicity of menthol in chromosome aberration and sister chromatid exchange assays using human lynphocytes *in vitro*. Toxicology *in Vitro* 5(4):337–340. [Funded by the Department Science and Technology, Government of India (SP/YS/L35/85)]

Rabinoff M, Caskey N, Rissling A, Park C (2007) Pharmacological and chemical effects of cigarette additives. American Journal of Public Health 97(11):1981–1991. [Funded by a pilot grant from the National Institute of Mental Health (NRSA training grant MH 14585)]

Roemer E, Tewes FJ, Meisgen TJ, Veltel DJ, Carmines EL (2002) Evaluation of the potential effects of ingredients added to cigarettes. Part 3: *In vitro* genotoxcity and cytotoxicity. Food and Chemical Toxicology 40:105–111. [No funding source(s) provided. Author affiliated with R.J. Reynolds Tobacco Company]

Ruch RJ, Sigler K (1994) Growth inhibition of rat liver epithelial tumor cells by monoterpenes does not involve Ras plasma membrane association. Carcinogenesis 15(4):787–789. [Funded by a grant from the American Institute for Cancer Research to RJ Reynolds Tobacco Company]

Russin WA, Hoesly JD, Elson CE, Tanner MA, Gould MN (1989) Inhibition of rat mammary carcinogenesis by monoterpenoids. Carcinogenesis 10(11):2161–2164. [Funded by a grant from the National Cancer Institute CA38128]

Schmeltz I, Schlotzhauer WS (1968) Benzo(a)pyrene, phenols and other products from pyrolysis of the cigarette additive, (d,1)-menthol. Nature 219(5152):370–371. [No funding source(s) provided. Authors affiliated with the U.S. Dept of Agriculture]

Sidell N, Taga T, Hirano T, Kishimoto T, Saxon A (1991) Retinoic acid-induced growth inhibition of a human myeloma cell line via down-regulation of IL-6 receptors. Journal of Immunology 146(11):3809–3814. [Funded by United States Public Health Service Grants A115251. A115332, CA30515. CA43503 and CA12800 from the National Institutes of Health and Grant-in-Aid for Specially Promoted Research from the Ministry of Education. Science and Culture. Japan]

Tatman D, Mo H (2002) Volatile isoprenoid constituents of fruits, vegetables and herbs cumulatively suppress the proliferation of murine B16 melanoma and human HL-60 leukemia cells. Cancer Letters 175(2):129–139. [Funded by Public Health Service grant CA 73418]

Wattenberg LW (1991) Inhibition of azoxymethane-induced neoplasia of the large bowel by 3-hydroxy-3,7,11-trimethyl-1,6,10-dodecatriene (nerolidol). Carcinogenesis 12(1):151–152. [Funded by grant SIG 5A from the American Cancer Society]

Werley MS, Coggins CRE and Lee PN (2007) Possible effects on smokers of cigarette mentholation: a review of the evidence relating to key research questions. Regulatory Toxicology and Pharmacology 47:189–203. [No funding source(s) provided. Authors affiliated with Philip Morris USA]

Yamamura H, Ugawa S, Ueda T, Morita A, Shimada S (2008) TRPM8 activation suppresses cellular viability in human melanoma. American Journal of Physiology: Cell Physiology 295(2):C296–C301. [Funded by Grants-in-Aid for Young Scientists from the Ministry of Education, Culture, Sports, Science and Technology and for Scientific Research (B) and Exploratory Research from the Japan Society for the Promotion of Sciences]

Zhang L, Barritt GJ (2004) Evidence that TRPM8 is an androgen-dependent Ca2+ channel required for the survival of prostate cancer cells. Cancer Research 64(22):8365–8373. [No funding source(s) provided. Authors affiliated with Flinders University]

B. Physiology

Menthol is widely used in drug products, foods, cosmetic products, and cigarettes, and generates a minty taste and a cooling sensation. The flavor and sensation may be pleasing, and can impact the way a smoker experiences a menthol cigarette. Menthol's effect on cooling, desensitization, anesthesia, and the potential effect on nicotine and tobacco specific nitrosamines (TSNAs) using both *in vitro* and *in vivo* studies in human and animal models can inform how researchers understand and policy-makers address menthol in cigarettes and its impact on individual behavior and public health outcomes, as well as effect of menthol on smoking topography.

This assessment focuses on the actions of menthol alone rather than tobacco smoke from menthol cigarettes.

Sensory Effects

Green and Schullery (2003) conducted a study that focused primarily on the bitterness stimulation induced by capsaicin and menthol. On average, capsaicin and menthol produced "moderate" bitterness in the edges and side of the tongue and weaker bitterness on the side and tip of the tongue. Sensory irritation from capsaicin was rated significantly higher at the tongue tip, whereas menthol coolness was rated higher in the edges and side of the tongue.

Kuhn et al. (2009) carried out an *in vitro* study on TRPM8, a cation channel activated by cold and menthol, and found that menthol and menthol derivatives were indistinguishable in their ability to evoke currents through channels in a Ca^{2+}-independent manner and by producing Ca^{2+}- dependent desensitization in human embryonic kidney (HEK-293) cells.

Sherkheli (2008) found that WS-12, a menthol derivative, is more potent and selective than menthol as a TRPM8 agonist in Xenopus laevis oocytes.

Ito et al. (2008) investigated the impact of menthol and icilin on airway smooth muscle contraction in guinea pigs. The study found that as a cold receptor agonist, menthol inhibited contractions elicited by MCh and high K^+ concentrations with a reduction in Ca^{2+}. Lowering the temperature to room temperature enhanced the relaxing effects of menthol on MCh-induced contractions. The result indicated that stimulation of an unknown cold receptor may be involved in the relaxation mediated by menthol in guinea pig tracheal smooth muscle.

Menthol gives a sense of cooling. Campero et al. (2009) used microneurography to search for C fibers (a type of sensory cell) in human skin that are activated by cooling and menthol. Menthol activated only Type 2 C fibers, which showed a strong reaction to harmless cooling and were strongly activated and sensitized to cooling by menthol.

Orani et al. (1991) found in guinea pigs that cooling of the larynx and application of l-menthol to the laryngeal lumen reduced ventilation. Application of menthol to the nasal cavity markedly enhanced the ventilatory inhibition. Although l-menthol did not actually reduce laryngeal temperature, the laryngeal lumen responded as though it did. In fact, l-menthol seems to be more effective in reducing ventilation than physical cooling.

Sant'Ambrogio et al. (1991, 1992) investigated the effect of l-menthol on laryngeal and upper airway cold receptors in dogs. The study found that l-menthol acted as a specific stimulant of laryngeal cold receptors. Trials with cold air and warm air plus l-menthol exposure on upper airway cold receptors greatly reduced ventilation in newborn dogs. The menthol-induced respiratory depression occured even earlier than the cold-induced effect. The faster onset of reflex response could be because the menthol stimulation of cold receptors was greater or because nasal cold receptors were involved in the menthol response.

By monitoring the action potentials of the ethmoidal nerve, Sekizawa (1996) characterized the responsiveness of nasal cold receptors to menthol and capsaicin in guinea pigs. Both cold air and l-menthol stimulated the ethmoidal afferent activity. Topical anesthesia of the nasal cavity with 2 percent lidocaine eliminated these responses. This study dovetails with those discussed earlier; it provides electrophysiological support for the breathing inhibition that other studies also found (Orani et al., 1991; Sant'Ambrogio et al., 1991; Sant'Ambrogio et al., 1992).

Mechanisms of Menthol Action

In an *in vivo* human study, Dessirier et al. (2001) assessed the responses of participants' tongues to menthol application. Repeated application of menthol produced desensitization as characterized by a progressive reduction in the ratings of the intensity of irritation across trials. This appeared to generalize, as menthol exposure also significantly weakened nicotine-evoked irritation. The desensitization and cross-desensitization was temporary, with a return to normal sensations after a rest period.

Cold temperatures and some chemical stimuli (like menthol) activate the TRPM8 receptor. Kuhn et al. (2009) found that prolonged menthol exposure desensitized TRPM8 receptors. Galeotti et al. (2002) found that menthol could induce analgesia in mice, regardless of the noxious stimulus used: thermal (hot-plate) or chemical (abdominal constriction test). The analgesic properties were mediated through a selective activation of ţ-opioid receptors.

An *in vivo* study demonstrated that menthol is an effective cough suppressant in chemically induced coughing in conscious guinea pigs (Laude et al., 1994).

Sekizawa et al. (1996) found that topical anesthesia of the nasal cavity eliminated the responsiveness of nasal cold receptors to cold air and l-menthol in guinea pigs. The desensitization and analgesic effect of menthol may reduce sensitivity of human response to irritation induced by smoking constituents.

Wright et al. (1997) found that menthol exposure promotes bronchodilatation both *in vitro* and *in vivo* in guinea pigs. The authors also proposed that menthol might act as an antagonist of calcium (Ca^{2+}) channels.

Sidell et al. (1990) demonstrated that exposure to menthol could block the depolarization-induced Ca^{2+} influx though both dihydropyridine (DHP)-sensitive and DHP-insensitive Ca^{2+} channels in LA-N-5 human neuroblastoma cells. Whether menthol blocks Ca^{2+} channels was concentration-dependent, rapid in onset, and readily reversible. In addition, applying menthol to neuroblastoma cells in culture resulted in morphologic differentiation and inhibition of cell growth that correlated with menthol's ability to block the dihydropyridine-insensitive Ca^{2+} current.

Lin et al. (2005) found menthol to have potential antitumor qualities. Menthol inhibited the growth of cancer cells in a dose- and time-dependent manner. Menthol inhibited topoisomerase I, IIĮ and IIù, but promoted the levels of NF-ţB gene expression. These data suggest that menthol may induce cytotoxicity through inhibiting gene expression of topoisomerase I, IIĮ and IIù and promoting the gene expression of NF-ţB in SNU-5 cells.

Metabolic Effects

MacDougall et al. (2003) found that menthol and synthetic congeners inhibited the microsomal oxidation of nicotine to cotinine (the primary metabolite of nicotine) in human liver microsomal testing systems. The data suggested that smoking menthol cigarettes may lead to inhibition of nicotine metabolism and allow the smoker to achieve prolonged exposure to nicotine.

Azzi et al. (2006) found menthol donor solution (0.08%) decreased the flux of 4-(methylnitrosamino)-1-(3-pyridyl)-1-butanone (NNK) and significantly increased the tissue reservoir formation in porcine esophageal mucosa. The magnitude of the reservoir formed was similar for control and menthol, but was significantly higher in the presence of both ethanol and menthol.

Squier et al. (2010) found that the presence of menthol significantly increased the uptake of both Nǫ-nitrosonornicotine (NNN) and nicotine over that of controls with no menthol in porcine buccal and floor of mouth mucosa. According to the authors, the presence of menthol might increase exposure of carcinogens and nicotine, which in turn might increase the risk of cancer and dependence, however there are no disease outcome data that support this hypothesis.

In a crossover study with 14 subjects, Benowitz et al. (2004) found that mentholation of cigarettes did not affect systemic intake of nicotine and carbon monoxide. Researchers reported that menthol smoking inhibits the metabolism of nicotine through slower oxidative metabolism to cotinine and slower glucuronide conjugation.

Effects of Menthol on Smoking Topography

Ahijevych & Parsley (1999) assessed smoking topography in a clinical research setting using a two-factor study design involving 95 women, half of whom smoked menthol cigarettes. Menthol smokers (n=49) had significantly larger puff volumes compared to nonmenthol smokers (n=46). Larger puff volumes can result in smokers' exposure to more chemicals.

Pickworth et al. (2002) found that mentholation of cigarettes had no effect on topography, with menthol smokers (n=18) and nonmenthol smokers (n=18) each taking approximately 8 puffs per commercial cigarette, and approximately 11 puffs per high nicotine yield cigarette and per low nicotine yield cigarette.

Using a two-factor factorial design and a sample of 37 women divided by menthol or nonmenthol cigarette use, Ahijevych et al. (1996) found nonmenthol smokers had a trend toward higher puff volumes as compared to menthol smokers (mean = 48.5 vs. 42.7 ml), however this did not reach signficance.

Jarvik et al. (1994) measured smoking topography in 20 smokers (10 were menthol smokers) and found menthol cigarettes decreased the average and total cumulative puff volumes and increased the mean puff flow rates of inhaled smoke. Researchers noted no significant differences in the depth of inhalation of the smoke or in the amount of insoluble smoke particulates delivered to or retained in the respiratory tract between the two types of cigarettes.

McCarthy et al. (1995) studied 29 male smokers who smoked either a regular or a menthol cigarette in two separate sessions one week apart. Researchers used commercial brands with comparable tar, nicotine, and CO content. When smoking the nonmenthol cigarettes, participants took 22 percent more puffs and had 13 percent higher mean volumes per puff than they did when smoking the menthol cigarettes.

The tobacco industry is aware that menthol has cooling, anaesthetic, and analgesic properties that moderate the harshness and irritation of tobacco. Yerger and McCandless (2011) reviewed publicly available tobacco industry documents and concluded that the documents suggest the amount of menthol in a cigarette is associated with how the cigarette is smoked and how satisfying it is to the smoker. According to these documents, menthol's physiological effects contribute to the sensory qualities of the smoke and affect smoking topography.

Industry Assessment of Menthol Effects

Heck (2009) found median blood carboxyhemoglobin values, total urinary 4-(methylnitrosamino)-1-(3-pyridyl)-1-butanol (NNAL), and urinary nicotine equivalents were not significantly different between the menthol and nonmenthol smokers.

Wang et al. (2010) found smoking menthol cigarettes does not increase daily exposure to smoke constituents as measured by nicotine equivalents (total and per cigarette), serum cotinine, and COHb after adjusting for cpd and the smoking behavior characteristics of the participants.

In its presentation to TPSAC, Altria Client Services presented analysis of the Total Exposure Study (TES) that also showed no differences between users of menthol and nonmenthol brands for a wide variety of biomarkers of exposure, biomarkers of potential harm, nicotine metabolite ratios, measures of smoker topography, and nicotine dependence, after adjustment for cpd and smoking behavior characteristics.

Conclusion

Menthol generates a minty taste and a cooling sensation. At lower concentrations menthol has a soothing effect, while it is irritating at high concentrations. Smokers experience the cooling sensation of menthol in cigarettes, and menthol is perceived as reducing the irritation and harshness of smoking. Several *in vitro* and *in vivo* studies investigated the sensory effects of menthol and discussed mechanisms for these effects. In addition, a few studies suggested that menthol might have a role on exposure and metabolism of nicotine and TSNAs.

Due primarily to menthol's sensory effects, the weight of evidence supports the conclusion that menthol in cigarettes in likely associated with altered physiological responses to tobacco smoke.

References

Ahijevych K, Garrett BE. (2004). Menthol pharmacology and its potential impact on cigarette smoking behavior. Nicotine & Tobacco Research 6(suppl 1):S17e28. [Funded by National Institute on Drug Abuse grant 10809 and General Clinical Research Center grant M01 RR00034]

Ahijevych K, Gillespie J, Demirci M, Jagadeesh, J. (1996). Menthol and nonmenthol cigarettes and smoke exposure in black and white women. Pharmacology Biochemistry and Behavior 53:355e60. [Funded by The Ohio State University Seed Grant and The Ohio State University General Clinical Research Center Grant MO1 RROO034]

Ahijevych K, Parsley LA. (1999). Smoke constituent exposure and stage of change in black and white women cigarette smokers. Addictive Behaviors 24:115e20. [Funded by an American Lung Association Research Grant, and General Clinical Research Center M01 RR00034]

Physiology: Table of Referenced Sources

Author Name(s)	Article Title	Year Pub.	Funded By	Type of Study	Subject Description (Including Special population(s))	Sample Size (N)	Authors' Results/Conclusion(s) related to Menthol* (excerpted directly from article)
Ahijevych K, Garrett BE.	Menthol pharmacology and its potential impact on cigarette smoking behavior.	2004	Funded in part by National Institute on Drug Abuse grant 10809 and General Clinical Research Center grant M01 RR00034	Literature Review	Not Applicable	Not Applicable	Menthol smokers have been shown to score higher on a measure of nicotine dependence, and Black smokers who prefer mentholated cigarette brands have lower quit rates than White smokers Industry findings also have shown that menthol is capable of increasing nicotine impact in cigarette smokers. These findings provide some support for increased tobacco addiction in mentholated cigarette smokers but are still inconclusive.
Ahijevych K, Gillespie J, Demirci M, Jagadeesh J.	Menthol and nonmenthol cigarettes and smoke exposure in black and white women.	1996	The Ohio State University Seed Grant and The Ohio State University General Clinical Research Center Grant MO1 RROO034	Cross sectional 2 factor factorial design	Black and White Women 19-59 years old, smoked "20 cpd	N=37 (18 Black, 19 White)	In the current study, lower CO boost with mentholated cigarettes suggests that factors beyond mentholation may affect differences in cotinine levels in black and white women.
Ahijevych K, Parsley LA.	Smoke constituent exposure and stage of change in black and white women cigarette smokers.	1999	American Lung Association Research Grant; General Clinical Research Center M01 RR00034	Two-factor design	Black and White Women	N=95 total women (48 black with 27 smoking menthol cigarettes, and 47 white with 22 smoking menthol cigarettes)	Black women had significantly higher beliefs about the negative aspects of smoking than did White women; menthol smokers had a shorter time to first cigarette, indicating greater nicotine dependence.

Author	Article Title	Year	Funded By	Type of Study	Subject Description	Sample	Authors' Results/Conclusion(s) related to
Azzi C, Zhang J, Purdon CH, Chapman JM, Nitcheva D, Hebert JR, Smith EW.	Permeation and reservoir formation of 4-(methylnitrosamino) -1-(3-pyridyl)-1-butanone (NNK) and benzo[a]pyrene (B[a]P) across	2006	MUSC/USC/HCC Department of Defense Funds, Phase VI, Cancer Prevention and Control Research Development Grant	Confocal microscopy studies	Porcine esophageal mucosa	Not Applicable	We have observed markedly different extents of permeation and reservoir formation for the tobacco carcinogens applied to porcine esophageal mucosa in the presence of ethanol and menthol.
	porcine esophageal tissue in the presence of ethanol and menthol.						
Benowitz NL, Herrera B, Jacob P 3rd.	Mentholated cigarette smoking inhibits nicotine metabolism.	2004	State of California Tobacco Related Disease Research Program Grant 1RT-0521, by U.S. Public Health Service Grants DA02277 and DA12393 awarded by the National Institute on Drug Abuse and CA32389 awarded by the National Cancer Institute, and by the General Clinical Research Center at San Francisco General Hospital Medical Center with the support of the Division of Research Resources, National Institutes of Health (RR-00083)	Cross Over	14 healthy cigarette smokers recruited through local papers. (7 African-Americans and 7 whites, 12 men and 2 women. Participants were selected as typically smoking 20 or more cigarettes per day and having a prior experience of smoking both mentholated and nonmentholated cigarettes.	N=14	Our finding of impaired metabolism of nicotine while mentholated cigarette smoking suggests that mentholated cigarette smoking enhances systemic nicotine exposure.

Physiology: Table of Referenced Sources (Continued)

Author Name(s)	Article Title	Year Pub.	Funded By	Type of Study	Subject Description (Including Special population(s))	Sample Size (N)	Authors' Results/Conclusion(s) related to Menthol* (excerpted directly from article)
Campero M, Baumann TK, Bostock H, Ochoa JL.	Human cutaneous c fibres activated by cooling, heating, and menthol.	2009	NIH Grant no. R01-NS48932	Not Applicable	18 adult volunteers over 4 years (11 males and 7 females) ages 17-52 years (mean age 27.3)	N=18	We propose that the Type 2 C fibres, although resembling Aį cold fibres in their repsosnes to innocuous cooling and menthol, have a more complex sensory function, colouring with a 'hot- burning' quality the perceptions of low and high temperatures.
Dessirier JM, O'Mahony M, Carstens E.	Oral irritant properties of menthol: sensitizing and desensitizing effects of repeated application and cross-	2001	Grant from the California Tobacco-Related Disease Research Program No. 6RT-0231	3 Experimental Design	Experiment 1: Healthy Males and females ages 18-43 yrs who were students and staff at University of California at Davis Experiment 2: Healthy	Experiment N=22 (6 males and 16 females) Experiment	These studies demonstrate 3 new properties of menthol as oral irritant chemical (a) exposure to menthol cross-desensitized irritation elicited by nicotine (b) When applied at a short (5-s) ISI, a significant proportion of subjects perceived the menthol irritation to increase briefly before desensitization appeared (c) when menthol was
	desensitization to nicotine.				Males and females ages 18-50 yrs who were students and staff at University of California at Davis, non smokers, and did not participate in Experiment 1. Experiment 3 was same as Exp 1 & 2	N=27 (5 males and 22 females)	reapplied following a rest period, most subjects appeared to exhibit recovery from desensitization.
Galeotti N, Di Cesare	Menthol: a natural analgesic	2002	No funding source(s) provided. Authors	Experimental	Not Applicable	Not Applicable	Menthol cross-desensitizes a class of capsaicinsensitive nociceptors, resulting in

Author	Article Title	Year	Funded By	Type of Study	Subject Description	Sample	Authors' Results/Conclusion(s) related to
Mannelli L, Mazzanti G, Bartolini A, Ghelardini C.	compound.		affiliated with University of Florence, Italy				analgesic activity. In rodents, menthol produced dose- dependent analgesic effects, postulated to work via activation of the K opioid system
Green BG, Schullery MT.	Stimulation of bitterness by capsaicin and menthol: differences between lingual areas innervated by the glossopharyngeal and chorda tympani nerves.	2003	Funded by a grant from the National Institutes of Health R01 DC 05002	Not Specified	Adults between ages of 18-45 yrs. old at Yale.	Exp 1: 15 (11 females and 4 males) Exp 2: 16 (9 females and 7 males)	Study suggests that Capsaicin and menthol are capable of stimulating a subset of taste neurons that respond to bitter substance and that the glossopharyngeal nerve may contain more such neurons than the chorda tympani nerve.
Heck JD.	Smokers of menthol and nonmenthol cigarettes exhibit similar levels of biomarkers of smoke exposure.	2009	No funding source(s) provided. Author affiliated with Lorillard Tobacco Company	Cross-sectional	male and female subjects 24 to 70 yrs of age, having a minimum smoking history of 3 pack-years, and reporting consumption of >15 menthol or nonmenthol cigarettes daily for the past year,	N=112 (54 menthol, 58 nonmenthol)	The present findings indicate that moderately heavy smokers of menthol and nonmenthol cigarettes of similar machine-generated smoke yield exhibit essentially identical levels of biomarkers of smoke constituent exposure.
Ito S, Kume H, Shiraki A, Kondo M, Makino Y, Kamiya K, Hasegawa Y.	Inhibition by the cold receptor agonists menthol and icilin of airway smooth muscle contraction.	2008	Grant-in-Aid for Young Scientists A, Scientific Research C, and the 21th Century COE Program from the Ministry of Education, Culture, Sports, Science, and Technology of Japan	*In Vitro*	Male Hartley guinea pigs	Not Specified	Findings support the use of menthol for reducing airflow limitation and chest congestion in patients with symptomatic airway diseases.

Physiology: Table of Referenced Sources (Continued)

Author Name(s)	Article Title	Year Pub.	Funded By	Type of Study	Subject Description (Including Special population(s))	Sample Size (N)	Authors' Results/Conclusion(s) related to Menthol* (excerpted directly from article)
Jarvik ME, Tashkin DP, Caskey NH, McCarthy WJ, Rosenblatt MR.	Mentholated cigarettes decrease puff volume of smoke and increase carbon monoxide absorption.	1994	California Tobacco Related Disease Research Program Grant #1 RT 0087; Medical Research Service, U.S. Departement of Veterans Affairs; Division of Lung Diseases, National Heart, Lung, and Blood Institute Contract NO-HR 46022	Comparative	Black and white male subjects with a self-reported history of smoking at least 15 cigarettes per day on a regular basis. Half were regular and half were menthol smokers.	N=20 (10 black, 10 white)	Compared to regular cigarettes, mentholated cigarettes produced a significantly greater boost in carbon monoxide measured as both blood carboxyhemoglobin and end-expired carbon monoxide, despite the fact that mentholated cigarettes decreased average and total cumulative puff volumes and increased mean puff flow rates of inhaled smoke.
Kühn FJ, Kühn C, Lückhoff A.	Inhibition of TRPM8 by icilin distinct from desensitization induced by menthol and menthol derivatives.	2009	the Deutsche Forschungsgemeinschaft Grant DFG KU 2271/1-1	Experimental	Not Applicable	Not Applicable	In this study we have demonstrated that the menthol derivatives WS-12, CPS-369, and CPS-154 act identically with menthol in terms of Ca2+-independent current activation andCa2+- dependent induction of desensitization on wild- type TRPM8 as well as on the S3 mutant.
Laude EA, Morice AH, Grattan TJ.	The antitussive effects of menthol, camphor and cineole in conscious guinea-pigs.	1994	No funding source(s) provided. Authors affiliated with University of Sheffield, UK	Experimental	Guinea Pigs	N=13	Menthol proved the most effective antitussive -- 10 and 30 micrograms/l produced a significant 28 and 56% reduction in cough frequency.
Lin JP, Lu HF, Lee JH, Lin JG, Hsia TC,	(-)-Menthol inhibits DNA topoisomerases I, II	2005	Grants CMC90-CM-01 and CMC91-CM-02 from the Research	Experimental	Human gastric SNU-5 cancer cells	Not Specified	(-)-Menthol may induce cytotoxicity through inhibiting gene expression of topoisomerase I, IIalpha and IIbeta and

Author	Article Title	Year	Funded By	Type of Study	Subject Description	Sample	Authors' Results/Conclusion(s) related to
Wu LT, Chung JG.	alpha and beta and promotes NF-		Section of China Medical University, Taichung City, Taiwan,				promoting the gene expression of NF-kappaB in SNU-5 cells.
	kappaB expression in human gastric cancer SNU-5 cells.		R.O.C.				
MacDougall JM, Fandrick K, Zhang X, Serafin SV, Cashman JR.	Inhibition of human liver microsomal (S)-nicotine oxidation by (-)- menthol and analogues.	2003	University of California Tobacco Related Disease Research Program (Grant 9RT-0196) and a Cornelius Hopper Diversity Award	Comparative, *In Vitro*	Not Specified	Not Specified	While highly potent inhibition of P450 2A6 was not observed for the menthol analogues examined, it is nevertheless possible that smoking mentholated cigarettes leads to inhibition of nicotine metabolism and allows the smoker to achieve a certain elevated dose of nicotine each day.
McCarthy WJ, Caskey NH, Jarvik ME, Gross TM, Rosenblatt MR, Carpenter C.	Menthol vs nonmenthol cigarettes: effects on smoking behavior.	1995	Cigarette and Tobacco Surtax Fund of the State of California through the Tobacco-Related Disease Research Program of the University of California, grant 1 RT-87	Controlled Clinical Trial, Comparative	Healthy male smokers	N=29	Whatever the mechanism by which menthol facilitates absorption of carbon monoxide (and probably nicotine), the study's repeated-measures data suggest that inferences about the genetic basis for observed racial differences in blood cotinine levels may be premature, and conjectures about the effects of menthol in cigarettes on smoking behavior may need to be modified.
Orani GP, Anderson JW, Sant'Ambrogio G, Sant'Ambrogio FB.	Upper airway cooling and l-menthol reduce ventilation in the guinea pig.	1991	National Heart, Lung, and Blood Institute Grant HL- 20122	Experimental	Guinea Pigs	N=23	Both cooling of the larynx and l-menthol in the laryngeal lumen reduce ventilation. Exposure of the nasal cavity to l-menthol markedly enhances this ventilatory inhibition; considering the stimulatory effect of l-menthol on cold receptors, these results suggest a predominant role of nasal cold receptors in this response.

Physiology: Table of Referenced Sources (Continued)

Author Name(s)	Article Title	Year Pub.	Funded By	Type of Study	Subject Description (Including Special population(s))	Sample Size (N)	Authors' Results/Conclusion(s) related to Menthol* (excerpted directly from article)
Pickworth WB, Moolchan ET, Berlin I, Murty R.	Sensory and physiologic effects of menthol and non- menthol cigarettes with differing nicotine delivery.	2002	National Institute on Drug Abuse intramural funds	Randomized Controlled Trial, Comparative	The menthol group was composed of 13 men and 5 women; 17 were African American, 1 was Caucasian. The nonmenthol group was composed of 14 men and 4 women; 3 were African American, 15	36 Menthol (n=18) and non-menthol (n=18) cigarette smokers)	Nicotine delivery, but not mentholation, influences cardiovascular and most subjective measures. These results illustrate the importance of threshold levels of nicotine on subjective responses to cigarette smoking.
					were Caucasian.		
Sant'Ambrogio FB, Anderson JW, Sant'Ambrogio G.	Effect of l-menthol on laryngeal receptors.	1991	National Heart, Lung, and Blood Institute Grant HL- 20122	Experimental	Dogs	N=11	L-menthol constitutes a specific stimulant of laryngeal cold receptors and could provide a useful tool for the study of their reflex effects.
Sant'Ambrogio FB, Anderson JW, Sant'Ambrogio G.	Menthol in the upper airway depresses ventilation in newborn dogs.	1992	National Institutes of Health Grant HL-20122	Experimental	Newborn dogs	N=8	However, a residual depressive effect of/-menthol was still present in 3 of 5 animals and was abolished by nasal anesthesia, suggesting the involvement of nasal cold receptors.
Sekizawa S, Tsubone H, Kuwahara M, Sugano S.	Nasal receptors responding to cold and l-menthol airflow in the guinea pig.	1996	JSPS Fellowships for Japanese Junior Scientists	*In Vitro*	Guinea Pigs	Not Specified	L-menthol noticeably stimulated the EN even after repeated capsaicin instillation into the nose, but these values were lower than those following the /-menthol stimulus before the 1st capsaicin treatment.
Sherkheli MA,	Menthol derivative	2008	IMPRS-CB, Research	Experimental	TRPM8 Ion channels	Not	The selectivity profile of WS-12, its

Author	Article Title	Year	Funded By	Type of Study	Subject Description	Sample	Authors' Results/Conclusion(s) related to
Gisselmann G, Vogt-Eisele AK, Doerner JF, Hatt H.	WS-12 selectively activates transient receptor potential melastatin-8 (TRPM8) ion channels.		Excellence School of Bochum and DAAD			Specified	several-fold higher potency and around two-fold increase in efficacy compared to menthol warrants its potential utility for therapy in chronic neuropathic pain states and as a diagnostic probe in prostate cancer.
Sidell N, Verity MA, Nord EP.	Menthol blocks dihydropyridine-insensitive Ca2+ channels and induces neurite outgrowth in human neuroblastoma cells.	1990	National Institutes of Health grants CA 43503, CA 30515, DK 36351, and DK 41585	Comparative	Human neuroblastoma cells	Not Specified	The parallel potency for blockade of DHP-insensitive Ca2+ influx with the biologic activity of menthol suggests a role for certain types of Ca2+ channels in triggering growth and morphologic changes in LA-N-5.
Squier, CA, MJ Mantz, PW Wertz.	Effect of menthol on the penetration of tobacco carcinogens and	2010	The Dows Institute for Dental Research, College of Dentistry, University of Iowa	Experimental	Porcine tissue	Not Specified	Menthol enhances penetration of NNN and nicotine through FM and BM *in vitro*, even after short exposure. Practical implications are for a potentially increased oral exposure to
	nicotine across porcine oral mucosa ex vivo.						carcinogens among users of menthol-flavored cigarettes and chewing tobacco.
Wang J, Roethig HJ, Appleton S, Werley M, Muhammad-Kah R, Mendes P.	The effect of menthol containing cigarettes on adult smokers' exposure to nicotine and carbon monoxide.	2010	No funding source(s) provided. Authors affiliated with Altria Client Services].	Cross-sectional, observational, ambulatory, multi-centre study	African-American and White adult males and females, 21 years old or older, in generally good health, from 31 states (39 investigative sites across the United States), were enrolled into one of 4 parallel	N=3341	Smoking mentholated cigarettes does not increase daily exposure to smoke constituents as measured by NE and COHb. These findings are consistent with the majority of epidemiological studies indicating no difference in smoking related risks between MS and NMS.

Physiology: Table of Referenced Sources (Continued)

Author Name(s)	Article Title	Year Pub.	Funded By	Type of Study	Subject Description (Including Special population(s))	Sample Size (N)	Authors' Results/Conclusion(s) related to Menthol* (excerpted directly from article)
					groups based on the smoking machine derived tar categories (i.e., 62.9 mg tar; 3.0– 6.9 mg tar; 7.0– 12.9 mg tar; and P13.0 mg tar) of the cigarettes they smoked.		
Wright CE, Laude EA, Grattan TJ, Morice AH.	Capsaicin and neurokinin A-induced bronchoconstriction in the anaesthetised guinea-pig: evidence for a direct action of menthol on isolated bronchial smooth muscle.	1997	No funding source(s) provided. Authors affiliated with University of Sheffield	Experimental	Dunkin-Hartley Guinea- pigs	N=24	Menthol attenuates both capsaicin and NKAinduced bronchoconstriction *in vivo* and relaxes KCl and ACh preconstricted bronchi *in vitro*. Menthol inhibition of NKA and capsaicin-induced bronchoconstriction could be, in part, explained by a direct action of menthol on bronchial smooth muscle.
Yerger VB, McCandless PM	Menthol sensory qualities and smoking topography: a review of tobacco industry	2011	Department of Health and Human Services Contract HHSN261201000035I, California Tobacco-Related Disease	Review of publicly available tobacco industry documents	Not Applicable	252 publicly available internal tobacco industry documents	Our review of industry studies suggests that the amount of menthol in a cigarette is associated with how the cigarette is smoked and how satisfying it is to the smoker.

Author	Article Title	Year	Funded By	Type of Study	Subject Description	Sample	Authors' Results/Conclusion(s)
	documents		Research Program, Grant #16RT-0149, and National Cancer Institute grant CA11371005				

* Note: these statements are taken directly from articles and may not include all relevant results/conclusions.

Azzi C, Zhang J, Purdon CH, Chapman JM, Nitcheva D, Hebert JR, Smith EW. (2006). Permeation and reservoir formation of 4-(methylnitrosamino)-1-(3-pyridyl)-1-butanone (NNK) and benzo[a]pyrene (B[a]P) across porcine esophageal tissue in the presence of ethanol and menthol. Carcinogenisis 27(1):137-45. [Funded by a MUSC/USC/HCC Department of Defense Funds, Phase VI, Cancer Prevention and Control Research Development Grant]

Benowitz NL, Herrera B, Jacob P 3rd. (2004) Menthol cigarette smoking inhibits nicotine metabolism. Journal of Pharmacology and Experimental Therapeutics 310(3):1208-15. [Funded by State of California Tobacco Related Disease Research Program Grant 1RT-0521, by U.S. Public Health Service Grants DA02277 and DA12393 awarded by the National Institute on Drug Abuse and CA32389 awarded by the National Cancer Institute, and by the General Clinical Research Center at San Francisco General Hospital Medical Center with the support of the Division of Research Resources, National Institutes of Health (RR-00083)]

Campero M, Baumann TK, Bostock H, Ochoa JL. (2009). Human cutaneous C fibers activated by cooling, heating and menthol. Journal of Physiology 587(Pt 23):5633-52. [Funded by NIH Grant no. R01-NS48932]

Dessirier JM, O'Mahony M, Carstens, E. (2001). Oral irritant properties of menthol sensitizing and desensitizing effects of repeated application of cross-desensitization to nicotine. Physiology & Behavior, 73:25-36. [Funded by a grant from the California Tobacco-Related Research Disease Program No. 6RT-0231]

Galeotti N, Di Cesare Mannelli L, Mazzanti G, Bartolini A, Ghelardini C. (2002). Menthol: a natural analgesic compound. Neuroscience Letters 322(3):145-8. [No funding source(s) provided. Authors affiliated with University of Florence, Italy]

Green BG, Schullery MT (2003). Stimulation of bitterness by capsaicin and menthol: Differences between linguaal areas innervated by the glossopharyngeal and chorda tympani nerves. Chemical Senses 28:45-55. [Funded by a grant from the National Institutes of Health R01 DC 05002]

Heck JD (2009) Smokers of menthol and nonmenthol cigarettes exhibit similar levels of biomarkers of smoke exposure. Cancer Epidemiology Biomarkers and Prevention 18(2):622-9. [No funding source(s) provided. Author affiliated with Lorillard Tobacco Company]

Ito S, Kume H, Shiraki A, Kondo M, Makino Y, Kamiya K, Hasegawa Y. (2008). Inhibition by the cold receptor agonists menthol and icilin of airway smooth muscle contraction. Pulmonary Pharmacology and Therapeutics21(5):812-7. [Funded by Grant- in-Aid for Young Scientists A, Scientific Research C, and the 21th Century COE Program from the Ministry of Education, Culture, Sports, Science, and Technology of Japan]

Jarvik ME, Tashkin DP, Caskey NH, McCarthy WJ, Rosenblatt MR (2004). Menthol cigarettes decrease puff volume of smoke and increase carbon monoxide absorption. Physiology & Behavior 1994;56:563e70. [Funded by California Tobacco Related Disease Research Program Grant #1 RT 0087; Medical Research Service, U.S. Departement of Veterans Affairs; Division of Lung Diseases, National Heart, Lung, and Blood Institute Contract NO-HR 46022]

Kühn FJ, Kühn C, Lückhoff A. (2009). Inhibition of TRPM8 by icilin distinct from desensitization induced by menthol and menthol derivatives. Journal of Biological

Chemistry 284(7):4102-11. [Funded by the Deutsche Forschungsgemeinschaft Grant DFG KU 2271/1-1]

Laude EA, Morice AH, Grattan, TJ. (1994) The antitussive effects of menthol, camphor and cineole in conscious guinea pigs. Pulmonary Pharmacology 7:179-184. [No funding source(s) provided. Authors affiliated with University of Sheffield, UK]

Lin JP, Lu HF, Lee JH, Lin JG, Hsia TC, Wu LT, Chung JG. (2005). (-)-Menthol inhibits DNA topoisomerases I, II alpha and beta and promotes NF-kappaB expression in human gastric cancer SNU-5 cells. Anticancer Research 25(3B):2069-74. [Funded by grants CMC90-CM-01 and CMC91-CM-02 from the Research Section of China Medical University, Taichung City, Taiwan, R.O.C.]

MacDougall JM, Fandrick K, Zhang X, Serafin SV, Cashman JR. (2003). Inhibition of human liver microsomal (S)-nicotine oxidation by (-)-menthol and analogues. Chemical Research in Toxicology 16(8):988-93. [Funded by the University of California Tobacco Related Disease Research Program (Grant 9RT-0196) and a Cornelius Hopper Diversity Award]

McCarthy WJ, Caskey NH, Jarvik ME, Gross, TM, Rosenblatt, MR, Carpenter, C. (1995). Menthol vs.nonmenthol cigarettes: effects on smoking behavior. American Journal of Public Health 1995;85:67e72. [Funded by the Cigarette and Tobacco Surtax Fund of the State of California through the Tobacco- Related Disease Research Program of the University of California, grant 1 RT-87]

Orani GP, Anderson JW, Sant'Ambrogio G, Sant'Ambrogio FB. (1991). Upper airway cooling and l-menthol reduce ventilation in the guinea pig. Journal of Applied Physiology 70:2080–2086. [Funded by the National Heart, Lung and Blood Institute Grant HL-20122.]

Pickworth WB, Moolchan ET, Berlin I, Murty R. (2002). Sensory and physiologic effects of menthol and non-menthol cigarettes with differing nicotine delivery. Pharmacology Biochemistry and Behavior. 71(1-2):55-61. [Funded by National Institute on Drug Abuse intramural funds]

Sant'Ambrogio FB, Anderson JW, Sant'Ambrogio G (1991) Effect of l-menthol on laryngeal receptors. Journal of Applied Physiology 70:788–793. [Funded by National Heart, Lung, and Blood Institute grant HL-20122]

Sant'Ambrogio FB, Anderson JW, Sant'Ambrogio G. (1992). Menthol in the upper airway depresses ventilation in newborn dogs. Respiration Physiology 89(3):299-307. [Funded by National Heart, Lung, and Blood Institute grant HL-20122]

Sekizawa SI, Tsubone H, Kuwahara M, Sugana S. (1996). Nasal receptors responding to cold and l-menthol airflow in the guinea pig. Respiration Physiology 103(3):211–219. [Funded by JSPS Fellowships for Japanese Junior Scientists, IMPRS-CB]

Sherkheli MA, Gisselmann G, et al. (2008) Menthol derivative WS-12 selectively activates transient receptor potential melastatin-8 (TRPM8) ion channels. Pakistan Journal of Pharmaceutical Sciences, 21(4):370–378. [Funded by IMPRS-CB, Research Excellence School of Bochum and DAAD]

Sidell N, Verity MA, Nord EP (1990) Menthol blocks dihydropyridine-insensitive Ca2+ channels and induces neurite outgrowth in human neuroblastoma cells. Journal of Cellular Physiology 142(2):410–419. [Funded by National Institutes of Health grants CA 43503, CA 30515, DK 36351 and DK 41585]

Squier CA, Mantz MJ, Wertz PW (2010) Effect of menthol on the penetration of tobacco carcinogens and nicotine across porcine oral mucosa ex vivo. Nicotine and Tobacco Research 12(7):763-7 [Funded by the Dows Institute for Dental Research, College of Dentistry, University of Iowa]

Wang J, Roethig HJ, Appleton S, et al. (2010): The effect of menthol containing cigarettes on adult smokers' exposure to nicotine and carbon monoxide. Regulatory Toxicology and Pharmacology 57:24–30. [No funding source(s) provided. Authors affiliated with Altria Client Services].

Wright CE, Laude EA, et al. (1997) Capsaicin and neurokinin A-induced broncho-constriction in the anaesthetised guinea-pig: evidence for a direct action of menthol on isolated bronchial smooth muscle. British Journal of Pharmacology 121(8):1645–1650. [No funding source(s) provided. Authors affiliated with University of Sheffield]

Yerger VB, McCandless PM. (2011) Menthol sensory qualities and smoking topography: a review of tobacco industry documents. Tobacco Control 20(suppl 2):ii37-43. [Funded by the Department of Health and Human Services Contract HHSN261201000035I, California Tobacco-Related Disease Research Program, Grant #16RT-0149, and National Cancer Institute grant CA113710-05]

C. Biomarkers

Biomarkers of exposure are used to objectively measure and evaluate levels of exposure to particular chemicals. Biomarkers that are used to evaluate smoke exposure include particular smoke constituents and/or their metabolites in biological specimens (e.g., exhaled air, saliva, blood, urine). Specifically, biomarkers assessed here include expired carbon monoxide (CO) and blood carboxyhemoglobin (COHb) for levels of CO exposure, cotinine and other nicotine equivalents in serum and urine for exposure to nicotine, and total NNAL in urine for exposure to TSNAs. Very limited data are available for other biomarkers of exposure and biomarkers of potential harm.

Biomarkers of Exposure to CO

Miller et al. (1994) measured the exhaled CO levels in male smokers (n = 12) who participated in three controlled-dose smoking sessions spaced one week apart. Exhaled CO levels increased along with menthol external dose. The authors proposed that these results suggested that menthol cigarette preference may account for some of the racial differences in smoking behavior and smoking-related outcomes.

In a cross-sectional study, Clark et al. (1996) found that, compared with White smokers (n=96), African American smokers (n=65) had significantly higher breath CO levels per cigarette smoked and per millimeter of the smoked tobacco rod after adjusting for race, cpd, and mean amount of each cigarette smoked.

Williams et al. (2007) examined expired CO for 89 smokers with schizophrenia and 53 control smokers two minutes after smoking an afternoon cigarette. Expired CO was higher in menthol compared with nonmenthol smokers, controlling for group, cpd, and race. The higher exhaled CO in menthol smokers suggests an increased intake of smoke from menthol cigarettes.

One study found menthol cigarettes were associated with decreased breath CO. Ahijevych et al. (1996) conducted a two-factor factorial trial with a sample of 37 women stratified by race and menthol or nonmenthol cigarette use. For CO boost, there was a significant main effect for race (African Americans > Whites) and a main effect for menthol or nonmenthol use (nonmenthol > menthol).

Benowitz et al. (2004) found that mentholation of cigarettes did not affect systemic intake of nicotine and CO in a crossover study with 14 smokers.

Biomarkers of Exposure to Nicotine

In a small, experimental study with 32 women, Ahijevych et al. (2002) examined the effect of selected factors of ethnicity, menthol cigarette preference, body composition and alcohol-use history on cotinine half-life. Being an African American menthol smoker, fewer years of alcohol use, and greater lean body mass explained 52.0 percent of the variance in cotinine half-life and was associated with a longer half-life. Among menthol smokers, baseline cotinine level and cotinine half-life were not significantly different between White and African American women.

Clark et al. (1996) found that, compared with White smokers (n=96), African American smokers (n=65) had significantly higher serum cotinine levels per cigarette smoked and per millimeter of smoked tobacco rod after adjusting for race, cpd, and mean amount of each cigarette smoked.

Using a sample of 359 participants, Mustonen et al. (2005) observed a positive correlation between cotinine and CO in all smokers and a correlation between cotinine and cpd in nonmenthol smokers. Among menthol smokers, cotinine and cpd correlations varied by gender and race. Results showed trends to higher cotinine levels in menthol smokers, although the differences were not statistically significant. The cotinine:cpd ratio was significantly higher among menthol smokers compared to nonmenthol smokers (p=0.004). A significant gender by race by menthol interaction existed on salivary cotinine level as well as cotinine:cpd ratio.

Williams et al. (2007) examined serum nicotine and cotinine for 89 smokers with schizophrenia and 53 control smokers two minutes after smoking an afternoon cigarette. Serum nicotine and cotinine levels were higher in smokers of menthol compared with nonmenthol cigarettes. There were no differences in 3-hydroxycotinine:cotinine ratios between groups when controlling for race. Further linear regression models showed that smoking menthol cigarettes was a significant predictor of nicotine and cotinine levels. The higher exhaled CO in menthol smokers described above suggests that the higher nicotine levels are at least partially related to increased smoke intake from menthol cigarettes. These authors suggested that menthol might be associated with increased health risks of smoking.

In a crossover study of 14 participants, Benowitz et al. (2004) found that mentholation of cigarettes did not affect systemic intake of nicotine. However, menthol cigarette smoking inhibited the metabolism of nicotine by slower oxidative metabolism to cotinine and by slower glucuronide conjugation.

White and African American Smokers

Perez-Stable et al. (1998) found higher levels of cotinine per cigarette smoked by African Americans (n=40) compared with Whites (n=39). Both slower clearance of cotinine and higher intake of nicotine per cigarette in African Americans explain this result.

Caraballo et al. (1998) provided evidence from a large national study (n=7182) that African American smokers have higher serum cotinine levels than do White or Mexican

American smokers, after adjustment for cpd, age, sex, body weight, number of smokers living in the home, and number of hours exposed at work to environmental tobacco smoke.

Using data from smokers in the the CARDIA longitudinal cohort study (n=1424), Wagenknecht et al. (1990) found signficantly higher serum cotinine levels in African American smokers as compared to White smokers. This difference remained significant after adjusting for cpd, nicotine content of the cigarette, years of smoking, inhalation frequency, and demographic factors. This difference was not explained by reporting bias or nicotine intake differences. The study suggested that the differences in serum cotinine levels may be due to innate differences between the races in the metabolism or excretion of nicotine or cotinine.

In a study of 91 adolescents seeking cessation treatment, Moolchan et al. (2006) found that African Americans (n=30) smoked significantly fewer cpd and had lower nicotine metabolite ratios when compared to White smokers (n=61). Consistent with metabolic variation, mean plasma cotinine:cpd ratio was significantly higher in African American compared to White adolescents. Results remained statistically significant when comparing menthol smokers by ethnicity. The data suggested that observed differences are due to factors other than menthol smoking and suggest that accounting for racial or ethnic differences is crucial for interpreting group differences.

Menthol and Nonmenthol Smokers

Using data from 1999–2002 NHANES (n=1520), Gan et al. (2008) found that serum cotinine levels were significantly higher in menthol smokers compared with nonmenthol smokers using a univariate model but not significantly higher using a multivariate model adjusted for gender, cpd, age, race, BMI, poverty status, Federal Trade Commission test nicotine content in each cigarette, and menthol or nonmenthol use.

In a sample of 37 white and African American women, Ahijevych et al. (1996) found no significant differences in nicotine boost by race and/or menthol or nonmenthol use.

In a community-based cross-sectional study (n=525), Muscat et al. (2009) found no significant differences in measures of smoking exposure (metabolites of nicotine or NNAL) by menthol status in either white or African American smokers.

Patterson et al. (2003) investigated the demographic, smoking status, and psychological predictors of nicotine boost in a clinical trial with 190 treatment-seeking smokers. Boost was assessed by comparing plasma nicotine levels before and after participants smoked one of their own brand of cigarettes as desired. Menthol or nonmenthol brand was not associated with the nicotine boost.

Using samples of 255 current smokers from the Southern Community Cohort Study participants, Signorello et al. (2009) found higher serum cotinine levels in African American compared with White smokers, particularly for women, and observed no increase in serum cotinine levels associated with menthol cigarette use after adjusting for age, race, sex, and cpd. The authors concluded that the differences in serum cotinine levels among smokers might be due to racial variation in exposure to and/or metabolism of tobacco smoke constituents.

Biomarkers of exposure to TSNAs

In a community-based cross-sectional study, Muscat et al. (2009) found no significant differences in measures of smoking exposure (metabolites of nicotine or NNAL). The NNAL-glucuronide(Gluc):NNAL ratio between smokers of menthol (n=67) and nonmenthol (n=80) cigarettes was 34 percent lower in Whites (P < 0.01) and 22 percent lower in African Americans; the difference in African Americans was not statistically significant.

In a study of 109 current smokers, Strasser et al. (2011) found faster nicotine metabolizers had greater total puff volume and total NNAL. Groups with more nonmenthol smokers (quartiles three and four) appeared to have higher mean NNAL than groups with fewer nonmenthol smokers (quartiles one and two) although the difference was not statistically significant.

Richie et al. (1997) found that urinary NNAL-Gluc:NNAL ratios, a likely indicator of NNAL glucuronidation and detoxification, were significantly greater in Whites (n=27) than in African Americans (n=34). The absolute levels of urinary NNAL, NNAL-Gluc, and cotinine were also greater in African Americans than in Whites when adjusted for the cpd. Dissimilarities in exposure or other sociodemographic or dietary factors did not explain observed racial differences. Also, it is unlikely that the dissimilarities are due to racial differences in preference for menthol cigarettes, because chronic administration of menthol to NNK-treated rats did not result in either increases in urinary total NNAL or decreases in NNAL-Gluc:NNAL ratios. Altogether, these results suggest that racial differences in NNAL glucuronidation may explain in part the observed racial differences in lung cancer risk.

Additional Evidence Based on Altria Total Exposure Study

FDA analyzed additional data from the Altria TES using unadjusted and adjusted regression models, which were collected from over 5,000 participants. The variables in the adjusted model consisted of gender, race, education, income, Hispanic ethnicity, BMI, number of years and cigarettes smoked, tar delivery category, and total puff volume. Biomarkers of exposure include urine level measures of total nicotine equivalents, total NNAL, total 1-hydroxypyrene (1-OHP), total 3-hydroxypropyl mercapturic acid (3-HPMA), total monohydroxy-3-butenyl mercapturic acids (MHBMA), total 1, 2-dihydroxybutyl mercapturic acid (DHBMA), and serum level measurements of cotinine, carboxyhemoglobin, and red blood cell 4-aminobiphenyl (4-ABP) hemoglobin (Hb) adducts. All biomarkers obtained from urine measurements were analyzed as cigarette-adjusted and creatinine-adjusted measures as well as totals. The analysis found no statistically significant differences between menthol and nonmenthol smokers in any biomarkers of exposure in the adjusted model. The observed statistically significant differences in biomarkers of exposure (unadjusted data) between menthol and nonmenthol smokers may be due to differences in demographic or smoking behavior characteristics between menthol and nonmenthol smokers. In both the total and creatinine-adjusted measures, menthol smokers showed significantly lower levels of exposure to nicotine equivalents (p<0.0001 and p=0.0002, respectively), NNAL (p<0.0001 and p=0.0002), 3-HPMA (p<0.0001 and p<0.0001), MHBMA (p<0.0001 and p<0.0001), and DHBMA (p<0.0001 and p<0.0001) in the unadjusted model. However, no per cigarette measure for these outcomes showed any statistically significant differences between menthol and nonmenthol smokers. Menthol smokers showed significantly higher levels of 1-OHP exposure per cigarette than nonmenthol smokers (p=0.0002) in the unadjusted model. However, no significant differences in exposure to 1-OHP per cigarette between menthol and nonmenthol smoker were observed in the adjusted model. The unadjusted 3-hydroxycotinine:cotinine ratio was significantly higher (indicating more rapid detoxification) in menthol smokers (p<0.0001). However, the significance of this difference did not persist after adjusting for demographic and smoking behavior variables. Neither the nicotine:cotinine ratio in the adjusted or unadjusted model showed any significant differences between menthol and nonmenthol smokers. The likely explanation for this result lies with differences between African American and other racial groups' cotinine levels.

In the TES, biomarkers of potential harm included urine level measures for 8-epi prostaglandin- F2Ɩ and 11-dehydrothromboxane-B2 and serum level measures of total bilirubin, white blood cells, C-reactive protein, fibrinogen, von Willebrand factor antigen, total, high density lipoprotein (HDL), low density lipoprotein (LDL), and oxidized LDL cholesterol, triglycerides, forced expiratory volume in one second (FEV1), and forced expiratory vital capacity (FVC). Urine measurements were analyzed as creatinine-adjusted measures as well as totals. In the unadjusted model, menthol smokers showed significantly lower levels of total cholesterol (p=0.0002), LDL cholesterol (p=0.0053), and triglycerides (p<0.0001), and higher levels of HDL cholesterol (p=0.0016). However, these differences were no longer significant after adjustment for demographic and smoking behavior variables. Menthol smokers also showed significantly lower unadjusted levels of 8-epi prostaglandin-F2 (p=0.0491), white blood cells (p=0.0002), and total bilirubin (p=0.0012), but higher levels of the van Willebrand antigen factor (p=0.0172). The only difference between menthol and nonmenthol smokers that remained statistically significant in the adjusted model was for 8-epi prostaglandin-F2 (p=0.0318). However, the effect of menthol on 8-epi prostaglandin-F2 reversed direction after adjustment for demographic characteristics and smoking behavior, with menthol smokers showing significantly higher levels of 8-epi prostaglandin of about 99 ng per 24 hour period higher for menthol smokers.

FDA also analyzed demographic, smoking, and biomarker levels for over 5000 smokers participating in the National Health and Nutrition Examination Survey (NHANES) from 1999- 2008. Researchers used linear regression, controlling for demographic, health, and smoking characteristics to analyze the associations between menthol cigarette use and biomarker levels. Menthol cigarette use was not associated with higher serum cotinine levels on a per cigarette basis. There was no statistically significant difference for NNAL levels for menthol smokers compared to nonmenthol smokers, although additional data are needed to more precisely estimate any association for this biomarker.

Menthol secondary data analysis (through RTI subcontracts) of the Hersey study examined the relationship in youth (n= 5,511) between smoking menthol cigarettes, salivary cotinine levels, and nicotine dependence. Controlling for age, sex, race or ethnicity, and the length, frequency, and level of smoking, descriptive and regression analysis found that menthol versus nonmenthol cigarette use was not significantly associated with salivary cotinine level models that included cpd smoked. Among youth who smoked for less than one year, a significant interaction exists between menthol use and the number of cigarettes smoked per day -- menthol cigarette use was associated with increased salivary cotinine levels among heavier smokers. Findings were similar for Whites and non-Whites.

Industry Assessment of Menthol Effects

Not all studies support the hypothesis that menthol cigarette smoking results in a greater absorption of tobacco smoke chemicals. In an industry-sponsored study, Heck (2009) found median blood carboxyhemoglobin values, total urinary 4-(methylnitrosamino)-1-(3-pyridyl)-1-butanol (NNAL), and urinary nicotine equivalents were not significantly different between the menthol and nonmenthol cigarette smokers. In an industry-sponsored study, Wang et al. (2010) found smoking menthol cigarettes does not increase daily exposure to smoke constituents as measured by nicotine equivalents (total and per cigarette), serum cotinine and COHb after adjusting for the number of cigarettes smoked per day and the smoking behavior characteristics of the participants. In its presentation to TPSAC, Altria Client Services presented analysis of the TES that also showed no differences between users of menthol and nonmenthol brands in the TES for a wide variety of biomarkers of exposure, biomarkers of potential harm, nicotine metabolite ratios, and measures of smoker topography and nicotine dependence after adjustment for the number of cigarettes per day and smoking behavior characteristics.

Conclusion

Although a few small studies have found that smoking menthol cigarettes may modulate exposure or metabolism of CO, nicotine, and/or TSNAs, several large, well-designed studies failed to find statistically significant differences in biomarkers between smoking menthol or nonmenthol cigarettes. Considering all available studies, but with more emphasis given to the findings of the large, well-controlled studies, the weight of evidence supports the conclusion that menthol in cigarettes is likely not associated with increased or decreased levels of biomarkers of exposure.

References

Ahijevych K, Gillespie J, et al. (1996) Menthol and nonmenthol cigarettes and smoke exposure in black and white women. Pharmacology, Biochemistry, and Behavior, 53(2):355–360. [Funded by The Ohio State University Seed Grant and The Ohio State University General Clinical Research Center Grant MO1 RR00034]

Ahijevych KL, Tyndale RF, Dhatt RK, et al. (2002) Factors influencing cotinine half-life during smoking abstinence in African American and Caucasian women. Nicotine and Tobacco Research, 4:423–431. [Funded by National Institute on Drug Abuse DA10809, DA 06889 and The Ohio State University General Clinical Research Center M01 RR00034, and Ohio State University Academic Primary Care Program, USDHHS Bureau of Health Professions 1 D12 HP00027]

Benowitz NL, Herrera B, et al. (2004) Menthol cigarette smoking inhibits nicotine metabolism. Journal of Pharmacology and Experimental Therapies, 310(3):1208–1215. [Funded by State of California Tobacco Related Disease Research Program Grant 1RT-0521, by U.S. Public Health Service Grants DA02277 and DA12393 awarded by the National Institute on Drug Abuse and CA32389 awarded by the National Cancer Institute, and by the General Clinical Research Center at San Francisco General Hospital Medical Center with the support of the Division of Research Resources, National Institutes of Health (RR-00083)]

Biomarkers: Table of Referenced Sources

Author Name(s)	Article Title	Year Pub.	Funded By	Type of Study	Subject Description (Including Special population(s))	Sample Size (N)	Authors' Results/Conclusion(s) related to Menthol* (excerpted directly from article)
Ahijevych K, Gillespie J, Demirci M, Jagadeesh J.	Menthol and nonmenthol cigarettes and smoke exposure in black and white women.	1996	The Ohio State University Seed Grant; The Ohio State University General Clinical Research Center Grant MO1 RR00034	Cross sectional 2 factor factorial design	Black and White Women 19-59 years old, smoked "20 cpd	N=37 (18 Black, 19 White)	In the current study, lower CO boost with mentholated cigarettes suggests that factors beyond mentholation may affect differences in cotinine levels in black and white women.
Ahijevych KL, Tyndale RF, Dhatt RK, Weed HG, Browning KK.	Factors influencing cotinine half-life during smoking abstinence in African American and Caucasian women.	2002	National Institute on Drug Abuse DA10809, DA 06889 and The Ohio State University General Clinical Research Center M01 RR00034, and Ohio State University Academic Primary Care Program, USDHHS Bureau of Health Professions 1 D12 HP00027	Analytic	African American and Caucasian women between 18-50 yrs. old who had smoked a minimum of 5 Cigarettes/day for at least 1 yr; no hx of liver/endocrine disease; not taking Rx or illicit drugs; not pregnant.	N=32 total women (16 African American and 16 White)	African American menthol smoking was a significant predictor of cotinine half-life in comparison to Caucasian non-menthol smoking.
Benowitz NL, Herrera B, Jacob P 3rd.	Mentholated cigarette smoking inhibits nicotine metabolism.	2004	State of California Tobacco Related Disease Research Program Grant 1RT-0521, by U.S. Public Health Service Grants DA02277 and DA12393 awarded by the National Institute on Drug Abuse and CA32389 awarded by the National Cancer Institute,	Cross Over	14 healthy cigarette smokers recruited through local papers. (7 African-Americans and 7 whites, 12 men and 2 women. Participants were selected as typically smoking 20 or more cigarettes per day	N=14	Our finding of impaired metabolism of nicotine while mentholated cigarette smoking suggests that mentholated cigarette smoking enhances systemic nicotine exposure.

Author Name(s)	Article Title	Year Pub.	Funded By	Type of Study	Subject Description (Including Special population(s))	Sample Size (N)	Authors' Results/Conclusion(s) related to Menthol* (excerpted directly from article)
			and by the General Clinical Research Center at San Francisco General Hospital Medical Center with the support of the Division of Research Resources, National Institutes of Health (RR-00083)		and having a prior experience of smoking both mentholated and nonmentholated cigarettes.		
Caraballo RS, Giovino GA, Pechacek TF, Mowery PD, Richter PA, Strauss WJ, Sharp DJ, Eriksen MP, Pirkle JL, Maurer KR.	Racial and ethnic differences in serum cotinine levels of cigarette smokers: Third National Health and Nutrition Examination Survey, 1988-1991.	1998	No funding source(s) were listed. Authors associated with Centers for Disease Control and Prevention, and Batelle Memorial Institute	Third National Health and Nutrition Examination Survey, 1988-1991	A nationally representative sample of persons aged 17 years or older (non-Hispanic blacks, non-hispanic whites, Mexican Americans) who participated in the survey	Of the 12 391 surveyed, data from 2136 subjects who reported smoking 1 cigarette or more in the past 5 days were included in the analyses. One of the analyses included data from both smokers and nonsmokers (n= 7182)	Blacks had higher cotinine levels than whites, even after ETS exposure and other factors were taken into account. The differences may be influenced by group-specific patterns of smoking behavior and may also be influenced by differences in nicotine pharmacokinetics and brand mentholation.
Clark PI, Gautam S, Gerson LW.	Effect of menthol cigarettes on biochemical	1996	A grant from the American Heart Association, Florida	Descriptive cross-sectional	University smoking research lab with 65 black and 96 white	N=161	After adjusting for race, cigarettes per day, and mean amount of each cigarette smoked, menthol was associated with higher

Biomarkers: Table of Referenced Sources (Continued)

Author Name(s)	Article Title	Year Pub.	Funded By	Type of Study	Subject Description (Including Special population(s))	Sample Size (N)	Authors' Results/Conclusion(s) related to Menthol* (excerpted directly from article)
	markers of smoke exposure among black and white smokers.		Affiliate		adult established smokers.		cotinine levels (p=0.03) and carbon monoxide concentrations (p=0.02).
Gan WQ, Cohen SB, Man SF, Sin DD.	Sex-related differences in serum cotinine concentrations in	2008	The Canadian Institutes of Health Research (IGH/ICRH), the Canadian Lung Association, and the	Retrospective survey	Data from the National Health and Nutrition Examination Survey (NHANES), 1999–2002;	N=1,520 participants for the present	Menthol can inhibit nicotine metabolism and, as such, may prolong the half-life of nicotine and cotinine.
	daily cigarette smokers.		Heart and Stroke Foundation of Canada. DDS is supported by a Canada Research Chair and a GlaxoSmithKline/Michael Smith/St. Paul's Hospital Foundation Professorship in COPD.		daily smokers • 20 years old who had smoked at least 100 cigarettes. Excluding those who used nicotine containing products other than cigarettes, and whose cotinine data were available.	analysis: 840 men and 680 women.	
Heck JD.	Smokers of menthol and nonmenthol cigarettes exhibit similar levels of biomarkers of smoke exposure.	2009	No funding source(s) provided. Author affiliated with Lorillard Tobacco Company	Cross-sectional	male and female subjects 24 to 70 yrs of age, having a minimum smoking history of 3 pack-years, and reporting consumption of >15	N=112 (54 menthol, 58 nonmenthol)	The present findings indicate that moderately heavy smokers of menthol and nonmenthol cigarettes of similar machine-generated smoke yield exhibit essentially identical levels of biomarkers of smoke constituent exposure.

Author Name(s)	Article Title	Year Pub.	Funded By	Type of Study	Subject Description (Including Special population(s))	Sample Size (N)	Authors' Results/Conclusion(s) related to Menthol* (excerpted directly from article)
					menthol or nonmenthol cigarettes daily for the past year,		
Miller GE, Jarvik ME, Caskey NH, Segerstrom SC, Rosenblatt MR, McCarthy WJ.	Cigarette mentholation increases smokers' exhaled carbon monoxide levels.	1994	California Tobacco-Related Disease Research Program Grant 1 RT 87	Empirical	Male smokers from the inpatient substance abuse ward at the Veterans Administration Medical Center, West Los Angeles. Subjects had to be free of pulmonary and respiratory disease, smoke a minimum of 15 cigarettes per day, and be free of psychotropic medication.	N=12	Exhaled carbon monoxide levels increased concomitantly with menthol dosage.
Moolchan ET, Franken FH, Jaszyna-Gasior	Adolescent nicotine metabolism:	2006	National Institute on Drug Abuse, Intramural Research Program	Comparative	Adolescent, tobacco- dependent volunteers 13-17 years of age	N=91 (61 African American,	Menthol was recently shown to inhibit nicotine metabolism, although it did not appear to influence cotinine metabolism; study chose to
M.	ethnoracial differences among dependent smokers.				recruited for a smoking cessation study between September 1999 and September 2003	30 White)	repeat the analyses comparing menthol smokers of both ethnicities. Results remained essentially unchanged, which suggests that the observed differences are due to factors other than menthol smoking

Biomarkers: Table of Referenced Sources (Continued)

Author Name(s)	Article Title	Year Pub.	Funded By	Type of Study	Subject Description (Including Special population(s))	Sample Size (N)	Authors' Results/Conclusion(s) related to Menthol* (excerpted directly from article)
Mustonen TK, Spencer SM, Hoskinson RA Jr, et al.	The influence of gender, race, and menthol content on tobacco exposure measures	2005	National Institute on Drug Abuse grant DA12165	Comparative	Boston-area participants in a randomized clinical trial of individualizing transdermal patch therapy treatment for cigarette smokers	N=307	The cotinine/CPD ratio was, however, higher among menthol smokers than nonmenthol smokers, M=23.3 (SD=13.6) versus M=19.4 (SD=9.4), F(1, 303)=8.2, p=.004. Post-hoc analyses indicated that White women smoking nonmenthol cigarettes have much lower cotinine values than do Black women smoking nonmenthol or menthol cigarettes (p=.05).
Patterson F, Benowitz N, Shields P, Kaufmann V, Jepson C, Wileyto P, Kucharski S, Lerman C.	Individual Differences in Nicotine Intake Per Cigarette.	2003	Transdisciplinary Tobacco Use Research Center Grant P50 CA84718 from the National Cancer Institute and National Institute on Drug Abuse and by USPHS Grants DD02277 and DA01696 from the National Institute on Drug Abuse	Not Specified	Male and female treatment-seeking smokers ages 18–75 years who reported smoking at least 10cpd.	N=190 (95 male, 95 female)	Among the smoking-related variables, cotinine level (r = 0.12; P = 0.09) and smoking rate (F= 2.26; P = 0.08) were marginally associated with boost, whereas nicotine/cotinine ratio (r = 0.11; P = 0.13), menthol/nonmenthol brand (t = 0.49; P = 0.63), cigarette type [i.e., light (t =1.6; P 1=0.11)], and nicotine dependence (r =s0.07, P = 0.31) were not.
Pérez-Stable EJ, Herrera B, Jacob P 3rd, Benowitz NL.	Nicotine metabolism and intake in black and white smokers.	1998	State of California Tobacco-Related Disease Research Program grant 1RT-0521, Public Health Service grants CA39260 and CA32389 awarded by the National Cancer Institute, DA02277 and	Comparative	A total of 40 black and 39 white smokers, average consumption of 14 and 14.7 cigarettes per day, respectively, of similar age (mean,	N=79	Higher levels of cotinine per cigarette smoked by blacks compared with whites can be explained by both slower clearance of cotinine and higher intake of nicotine per cigarette in blacks. Greater nicotine and therefore greater tobacco smoke intake per cigarette could, in part, explain some of the ethnic differences in smoking-related

Author Name(s)	Article Title	Year Pub.	Funded By	Type of Study	Subject Description (Including Special population(s))	Sample Size (N)	Authors' Results/Conclusion(s) related to Menthol* (excerpted directly from article)
			DA01696 awarded by the National Institute on Drug Abuse, HS07373 awarded by the Agency for Health		32.5 and 32.3 years, respectively) and body weight (mean, 73.3 and 68.8 kg, respectively).		disease risks.
			Care Policy and Research, 1P30 AG15272 awarded by the National Institute on Aging, the National Institute of Nursing Research, and the Office of Research on Minority Health, and carried out in part in the General Clinical Research Center at San Francisco General Hospital Medical Center with support of the Division of Research Resources, National Institutes of Health (RR-00083).				
Richie JP Jr, Carmella SG, et al.	Differences in the urinary metabolites of the tobacco- specific lung carcinogen 4-(methylnitrosamin o)-1-(3-	1997	Grants CA-32617 and CA- 29580 from the National Cancer Institute	Metabolic epidemiological study	different biomarkers of NNK exposure and metabolism, including the urinary metabolite 4-(methylnitrosamino)- 1-(3-pyridyl)-1-	N=61 (34 black and 27 white)	Urinary NNAL-Gluc:NNAL ratios, a likely indicator of NNAL glucuronidation and detoxification, were significantly greater in whites than in blacks ($P < 0.02$). In addition, two phenotypes were apparent by probit analysis representing poor (ratio < 6) and extensive (ratio > or = 6) glucuronidation groups. The proportion of

Author Name(s)	Article Title	Year Pub.	Funded By	Type of Study	Subject Description (Including Special population(s))	Sample Size (N)	Authors' Results/Conclusion(s) related to Menthol* (excerpted directly from article)
	pyridyl)-1-butanone in Black and White smokers.				butanol (NNAL) and the presumed detoxification product [4-(methylnitrosamino)-1- (3-pyridyl)but-1-yl]-beta- O-D-glucosiduronic acid (NNAL-Gluc), were examined along with questionnaire data on lifestyle habits and diet in a metabolic epidemiological study of		blacks falling into the former, potentially high- risk group was significantly greater than that of whites ($P < 0.05$). The absolute levels of urinary NNAL, NNAL-Gluc, and cotinine were also greater in blacks than in whites when adjusted for the number of cigarettes smoked. None of the observed racial differences could be explained by dissimilarities in exposure or other sociodemographic or dietary factors. Also, it is unlikely that the dissimilarities are due to racial
					34 black and 27 white healthy smokers.		differences in preference for mentholated cigarettes, because chronic administration of menthol to NNK-treated rats did not result in either increases in urinary total NNAL or decreases in NNAL-Gluc:NNAL ratios. Altogether, these results suggest that racial differences in NNAL glucuronidation, a putative detoxification pathway for NNK, may explain in part the observed differences in cancer risk.
Signorello LB, Cai Q, Tarone RE,	Racial differences in serum cotinine	2009	Grant R01 CA092447 from the National Cancer Institute	Comparative	Current smokers sampled from Southern	N=255	Differences in cotinine levels among smokers suggest racial variation in exposure to and/or metabolism of tobacco

Author Name(s)	Article Title	Year Pub.	Funded By	Type of Study	Subject Description (Including Special population(s))	Sample Size (N)	Authors' Results/Conclusion(s) related to Menthol* (excerpted directly from article)
McLaughlin JK, Blot WJ.	levels of smokers.				Community Cohort Study participants (65 black men, 65 black women, 63 white men, 62 white women)		smoke constituents, but our findings do not support a role for menthol preference in this disparity.
Strasser AA, Malaiyandi V, Hoffmann E, Tyndale RF, Lerman C.	An association of CYP2A6 genotype and smoking topography.	2007	Grants from the National Cancer Institute and the National Institutes on Drug Abuse at the National Institutes of Health: P50 CA/DA84718, CA143187, U01 DA020830, R01 CA120594 and R01 CA130961; and Canadian Institutes of Health Research: MOP86471	Experimental	Treatment-seeking smokers	N=120	Smoking topography variables did not differ significantly by level of nicotine dependence or cigarette mentholation (p values >.2).
Wagenknecht LE, Cutter GR, Haley NJ, Sidney S, Manolio TA, Hughes GH, Jacobs DR.	Racial differences in serum cotinine levels among smokers in the Coronary Artery Risk Development in (Young) Adults study.	1990	NHLBI Contracts N01-HC- 48047, N01-HC-48048, N01-HC-48049, and N01- HC-48050	Multicenter	18-30 year old, Black and White, men and women participating in the Coronary Artery Risk Development in (Young) Adults Study	N=5,115	Mentholated cigarettes, smoked by 89 percent of Black smokers but only 30 percent of White smokers, might account for underreporting of inhalation frequency because of the anesthetic effect that menthol provides.

Biomarkers: Table of Referenced Sources (Continued)

Author Name(s)	Article Title	Year Pub.	Funded By	Type of Study	Subject Description (Including Special population(s))	Sample Size (N)	Authors' Results/Conclusion(s) related to Menthol* (excerpted directly from article)
Wang J, Roethig HJ, Appleton S, et al.	The effect of menthol containing cigarettes on adult smokers' exposure to nicotine and carbon monoxide.	2010	No funding source(s) provided. Authors affiliated with Altria Client Services Inc, Center for Research and Technology	Cross-sectional, observational, ambulatory, multi-centre study	The 3341 African-American and White adult cigarette smokers included in this analysis were from the TES study, which was a cross-sectional, observational, ambulatory, multi-centered study. Adult males and females, 21 years old or older, in generally good health, from 31 states	N=3,341	Analyses of variance revealed no statistically significant effects of mentholated cigarettes on NE/24 h, COHb, serum cotinine and NE/cigarette. On average MS smoked 15.0 and NMS 16.8 cigarettes/day. The unadjusted mean differences were as follows: MS had lower NE/24 h (5.4%) and COHb (3.2%), higher serum cotinine (3.0%) and NE/cigarette (5.7%) than NMS. African-Americans MS smoked 40% fewer cigarettes, showed lower NE/24 h (24%) and COHb (10%) and higher NE/cig (29%) and serum cotinine (8%) levels than their White counterparts. Conclusions: Smoking mentholated cigarettes does not increase daily exposure to smoke constituents as measured by NE and COHb. These findings are consistent with the majority of epidemiological studies indicating no difference in smoking related risks between MS and NMS.
Williams JM, Gandhi KK, Steinberg ML, Foulds J, Ziedonis DM, Benowitz, NL.	Higher nicotine and carbon monoxide levels in menthol cigarette smokers with and without schizophrenia.	2007	Funded by National Institute on Drug Abuse grants DA140090, DA018203, and DA15978, DA015537, DA02277 and DA12393, and a grant from the New	Lab study	Expired carbon monoxide (CO) and serum nicotine and cotinine were measured in 89 smokers with schizophrenia and	N=142	Serum nicotine levels (27 vs. 2ng/ml, p=.010), serum cotinine levels (294 vs. 240ng/ml, p=.041), and expired CO (25 vs. 21ppm, p=.029) were higher in smokers of menthol compared with nonmenthol cigarettes, with no differences in 3-hydroxycotinine/cotinine ratios between

Author Name(s)	Article Title	Year Pub.	Funded By	Type of Study	Subject Description (Including Special population(s))	Sample Size (N)	Authors' Results/Conclusion(s) related to Menthol* (excerpted directly from article)
			Jersey Department of Health and Senior Services, Office of the State Epidemiologist, through funds from New Jersey Comprehensive Tobacco Control Program		53 control smokers immediately after smoking an afternoon cigarette		groups when controlling for race. Backward stepwise linear regression models showed that, in addition to having a diagnosis of schizophrenia, smoking menthol cigarettes was a significant predictor of nicotine and cotinine levels.

* Note: these statements are taken directly from articles and may not include all relevant results/conclusions.

Caraballo RS, Giovino GA, et al. (1998) Racial and ethnic differences in serum cotinine levels of cigarette smokers—Third National Health and Nutrition Examination Survey, 1988–1991. JAMA, 280(2):135–139. [No funding source(s) were listed. Authors associated with Centers for Disease Control and Prevention, and Batelle Memorial Institute]

Clark PI, Gautam S, et al. (1996) Effect of menthol cigarettes on biochemical markers of smoke exposure among black and white smokers. Chest, 110(5):1194–1198. [Funded in part by a grant from the American Heart Association, Florida Affiliate]

Gan WQ, Cohen SB, et al. (2008) Sex-related differences in serum cotinine concentrations in daily cigarette smokers. Nicotine and Tobacco Research, 10(8):1293– 1300. [Funded by ICEBERGS (Interdisciplinary Capacity Enhancement: Bridging Excellence in Respiratory Disease and Gender Studies), which is funded by the Canadian Institutes of Health Research (IGH/ICRH), the Canadian Lung Association, and the Heart and Stroke Foundation of Canada. Also by a Canada Research Chair and a GlaxoSmith Kline/Michael Smith/St. Paul's Hospital Foundation Professorship in COPD]

Heck JD (2009) Smokers of menthol and nonmenthol cigarettes exhibit similar levels of biomarkers of smoke exposure. Cancer Epidemiology, Biomarkers and Prevention, 18(2):622–629. [No funding source(s) provided. Author affiliated with Lorillard Tobacco Company]

Miller GE, Jarvik ME, et al. (1994) Cigarette mentholation increases smokers' exhaled carbon monoxide levels. Experimental and Clinical Psychopharmacology, 2(2):154–160. [Funded by California Tobacco-Related Research Program Grant 1 RT 87]

Moolchan ET, Franken FH, Jaszyna-Gasior M (2006) Adolescent nicotine metabolism: ethnoracial differences among dependent smokers. Ethnicity and Disease, 16:239–243. [Funded by National Inisttute on Drug Abuse Intramural funds]

Mustonen TK, Spencer SM, Hoskinson RA Jr, et al. (2005) The influence of gender, race, and menthol content on tobacco exposure measures. Nicotine and Tobacco Research, 7:581–590. [Funded by National Institute on Drug Abuse grant DA12165]

Patterson, F., Benowitz, N, Shields, P, et al. (2003) Individual Differences in Nicotine Intake Per Cigarette. Cancer Epidemiology, Biomarkers, and Prevention, 12:468–471. [Funded by Transdisciplinary Tobacco Use Research Center Grant P50 CA84718 from the National Cancer Institute and National Institute on Drug Abuse and by USPHS Grants DD02277 and DA01696 from the National Institute on Drug Abuse]

Perez-Stable EJ, Herrera B, et al. (1998) Nicotine metabolism and intake in Black and White smokers. JAMA, 280(2):152–156. [Funded by State of California Tobacco-Related Disease Research Program grant 1RT-0521, Public Health Service grants CA39260 and CA32389 awarded by the National Cancer Institute, DA02277 and DA01696 awarded by the National Institute on Drug Abuse, HS07373 awarded by the Agency for Health Care Policy and Research, 1P30 AG15272 awarded by the National Institute on Aging, the National Institute of Nursing Research, and the Office of Research on Minority Health, and carried out in part in the General Clinical Research Center at San Francisco General Hospital Medical Center with support of the Division of Research Resources, National Institutes of Health (RR-00083)]

Richie JP Jr, Carmella SG, et al. (1997) Differences in the urinary metabolites of the tobacco-specific lung carcinogen 4-(methylnitrosamino)-1-(3-pyridyl)-1-butanone in Black and

White smokers. Cancer Epidemiology, Biomarkers, and Prevention, 6(10):783–790. [Funded by Grants CA-32617 and CA-29580 from the National Cancer Institute]

Signorello L, Cai Q, et al. (2009) Racial differences in serum cotinine levels of smokers. Disease Markers, 27(5):187–192. [Funded by grant R01 CA092447 from the National Cancer Institute]

Strasser AA, Benowitz NL, Pinto AG (2011). Nicotine metabolite ratio predicts smoking topography and carcinogen biomarkers. Cancer Epidemiol Biomarkers, Prev. 20: 234-238. [Funded by grants from the National Cancer Institute and the National Institutes on Drug Abuse at the National Institutes of Health: P50 CA/DA84718, CA143187, U01 DA020830, R01 CA120594 and R01 CA130961; and Canadian Institutes of Health Research: MOP86471]

Wagenknecht LE, Cutter GR, et al. (1990) Racial differences in serum cotinine levels among smokers in the Coronary Artery Risk Development in (Young) Adults study. American Journal of Public Health, 80(9):1053–1056. [Funded by NHLBI Contracts N01-HC-48047, N01-HC-48048, N01-HC-48049, and N01-HC-48050]

Wang J, Roethig HJ, Appleton S, et al. (2010) The effect of menthol containing cigarettes on adult smokers' exposure to nicotine and carbon monoxide. Regulatory, Toxicology, and Pharmacology, 57:24–30. [No funding source(s) provided. Authors affiliated with Altria Client Services Inc, Center for Research and Technology]

Williams JM, Gandhi KK, Steinberg ML, Foulds J, Ziedonis DM, Benowitz, NL (2007) Higher nicotine and carbon monoxide levels in menthol cigarette smokers with and without schizophrenia. Nicotine and Tobacco Research, 9(8):873–881. [Funded by National Institute on Drug Abuse grants DA140090, DA018203, and DA15978, DA015537, DA02277 and DA12393, and a grant from the New Jersey Department of Health and Senior Services, Office of the State Epidemiologist, through funds from New Jersey Comprehensive Tobacco Control Program]

D. Patterns of Use

Approximately one-fourth of all cigarettes sold in the United States are menthol (Giovino, 2004). An understanding of menthol cigarette usage patterns can guide health providers, public health professionals, and policy makers to develop effective strategies to reduce smoking prevalence and smoking-attributable morbidity and mortality. Nationwide, there are significant disparities among cigarette use, with higher prevalence among certain racial/ethnic groups and among those of lower socioeconomic status (U.S. Department of Health and Human Services, 2012). Similarly, there are different demographic distribution and characteristics of menthol and nonmenthol smokers. Understanding these patterns of use and relationships are critical to addressing the public health needs of these groups. This section evaluated studies of national survey data examining the patterns of use of menthol cigarettes as compared to nonmenthol cigarettes.

Tobacco Use Supplement to the Current Population Survey (CPS-TUS)

The CPS-TUS had a nationally representative sample of respondents and a high response rate with comprehensive demographic data collection. The survey also assumed no switching between cigarette types during subjects' lifetimes, which could also lead to misclassification.The use of mixed interview procedures (most by telephone and some by personal interview) may have affected responses, which may or may not be substantial. Proxy respondents were included which may have affected the reliability of data, particularly on menthol cigarette use. In addition, a relatively small number of minority population subjects (i.e., Asian American/Pacific Islanders and American Indian/Alaska Natives) could limit the ability to provide meaningful estimates of these minority groups.

Alexander et al. (2010) analyzed data from the 2006/2007 CPS-TUS on 30,176 current smokers who were at least 18 years old to examine the relationships among occupational status, menthol smoking preference and employer-sponsored smoking cessation programs and policies on quitting behaviors. The authors of the study found that menthol smokers were more likely to be females compared with nonmenthol smokers (55.1% vs. 43.4%), The authors also found that menthol smokers were more likely to be African American (30.2% vs. 4.4%), less educated (i.e., less than high school) (20.2% vs. 17.9%), never married (35.5% vs. 28.4%), residing in the northeast region (21.1% vs. 15.4%), and service employees (23.2% vs. 18.4%) compared with nonmenthol smokers.

Fagan et al. (2010) analyzed data from the 2003 and 2006/2007 CPS-TUS on 46,273 daily current smokers who were at least 18 years old survey to examine the associations between usual cigarette type (i.e., menthol or nonmenthol) and markers for nicotine dependence and also between cigarette type and quitting behaviors. The study found differences in demographics between menthol and nonmenthol daily current smokers. Menthol smokers were more likely to be females (58.0% vs. 47.3%), younger adults (age 18 to 30 years) (27.4% vs. 24.2%), African American (26.9% vs. 3.5%), never married (32.9% vs. 25.3%), less educated (less than high school diploma or GED) (17.1% vs. 14.5%), and have an annual income of less than $10,000 (13.0% vs. 9.6%) compared to nonmenthol smokers. Among menthol smokers, there were also more respondents who were administrative and office workers, worked in service sectors, unemployed, living in northeastern and midwestern regions, and residing in metropolitan areas compared with nonmenthol smokers. The study also found that menthol smokers reported smoking a mean of 13 cpd compared with 15 cpd among nonmenthol smokers ($p < 0.001$).

Fernander et al. (2010) analyzed data on 66,145 current smokers from the 2003 and 2006/2007 CPS-TUS who were at least 18 years old to examine the relationship between age of cigarette smoking initiation and cigarette purchasing patterns of menthol cigarettes among current smokers. The study found that 24.6 percent of current smokers reported using menthol cigarettes, whereas 70.9 percent reported using nonmenthol cigarettes. The study also found that menthol smokers were more likely to be female (54.8% vs 43.7%), African American (28.7% vs. 3.9%), younger (i.e., 18-24 years old: 17.3% vs. 14.1%), and less educated compared with nonmenthol smokers.

Trinidad et al. (2010) analyzed data from the 2003 and 2006/2007 CPS-TUS involving 283,443 respondents 20-65 years old at the time of the survey. The study showed that a much larger proportion of African American current smokers reported usually smoking menthol cigarettes (69.8% ± 1.6%) compared to other racial groups (20.1% for White; 25.4% for Hispanic/Latino smokers).

Lawrence et al. (2010) analyzed data from the 2003 and 2006/2007 CPS-TUS and presented results of data on 69,193 smokers 18 years old or over. They found that, overall, 27.6 percent of current smokers smoked menthol cigarettes. Of African American current smokers, 73.6 percent smoked menthol cigarettes followed by 27.9 percent of Hispanic, 26.2

percent of Asian American/Pacific Islander, 22.5 percent of American Indian/Alaska Native, and 21.1 percent of White current smokers. The prevalence of smoking menthol cigarettes was highest in the following sociodemographic categories (in order of proportion): African American, born in a US territory, unemployed, annual family income of less than $10,000, residence in the Northeast, never married, consumption of less than 10 cpd, education level of 9-11 years, 18-24 years old, female, smoking on some days, start of regular smoking after age 18, residence in a metropolitan area, and no use of other forms of tobacco. African American smokers were 10-11 times more likely to smoke menthol cigarettes than White smokers were. Most non-White smokers, with the exception of American Indian/Alaska Natives, and women were also more likely to smoke menthol cigarettes than White smokers and male smokers. African American smokers 18-24 years old were four times more likely to smoke menthol cigarettes compared with African American smokers 65 years old or over.

National Youth Tobacco Survey (NYTS)

The NYTS had a nationally representative sample from public and private schools with a response rate of 80 percent and oversampled African American, Hispanic, and Asian American students. The survey included two types of data on menthol cigarette use – exclusive brand (Newport or Kool) and self-reported menthol cigarette use. However, the sample size was smaller due to restrictions on the study population, with assumptions made regarding no switching between cigarette brands. Smoking status was based on self-report. Generalizability may be limited since study subjects were students enrolled in regular public and private schools; students in non-traditional schools, such as schools for special education, were excluded from the study. Furthermore, there were insufficient numbers of Asian Americans and Hawaiian/Pacific Islanders (H/PI). The data reflect smoking status in the past 30 days (which is typical for smoking surveys) and did not have information on temporal effects or switching patterns. The response rates were reasonable (84% in 2000 and 75% in 2002), with assessment of the possible misclassification by comparing respondents' reports of menthol use.

Appleyard et al. (2001) analyzed data from the 2000 NYTS of 35,828 middle and high school students in public and private schools across the country to estimate the prevalence of cigarette smoking and describe smoking behaviors among H/PI youth. This study found among those who reported smoking in the past 30 days, 42 percent reported that they smoked menthol cigarettes. While 74 percent of African American youth said their usual brand of cigarette was a menthol brand, 58 percent of Asian Americans, 51 percent of Hispanics, 46 percent of H/PI, and 32 percent of Whites indicated the same. This study is one of only a few studies that focused on Asian American and H/PI youth.

Wackowski et al. (2007) conducted a cross-sectional study to examine the rates of menthol smoking and measures of nicotine dependence using data on 1,345 current established smokers in grade 9 – 12 who participated in the 2004 NYTS. This study found that approximately 46 percent of all current established cigarette smokers (e.g., those who smoked in the past 30 days and smoked at least 100 cigarettes during their lifetime) were menthol smokers. Overall, 21.7 percent of 9 – 12 grade students were current cigarette smokers and 13.8 percent were current established cigarette smokers. Prevalence of smoking significantly increased by grade among both current and current established smokers and differed by race or ethnicity, with prevalence being highest among White students. Approximately 24 percent of current established smokers indicated smoking a menthol exclusive brand (a brand that is only available in menthol, such as Newport (until 2010) or Kool) and 44 percent reported that they usually smoked menthol cigarettes. Of African American smokers, 88.4 percent reported that they regularly smoked menthol cigarettes, as compared to 54.2 percent Hispanic smokers, 49.7 percent of Asian American smokers, and 43.8 percent of White smokers who reported regularly smoking menthol cigarettes.

Hersey et al. (2006) analyzed data from the 2000 and 2002 NYTS on students in grades 6-12 in public and private schools at the time of the survey who reported to be current smokers (smoking cigarettes on one or more of the past 30 days) and who reported that they had a usual brand of cigarettes. This study reported that between 2000 and 2002, the percentage of smokers who regularly smoked menthol cigarettes increased significantly ($p<0.05$) from 40.0 percent to 47.4 percent - an increase of 18.5 percent. Menthol cigarette use significantly increased among middle school smokers (from 51.6% to 59.6%, $p<0.05$). Menthol cigarettes were most popular among younger and newer smokers. Overall, 51.8 percent of teens who had smoked for less than one year smoked menthol cigarettes, compared with 43.6 percent of those who had smoked for a year or more. For Hispanic and White youth, the prevalence of menthol cigarette use was higher among middle school students than among high school students. Among Hispanic youth, 62.9 percent of smokers in middle school, compared with 52.4 percent of smokers in high school, smoked menthol cigarettes. Among Whites, 53.1 percent of smokers in middle school, compared with 37.4 percent of smokers in high school, smoked menthol cigarettes. Among African American students, smokers in middle school (87.5%) and in high school (86.8%) smoked predominantly menthol cigarettes.

Hersey et al. (2010) analyzed data from the 2006 NYTS to examine the reliability of youth self- reported menthol cigarette use. They analyzed data from 4,738 students in grades 6-12 in the spring of 2006 who reported that they had smoked in the past 30 days, had a usual brand of cigarette, and could identify whether the usual brand was menthol or nonmenthol. The study found that among youth smokers who reported a usual brand, 51.7 percent of middle school smokers and 43.1 percent of high school smokers consistently reported that their usual brand was menthol. The proportion of middle school smokers whose usual brand was menthol was higher among those who smoked for one year or more (54.7%) than among those who smoked for less than a year (42.2%). Among high school youth, these percentages were similar for smokers who had smoked for less than and for more than one year (42.8% vs. 43.1%).

This study also found that menthol cigarette use was very high among minority youth – 80.6 percent of African American middle school smokers and 84.8 percent of African American high school smokers reported that their usual brand was menthol. Among Asian Americans, a menthol brand was used by 57.4 percent of middle school smokers and 43.6 percent of high school smokers. Among Hispanics, 57.9 percent of middle school smokers and 56.4 percent of high school smokers reported that they smoked menthol cigarettes. In non-Hispanic Whites, the proportion of menthol smokers was higher among middle school students (43.1%) than among high school students (37.6%). Misclassification of menthol or nonmenthol cigarette use was up to 12 percent among new smokers (i.e., smoked < 6 cigarettes over lifetime; about 19 percent of smokers) compared to 2 percent among established smokers (who had smoked for at least 12 months).

National Health Interview Survey – Cancer Control Supplement (NHIS – CCS)

The NHIS-CCS had a nationally representative sample with information on smoking habits. The relatively small sample size limited subgroup analysis, and data may not have been representative of the population under 25 years old and over 64 years old due to the selection of the study population. There was also a potential for misclassification, as former smokers were defined as not currently smoking, which could have classified those who quit as recently as one week before as former smokers. There was also no description of how the predicted prevalence was calculated or what imputation method was used for assigning missing data on income. There was no validation or comparison between imputed and non-imputed data.

Cubbin et al. (2010) analyzed data from the 2005 NHIS – CCS. Among 7,688 former smokers and current everyday smokers who were 25-64 years old and provided information on the brand of cigarettes they used, the prevalence of menthol cigarette use was significantly higher in African American female and male current everyday smokers (77.9% and 69.7%, respectively) and former smokers (72.7% and 66.0%, respectively) compared with their Hispanic and White counterparts (14.6% and 35.6% in current smokers, respectively; 14.5% and 34.9% in former smokers, respectively).

Mendiondo et al. (2010) analyzed data from the 2005 NHIS – CCS survey. The study found that among 6,055 current menthol smokers, 55.6 percent were female (41.7% in 5,949 nonmenthol smokers), 33.1 percent were African American (3.8% in nonmenthol smokers), 20.8 percent resided in the Northeast (15.0% in nonmenthol smokers), 22.2 percent had less than a high school education (20.2% in nonmenthol smokers), 27.1 percent had an annual income of less than $20,000 (21.9% in nonmenthol smokers). Among former menthol smokers, 60.7 percent were female (39.9% in the nonmenthol group), and 19.1 percent were African American (3.6% in the nonmenthol group).

Stahre et al. (2010) analyzed data from the 2005 NHIS – CCS (n = 31,428). They found that 42 percent of the study subjects reported being either a current (n = 6,511 or 21%) or former (n = 6,774 or 21%) smoker. Of 12,004 study subjects for which menthol cigarette status was known, approximately 26 percent of current smokers smoked menthol cigarettes and 22 percent of former smokers had used menthol. Overall, menthol smoking prevalence was significantly different by gender, region, race, marital status, and quantity of cigarettes smoked per day. African American smokers had the highest prevalence of menthol cigarette use (76% for current smokers; 63% for former smokers) compared with White and other racial groups (20% and 33% in current White and Asian American smokers, respectively; 21% and 30% in former White and Asian American smokers, respectively). More female smokers (33% for both current and former smokers) used menthol than male smokers did (22% for current smokers and 18% for former smokers). Participants 18-24 years old had the highest prevalence of menthol use for both current and former smokers (32% and 34%) compared with other age groups (23-28% for current smokers; 19-28% for former smokers). Among both current and former smokers, menthol smokers smoked fewer cigarettes per day (15 for current smokers and 17 for former smokers) compared with nonmenthol smokers (17 for current and 19 for former smokers).

National Survey on Drug Use and Health (NSDUH)

The NSDUH is an annual nationwide household survey with a nationally representative sample of population 12 years old or over. This study was of a nationally representative sample with a reasonable response rate of 75 percent. However, smoking status was based on self-report, and there was a small sample size for certain racial groups (Asian American and American Indian/Alaska Native).

O'Connor et al. (2005) analyzed data from the 2002 NSDUH and reported that Newport (exclusively menthol brand at time of study) was the dominant brand among African American smokers under age 26 years old. Among 12–17 year olds, 54.1 percent smoked Newport Full Flavor (FF) and 13.5 percent smoke Newport Lights, while among 18–25 year olds, 70.6 percent smoke Newport FF and 9.1 percent smoke Newport Lights. By contrast, only 36.7 percent of African American smokers over age 26 smoked Newport FF and 4.2 percent smoked Newport Lights. Since this study was reported in the form of a Letter to the Editor, details of the study were limited and there was no description of the study population.

Rock and associates (2010) analyzed combined data from the 2004 – 2008 NSDUH to assess menthol cigarette use among current smokers. Rock reported that 35.7 percent of current smokers 12 years old or over smoked menthol cigarettes. In this population, more than half of menthol smokers were females (52.2%) compared with 43.0 percent of nonmenthol smokers. About 29.4 percent of all menthol smokers were African American, which was almost 10 times the percentage of nonmenthol smokers who were African American (3.0%). For Hispanic and Asian American smokers, the percentages of menthol and nonmenthol smokers were approximately the same. White smokers represented more than half of the menthol smokers (54%). Approximately 71.2 percent of all menthol smokers were adults 26 years old and over, 23.0 percent were young adults 18-25 years old, and 5.8 percent were youth 12-17 years old compared with 77.5 percent, 19.2 percent, and 3.4 percent of all nonmenthol smokers of the same age groups, respectively.

National Health and Nutrition Examination Survey (NHANES)

FDA analyzed demographic characteristics of over 5,000 smokers participating in NHANES from 1999-2008. Unlike the previously discussed surveys, menthol use data were collected through barcode scanning of the participants' cigarette packs. Thus, there is no opportunity for misclassification. As has been reported previously, menthol cigarette use was more common in female smokers than male smokers and in African American smokers compared to White smokers.

Conclusion

Multiple large scale surveys and studies of nationally representative populations show consistency in the patterns of use of menthol cigarettes. The five studies that reported from CPS-TUS data found that menthol cigarette use was more common among smokers who were female, African American, had a lower education, and younger (Alexander et al., 2010; Fagan et al., 2010; Fernander et al., 2010; Lawrence et al., 2010; Trinidad et al., 2010). The four studies that reported from NYTS data found that menthol cigarette use was more common among smoking students who were African American and Hispanic, and that there was an inverse relationship by grade (Appleyard et al., 2001; Hersey et al., 2006; Hersey et al., 2010; Wachowski et al., 2007). The three studies that reported on data from the NHIS found that menthol cigarette use was more common among smokers who were female, African American and had lower education (Cubbin et al., 2010; Mendiondo et al., 2010; Stahre et al., 2010). The two studies that reported on NSDUH data found that menthol cigarette use was more common among smokers who were African American, female, and under age 26 (O'Connor et al., 2005; Rock et al., 2010). The FDA analysis of NHANES data found that menthol cigarette smokers were more likely to be female and African American. The varied nature of these studies and the large number of analyses performed on this data, which provide consistent findings, enable researchers to draw clear conclusions. Most of the surveys relied on self-reported data to categorize menthol and nonmenthol smokers. Use of such self-reported data are standard in the research field. Although studies that relied on self-report of menthol or nonmenthol use may have potential misclassifications, this is not necessarily a problem. As noted by Caraballo et al. (2011), it is likely that this type of bias is fairly constant over time. Data support that (1) a majority of African American smokers reported menthol cigarette use and other minority groups were more likely to smoke menthol cigarettes than White smokers, (2) younger smokers had the highest rate of smoking menthol cigarettes, (3) female smokers were more likely to smoke menthol cigarettes, and (4) menthol smokers were more likely to have lower education levels and lower incomes compared with nonmenthol smokers. From published studies and FDA analysis of the 1999–2008 NHANES data with nationally representative samples, the weight of evidence supports the conclusion that menthol in cigarettes is associated with particular patterns of smoking.

References

Alexander LA, Crawford T, Mendiondo MS (2010). Occupational status, work-site cessation programs and policies and menthol smoking on quitting behaviors in US smokers. Addiction 105(suppl. 1):95–104. [No funding source(s) provided. Authors are affiliated with the University of Kentucky]

Appleyard J, Messeri P, Haviland ML (2001) Smoking among Asian American and Hawaiian/Pacific Islander youth: data from the 2000 National Youth Tobacco Survey. Asian American & Pacific Islander Journal of Health 9(1):5-14. [Funded by the American Legacy Foundation]

Caraballo, RS & Asman, K (2011). Epidemiology of menthol cigarette use in the United States. Tobacco Induced Diseases, 9 (Suppl 1): S1. [No funding source(s) provided. Authors affiliated with the Centers for Disease Control and Prevention]

Cubbin C, Soobader M-J, LeClere FB (2010) The intersection of gender and race/ethnicity in smoking behaviors among menthol and non-menthol smokers in the United States. Addiction 105(suppl. 1):32–8. [Funded by Research Network on Disparities]

Fagan P, Moolchan ET et al. (2010) Nicotine dependence and quitting behaviors among menthol and non-menthol smokers with similar consumptive patterns. Addiction 105(suppl. 1):55–74. [Funded by the National Cancer Institute, Virginia Commonwealth University and the Massey Cancer Center]

Patterns of Use: Table of Referenced Sources

	Article Title	Year Pub.	Funded By	Type of Study	Subject Description (Including Special population(s))	Sample Size (N)	Authors' Results/Conclusion(s) related to Menthol* (excerpted directly from article)
Alexander LA, Crawford T, Mendiondo MS	Occupational status, work-site cessation programs and policies and menthol smoking on quitting behaviors in US smokers. Addiction 105(suppl. 1):95–104.	2010	No funding source(s) provided. Authors are affiliated with the University of Kentucky	Cross-sectional survey (2006 Tobacco Use Supplement to the Current Population Survey)	Current smokers age 18 and older	N=30,176	...there were no differences for menthol versus non-menthol smokers on quitting behaviors [odds ratio (OR) = 0.98; 95% confidence interval (CI) = 0.83, 1.15]. When occupational status and work-place smoking policies are controlled for, smokers of menthol cigarettes in the United States appear to have similar self-reported life-time rates of attempts to stop smoking to non-menthol smokers.
Appleyard J, Messeri P, Haviland ML.	Smoking among Asian American and Hawaiian/Pacific Islander youth: data from the 2000 National Youth Tobacco Survey.	2001	American Legacy Foundation	National Youth Tobacco Survey	Asian American and Hawaiian/ Pacific Islander youth	N=35,828.The schools response Rate was 90% and the student response rate was 93%, resulting in an overall response rate of 84%.	While many studies have documented the high prevalence of Menthol cigarette use among African Americans, NYTS 2000 data reveal that smoking mentholated cigarettes is also common among Asian American youth. Overall, 74% of African Americans and 58% of Asian Americans reported that their usual brand of cigarette is menthol brand.
Caraballo, RS & Asman, K	Epidemiology of menthol cigarette use in the United States.	2011	No funding source(s) provided. Authors affiliated with the Centers for Disease Control and Prevention	Review and secondary analyses of national surveys	NSDUH: adolescents aged 12-17 years old who smoked in the past month and adult smokers (aged 18	NSDUH: 9,595 adolescents; 62,010 adults NYTS: 1,978	Menthol cigarettes are disproportionately smoked by adolescents, blacks/African Americans, adult females, those living in the Northeast of the United States and those with family incomes lower than $50,000. Based on self-reports of menthol cigarette use,

	Article Title	Year Pub.	Funded By	Type of Study	Subject Description (Including Special population(s))	Sample Size (N)	Authors' Results/Conclusion(s) related to Menthol* (excerpted directly from article)
					years or older) who smoked in the past month NYTS: middle school (MS) and high school (HS) students with school year, past 30	MS students and 6,163 HS students MTF: 20,863 8th	menthol cigarette use among smokers have increased from 2004 to 2008.
					day smoking, brand use, and menthol information. MTF: current smokers in 8th, 10th and 12th grade NHANES: 20 years and older who had Smoked and were non- Hispanic white, non-Hispanic black/African American, or Mexican American	graders; 30,722 10th graders; 40,914 12th Graders NHANES: 1571 individuals with UPC information	
Cubbin C, Soobader M-J, LeClere FB	The intersection of gender and race/ethnicity in smoking behaviors among menthol and non-menthol smokers in the United	2010	Research Network on Disparities	Cross-sectional National survey (2005 National Health Interview Survey and Cancer Control	Black, Hispanic and white men and women, 25-64 years old	N= 7688 Size	After adjusting for age, income and education, black (compared with Hispanic and white) and female (compared with male) smokers were more likely to choose menthol cigarettes. There was only one statistically significant difference in age of initiation, cigarettes smoked per day, quit attempts or time since quitting between menthol and

Patterns of Use: Table of Referenced Sources (Continued)

	Article Title	Year Pub.	Funded By	Type of Study	Subject Description (Including Special population(s))	Sample	Authors' Results/Conclusion(s) related to Menthol* (excerpted directly from article)
	States.			Supplement)			non-menthol smokers: white women who smoked menthol cigarettes reported longer cessation compared with those who smoked non-menthol cigarettes.
Fagan P, Moolchan ET et al.	Nicotine dependence and quitting behaviors among menthol and non-menthol smokers with similar consumptive patterns.	2010	The National Cancer Institute, Virginia Commonwealth University and the Massey Cancer Center	Cross-sectional survey (2003 and 2006/07 Tobacco Use Supplements to the Current Population Surveys)	Civilian non-institutionalized daily smokers aged 18 years and above.	N=11,671 (menthol smokers) N=33,644 (nonmenthol smokers) N=958 (no usual type)	...among adults, daily menthol smokers consuming six to 10 cigarettes per day were more likely than non-menthol smokers consuming six to 10 cigarettes per day to smoke their cigarette within the first 5 minutes after waking.
Fernander A, Rayens ML, et al.	Are age of smoking initiation and purchasing	2010	No funding source(s) provided. Authors affiliated with the	Cross-sectional survey (2003 and 2006/07	Civilian non-institutionalized individuals aged 18	N= 16,294 (menthol smokers)	The multivariate logistic model only marginally revealed that age of smoking initiation predicted menthol smoking: findings are suggestive that
	patterns association with menthol smoking?		University of Kentucky	Tobacco Use Supplement to the Current Population Survey)	years and above.	N= 46,899 (non-menthol smokers)	the longer the delay of initiation the more likely that an individual smoked menthol cigarettes [odds ratio (OR) = 1.01; 95% confidence interval (CI): 1.00–1.01]. Menthol smokers in the United States are more likely to be female, younger, from ethnic minority groups, and to have a high school education
Giovino GA, et al.	Epidemiology of menthol cigarette	2004	No funding source(s) provided. Authors	Review article	Not applicable	Not applicable	The epidemiological literature on menthol cigarettes and cancer risk is inconclusive

	Article Title	Year Pub.	Funded By	Type of Study	Subject Description (Including Special population(s))	Sample	Authors' Results/Conclusion(s) related to Menthol* (excerpted directly from article)
	use		affiliated with the Roswell Park Cancer Institute, Kaiser Permanente Medical Care Program, Substance Abuse and Mental Health Services Administration, University of Michigan, American Legacy Foundation, Centers for Disease Control and Prevention				regarding whether these cigarettes confer a risk for cancer above that of nonmentholated varieties. Available data indicate that mentholated cigarettes are at least as dangerous as their nonmentholated counterparts. In addition, because mentholation improves the taste of cigarettes for a substantial segment of the smoking population and appears to mask disease symptoms, this additive may facilitate initiation or inhibit quitting.
Hersey JC, Ng SW, Nonnemaker JM, Mowery P, Thomas KY, Vilsaint MC, Allen JA, Haviland ML.	Are menthol cigarettes a starter product for youth?	2006	American Legacy Foundation and RTI International	2000 and 2002 NYTS, School-based, national survey	Data from the 2000 NYTS and from the 2002 NYTS.The survey used a three-stage cluster sample design that oversampled African American, Hispanic, and Asian students. The NYTS was administered to	N=5,512 youth (2000 NYTS) and 3,202 youth (2002 NYTS)	Additionally, youth who smoked menthol cigarettes had significantly higher scores on a scale of nicotine dependence compared with nonmenthol smokers, controlling for demographic background and the length, frequency, and level of smoking..
Hersey JC, Nonnemaker JM, Homsi G.	Menthol cigarettes contribute to the appeal and addiction potential of smoking for	2010	American Legacy Foundation	Survey (2006 National Youth Tobacco Survey)	Middle and high school students who smoked in the past 30 days who reported that they had a usual brand of cigarette and who	N=1458 (menthol smokers) N=1710 (nonmenthol smokers)	A logistic regression model of dependence, controlling for background (i.e., school level, gender, and race/ethnicity) and smoking level (i.e., years, frequency, and level of smoking) found that smoking menthol cigarettes was significantly associated with reduced time to needing a cigarette among

Patterns of Use: Table of Referenced Sources (Continued)

	Article Title	Year Pub.	Funded By	Type of Study	Subject Description (Including Special population(s))	Sample	Authors' Results/Conclusion(s) related to Menthol* (excerpted directly from article)
	youth.				could identify whether the usual brand was menthol or nonmenthol.		smokers with a regular brand (odds ratio [OR]: 1.86, $p = .003$) and among established smokers (OR: 2.06, $p = .001$).
Lawrence DL, Rose A et al.	National patterns and correlates of menthol cigarette use in the United States.	2010	National Cancer Institute	Cross-sectional survey (2003 and 2006/07 Tobacco Use Supplements to the Current Population Survey)	Smokers at least 18 years old.	N=63,193	Use of mentholated cigarettes was higher among women than among men. Additional significant factors associated with mentholated cigarette smoking included being unmarried (never married: OR: 1.21, 99% CI: 1.09–1.34; divorced/separated: OR: 1.13, 99% CI: 1.03–1.23), being born in a US territory (OR: 2.01, 99% CI: 1.35–3.01), living in a non-
Mendiondo MS, Alexander LA, Crawford T	Health profile differences for menthol and non- menthol smokers: findings from the National Health Interview Survey.	2010	No funding source(s) provided. Authors affiliated with the University of Kentucky	Cross-sectional survey (2005 National Health Interview Survey and its cancer control supplement	civilian, non-institutionalized adults at least 18 years old	N=5949	Overall, current menthol and non-menthol smokers have similar health profiles. However, menthol smokers reported smoking fewer cigarettes per day than their non-menthol counterparts.
O'Connor RJ.	What brands are US smokers under 25 choosing?	2005	No funding source(s) provided. Authors affiliated with Roswell Park Cancer Center	Online Analysis	Data on the cigarette brand preferences of smokers in the 2002 US National Survey on Drug Use and	12–17 years (n = 2290), 18–25 years (n = 7321), 26+ years (n = 5238).	The youth market in the USA appears dominated by varieties of the major advertised brands; other products make up a more modest percentage of the market. Conversely, the adult market is much more diffuse, with the major varieties

	Article Title	Year Pub.	Funded By	Type of Study	Subject Description (Including Special population(s))	Sample	Authors' Results/Conclusion(s) related to Menthol* (excerpted directly from article)
					Health from three age groups: 12–17, 18–25 years, and 26+ years.		commanding smaller overall percentages of the market. Light varieties appear to be popular choices for younger smokers. Similar investigations in other countries could shed further light on younger smokers' brand choices, particularly in those countries that have banned descriptors such as "Light'' and "Mild".
Rock VJ, Davis SP, Thorne SL, et al.	Menthol cigarette use among racial and ethnic groups in the United States, 2004- 2008.	2010	No funding source(s) provided. Authors affiliated with the Centers for Disease Control and Prevention	Cross-sectional survey (2004–2008 National Survey on Drug Use and Health)	Current smokers age 12 and over	N=71,605	Over half of menthol cigarette smokers were female (52.2%), and approximately 29.4% of all menthol smokers were Black, which was almost 10 times the percentage of nonmenthol smokers who were Black (3.0%, $p < .01$). Prevalence of past month menthol cigarette use was highest among current smokers aged 12–17 years (44.7%) and decreased as age group increased.
Stahre M, Okuyemi KS et al.	Racial/ethnic differences in menthol cigarette smoking, population quit ratios and utilization of evidence-based tobacco cessation treatments.	2010	Department of Veterans Affairs, Veterans Health Administration, Office of Research and Development and Health Services Research and Development	Cross-sectional survey (2005 National Health Interview Survey (NHIS) Cancer Control Supplement)	Current or former smokers, age 18 and over	N= 6511 (smoker) N= 6774 (former smoker)	Overall menthol smoking prevalence was significantly different by sex, region of the United States, race, marital status and average number of cigarettes smoked per day for both current and former smokers and age for former smokers only. For current and former smokers, non-menthol smokers reported a higher number of cigarettes smoked per day on average than menthol smokers. Menthol smoking status was not associated with differences in utilization of quit aids.

Patterns of Use: Table of Referenced Sources (Continued)

	Article Title	Year Pub.	Funded By	Type of Study	Subject Description (Including Special population(s))	Sample	Authors' Results/Conclusion(s) related to Menthol* (excerpted directly from article)
Trinidad DR, Gilpin EA, Lee L, Pierce JP.	Do the majority of Asian-American and African-American smokers start as adults?	2004	Grant no. MRSGT 07-277- 01 from the American Cancer Society, no. 15RT- 0238 from the Tobacco- Related Disease Research Program of the University of California Office of the President and contract no.28XS017 from the National Cancer Institute; the Tobacco Research Network on Disparities funded by the National Cancer Institute and the American Legacy Foundation	Comparative	Adults aged 26 to 50 years. Asians/Pacific Islanders (A/PI), African Americans (AA), Hispanics/Latinos (H/L) and non-Hispanic whites (WH).	N=130,356	Significant ethnic disparities in relation to when people start smoking, with the majority of A/PIs and AAs initiating as young adults. The findings suggest that prevention strategies should begin at a young age and continue throughout young adulthood, especially among ethnic minority populations.
U.S. Department of Health and Human Services	Preventing tobacco use among youth and young adults: a report of the Surgeon General	2012	U.S. Deparment of Health and Human Services	Review	Not applicable	Not applicable	[Not applicable]
Wackowski O, Delnevo CD.	Menthol cigarettes and indicators of tobacco dependence	2007	No funding source(s) provided. Authors are associated with the University of Medicine	Survey	U.S. high school students, School-based, national survey	N=1345 current smokers in grades 9-12	Menthol cigarette smoking was associated with two dependence measures and may be more addictive than regular cigarettes in young smokers.

* Note: these statements are taken directly from articles and may not include all relevant results/conclusions.

Fernander A, Rayens ML, et al. (2010) Are age of smoking initiation and purchasing patterns association with menthol smoking? Addiction 105(suppl. 1): 39–45. [No funding source(s) provided. Authors affiliated with the University of Kentucky]

Giovino, GA, Sidney, S, Gfroerer, JC, O'Malley, PM, Allen, JA. et al. (2004) Epidemiology of menthol cigarette use. Nicotine and Tobacco Research 6 Suppl 1:S67-S81. [No funding source(s) provided. Authors affiliated with the Roswell Park Cancer Institute, Kaiser Permanente Medical Care Program, Substance Abuse and Mental Health Services Administration, University of Michigan, American Legacy Foundation, Centers for Disease Control and Prevention]

Hersey JC, Ng SW, et al. (2006) Are menthol cigarettes a starter product for youth? Nicotine and Tobacco Research 8(3):403–13. [Funded by the American Legacy Foundation]

Hersey JC, Nonnemaker JM & Homsi G. (2010) Menthol cigarettes contribute to the appeal and addiction potential of smoking for youth. Nicotine and Tobacco Research 12(suppl. 2):S136-146. [Funded by the American Legacy Foundation]

Lawrence DL, Rose A et al. (2010) National patterns and correlates of menthol cigarette use in the United States. Addiction 105(suppl. 1):13–31. [Funded by the National Cancer Institute]

Mendiondo MS, Alexander LA, Crawford T (2010) Health profile differences for menthol and non-menthol smokers: findings from the National Health Interview Survey. Addiction 105(suppl. 1):124-40. [No funding source(s) provided. Authors affiliated with the University of Kentucky]

O'Connor RJ (2005) What brands are US smokers under 25 choosing? Tobacco Control 14:213-8. [No funding source(s) provided. Authors affiliated with Roswell Park Cancer Center]

Rock VJ, Davis SP, Thorne SL, et al. (2010) Menthol cigarette use among racial and ethnic groups in the United States, 2004-2008. Nicotine and Tobacco Research 12(suppl. 2):S117-24. [No funding source(s) provided. Authors affiliated with the Centers for Disease Control and Prevention]

Stahre M, Okuyemi KS et al. (2010) Racial/ethnic differences in menthol cigarette smoking, population quit ratios and utilization of evidence-based tobacco cessation treatments. Addiction 105(suppl. 1):75–83. [Funded by Department of Veterans Affairs, Veterans Health Administration, Office of Research and Development and Health Services Research and Development]

Trinidad DR, Perez-Stable EJ, Messer K, et al. (2010) Menthol cigarettes and smoking cessation among racial/ethnic groups in the United States. Addiction 105:84-94. [Funded by grant no. MRSGT 07-277-01 from the American Cancer Society, no. 15RT-0238 from the Tobacco-Related Disease Research Program of the University of California Office of the President and contract no.28XS017 from the National Cancer Institute; the Tobacco Research Network on Disparities funded by the National Cancer Institute and the American Legacy Foundation]

U.S. Department of Health and Human Services (2012). Preventing tobacco use among youth and young adults – A report of the Surgeon General. Rockville, MD.

Wackowski O, Delnevo CD (2007) Menthol cigarettes and indicators of tobacco dependence among adolescents. Addictive Behaviors 32:1964–9. [No funding source(s) provided. Authors are associated with the University of Medicine and Dentistry of New Jersey]

E. Marketing and Consumer Perception of Risk

Marketing plays a role in promoting consumer products, and touches each of us every day, whether we see a television commercial for children's cereal, a billboard for car insurance, or hear a radio ad for pet food. These ads influence consumer choices, and the tobacco industry uses proven marketing tools to market tobacco as well. In order to determine how marketing influences smokers, FDA examined data on trends in the marketing of menthol cigarettes. In addition, this chapter reviews consumer perceptions of menthol cigarettes. In particular, this chapter reviews marketing articles related to trends in brand preference and marketing strategies used to promote menthol cigarettes as well as consumer perceptions literature related to the risks and benefits of using menthol cigarettes, in an effort to determine what role, if any, marketing plays in the use of menthol cigarettes and the relationship between consumer perceptions and the use of menthol. Of particular interest is whether these relationships are present among subpopulations (e.g., youth, African Americans, Hispanics, women).

Marketing

Brand Preference

Understanding trends in brand preference allows for contextualization of use patterns, advertising strategies, beliefs, and the process of establishing brand loyalty. The data overwhelmingly support distinct trends in adolescent brand preference, with a much more heavily concentrated preference evident among adolescents than adults (Cummings et al., 1997, Pollay et al., 1996). The majority of teens report Marlboro as their preferred brand, followed by Newport and Camel (CDC, 1994; CDC, 1992; Cummings et al., 1997; Johnston et al., 1999; O'Connor, 2005). Newport's popularity among teens doubled from 1989-1996, from 8.3 percent to 16.4 percent (Johnston et al., 1999; Kaufman et al., 2004).

Research suggests adolescent brand preference is not a mere imitation of adult brand preference (Cummings et al., 1997; Pollay, 1996). Cummings et al. (1997) found that adult and adolescent brand preferences differ within communities, suggesting something other than modeling is influencing adolescent brand preference. Pollay et al. (1996) found that analysis of brand and behavior survey along with market share and ad expenditure data supported econometric studies that report teens' brand preference is three times more sensitive to cigarette ads than adults. This is further supported by teens overwhelming preference for the top three most heavily advertised brands (American Legacy Foundation, 2007; Arnett et al., 1998; CDC, 2009; CDC, 1992; Pollay et al., 1996). National surveys typically do not tease out sub-brand preference (e.g., Marlboro Menthol), which may cause difficulties in making an absolute judgment about menthol versus nonmenthol brand preference; menthol sub-brands make up only a small percentage of the market for Marlboro and Camel. Until 2010, Newport was an exclusively menthol brand. Thus, Marlboro and Camel are most often reported as nonmenthol brands and Newport as a menthol brand.

Evidence suggests differences in brand preference by age, race or ethnicity, and region. Brand loyalty begins in adolescence. The number of teens who report they do not have a brand preference declines dramatically with age (Johnston, et al., 1999). Data indicates that preference for certain nonmenthol cigarettes (Marlboro and Camel) neither changes with age (Mowry, 2004), nor rises in popularity (Johnston et al., 1999). Newport use suggests a different trajectory of preference. Data suggest that preference for Newport declines with age, with 22 percent of 8th graders reporting a preference for Newport and 13 percent of 12th graders reporting this preference (CDC, 1994; CDC et al., 1992; Johnston et al., 1999). O'Connor (2005) found Newport's popularity declines dramatically after age 26. According to the 2010 National Survey on Drug Use and Health, the decline in preference for Newport by age is found across races and ethnicities. Whereas 78.7 percent of African American smokers and 24.8 percent of Hispanic smokers 12-25 years old report using Newport cigarettes, only 48.4 percent of African American smokers and 13 percent of Hispanic smokers ages 26+ report using Newports. Newport preference among Caucasians declines from 11.4 percent in 12-25 year olds to 3.3 percent in smokers 26+ years old. Newport is overwhelmingly preferred by African Americans, with 41 percent of African American adults and 75 percent of African American youth reporting preference for Newport cigarettes (Cummings et al., 1987; Cummings, 1997; Johnston et al., 1999; O'Connor, 2005). Johnston et al. (1999) found a slight preference for the Newport brand among Hispanic youth. Additionally, some evidence suggests regional differences, with more cigarette smokers reporting a preference for Newport in the Northeast than in the West (OAS, 2003; CDC, 1994; Johnston et al., 1999). These regional differences in Newport use exist for African American, White, and Hispanic smokers. CDC reports from 1994 suggest regional preferences for Newport combined with a decrease in overall advertisement expenditures for Newport may have resulted from a heavier reliance on a regional marketing strategy than a national strategy. Differences in menthol versus nonmenthol brands by age, race, and region may suggest differences in marketing strategies, as described below.

Marketing Strategies

Similar to other consumer products, evidence indicates tobacco companies employ targeted marketing strategies to attract consumers to their brands. These strategies include using market research with target audiences to inform product placement and marketing, strategic placement of advertising, partnerships with relevant national and community organizations, and use of specific promotions to encourage use. Samji (2008) reviewed a collection of several thousand cigarette advertisements from 1920-1954 and that found these ads attempt to convey a health benefit through endorsements by physicians, with menthol advertising suggesting a therapeutic, soothing benefit. Anderson (2011) reviewed industry documents that further revealed cigarette marketing on a health platform conveying to consumers that menthol cigarettes were healthier than nonmenthol.

Research indicates tobacco companies with menthol brands use a marketing mix and concepts that target African Americans (Altman et al., 1991; Balback et al., 2003; Boley et al., 2010; Cummings et al., 1987; Glantz et al., 2006; Landrine et al., 2005; Laws et al., 2002; Sutton et al., 2004; White et al., 2006). This is reflected in advertising placement, with magazines with primarily African American readership containing more menthol advertisements than nonmenthol advertisements and more menthol advertisements than those magazines with primarily White readership (Balbach et al., 2003; Cummings et al., 1987; Landrine et al., 2005) and more outdoor menthol advertisements in African American neighborhoods than neighborhoods of other races/ethnicities (Altman et al., 1991; Henriksen et al., 2011; Laws et al., 2002; Seidenberg et al., 2010). A review of publicly available tobacco industry documents conducted by Yerger, Przewoznik, and Malone (2007) describes the tobacco industry's use of free sampling, mobile vans, event sponsorships, and special inner-city sales programs to promote sales of menthol brands to African American communities. Anderson (2011) identified a similar pattern. An observational study conducted in Hawaii to examine the number of ads inside and outside of retail establishments found Kool, the most heavily used brand by middle schoolers, to have the most ads inside and outside retail establishments (Glantz et al., 2006). Industry documents and observational reviews suggest themes that reflect an urban, "cool" lifestyle have been used in advertising campaigns and product names to promote menthol cigarettes to the African American community (Gardiner, 2004: Sutton et al., 2004).

Connolly et al. (2011) found evidence of similar targeted marketing strategies in Japan which were used to increase the preference for menthol cigarettes among women. The study found that by 2000, half of all female smokers were smoking menthol cigarettes and that menthol use among adolescents was significantly higher than in the general population of smokers. While the Japanese National Health and Nutrition Survey did not measure cigarette use by brand and subbrand, evidence indicated that smoking rates increased significantly among the younger female cohort (20-29 years old) between 1989 and 2004, when menthol cigarettes were introduced into the Japanese market. The authors determined this rise in smoking among women was being driven in large part by the uptake in smoking by young girls—who, according to the youth smoking measure, are smoking primarily menthol cigarettes. The authors supported this data with illustrations from industry documents that detail marketing strategies to promote a lighter, more feminine cigarette to women in Japan. The marketing strategies appear to build on social and cultural norms and rely on brand extension strategies of already popular brands (e.g., Marlboro).

Researchers who reviewed publicly available tobacco industry documents reported evidence of tobacco companies conducting extensive market research with African Americans to better understand trends, attitudes, preferences, and behaviors and target their marketing strategies accordingly (Boley et al., 2010; Cruz et al., 2010; Gardiner, 2004; Johnson et al., 2008; Sutton et al., 2004). Johnson et al. (2008) and Gardiner (2004) also noted industry documents that suggest players in the tobacco industry formed strategic partnerships with national and community African American organizations to gain support for their menthol brands. Klausner's (2011) review of industry documents suggests this targeted marketing strategy occurred after manufacturers realized certain smokers, including African Americans, were disproportionately smoking menthol cigarettes. In the 1970s and 1980s, tobacco companies began using targeted marketing strategies to promote smoking behavior trends that were noted around this time. The studies of industry documents have limitations, though, that should be considered when evaluating their validity and reliability[1].

Mazis et al. (1992) conducted a study to examine the relationship between perceived age and attractiveness of models in tobacco advertisements in magazines. They found that models who were judged to be younger were rated as more attractive by participants. The authors noted that ads with models perceived as younger appeared more often in magazines with younger readerships. They also found that menthol ads featured models with a younger perceived age (25.7 years old) than those featured in nonmenthol ads (31.9 years old). The authors concluded, however, that given the limited number of ads with a clearly portrayed model, tobacco companies were probably not using younger models as a primary marketing strategy to attract youth.

White et al. (2006) found differences by brand in the use of promotional coupons as a marketing strategy, even when controlling for household income. They analyzed data from the 2002 California Tobacco Survey, including a question asking about how often the consumer took advantage of advertising promotions and about how often the consumer sees such promotions when purchasing cigarettes. The authors found that smokers of Newport and Kool cigarettes (both menthol brands) used coupons more often than those who purchased Marlboro and Camel cigarettes (both nonmenthol brands). Additionally, they found that African Americans who smoked menthol cigarettes (65%) used coupons more often than African Americans who smoked nonmenthol cigarettes (28%). The study also found that those who saw promotions more frequently were more likely to take advantage of them. This data suggest menthol smokers take advantage of price promotions more often than nonmenthol smokers. However, this study analyzed data only from California, so the results may not be representative of promotion use patterns in the rest of the United States.

Henrisken et al. (2011) examined variations in the price and availability of promotions of menthol and nonmenthol cigarettes as a function of neighborhood demographics. Researchers coded the presence of advertised promotions and lowest pack price in over 400 stores in 31 neighborhoods in California. Researchers found that 25 percent of the advertisements recorded were for menthol cigarettes. Menthol advertisements were particularly common in areas with higher proportions of African Americans and youth 10-17 years old. The proportion of stores that advertised promotions for Newport (menthol), Marlboro Menthol, and Marlboro (nonmenthol) were 27 percent, 51.4 percent, and 75 percent, respectively. When analyzed further, researchers found that for every 10 percent increase in the proportion of African American students in the neighborhood, the odds of a store advertising promotions for Newport were 1.5 times greater. Similarly, for every 10 percent increase in the proportion of youth 10-17 years old in the neighborhood, the odds of a store advertising promotions for Newport was 5.3 times greater. Although like others who have observed Newport are priced higher than Marlboro (nonmenthol), the authors reported that average price per pack for Newport appeared to be related to the racial makeup of neighborhoods, with the price of Newport decreasing $.12 for each 10 percent point increase in African American students. The amount of discount for Newport did not appear to be related to neighborhood demographics. No relationship between neighborhood demographics, promotions advertised, and/or price was found for Marlboro Menthol or Marlboro (nonmenthol).

Some data suggest differences in the influence of advertising receptivity on smoking behavior based on smoking status, gender, race or ethnicity, and age. Although there does not appear to be a validated measure of tobacco industry marketing exposure and receptivity, researchers define ad receptivity as the influence of tobacco marketing on an individual's attitudes, preferences, and behaviors (Evans, 1995). In the case of tobacco advertising, one hypothesis suggests that an individual's receptivity to advertising may predict initiation, preference, and continued use. Sargent et al. (2009) suggest the influence of advertising receptivity on initiation may vary by smoking status, whereby those who have not yet initiated smoking may be more influenced by smoking in movies than tobacco advertisements and promotions. Upon initiation, however, teens may become more receptive to tobacco advertising, and receptivity to tobacco marketing may further stimulate experimentation. Choi et al. (2002) also found that adolescents who were experimenters and were found to be highly receptive to advertising were 70 percent more likely to become established smokers at follow-up than those who were minimally receptive. Several studies included in the Lovato et al.

(2003) review found gender differences in receptivity, whereby advertising receptivity was influential for girls but not boys. Research also suggests susceptible never smoking African Americans and Hispanics may be less likely to be receptive to tobacco advertising than never smoking White adolescents (Chen et al., 2002; West et al., 2007). Chen et al. (2002) only found a statistically significant relationship between receptivity and smoking for White and Hispanic youth. Evans (1995) found younger adolescents scored higher on measures of ad receptivity than older adolescents. Studies of advertising receptivity did not examine differences between menthol smokers and nonmenthol smokers nor were differences in receptivity to menthol versus nonmenthol advertisements studied.

Consumer Perceptions

Richter et al. (2006) conducted focus groups and found differences in perceived risk by race.

While White participants reported menthol cigarettes to be safer than nonmenthol cigarettes, African American participants believed there were no differences in risk between types of cigarettes. Hispanic participants were twice as likely as White participants to rank menthol cigarettes as safer than light cigarettes. African Americans reported the highest preference for menthol cigarettes, and Hispanic participants reported a slight preference. Researchers did not control for the type of cigarette smoked—menthol or nonmenthol—in the analysis. Richter (2008) held a follow up set of focus groups with African Americans in Atlanta and found the discussion around risk and harm to yield mixed results among the different focus groups. While some participants reported menthol cigarettes were less harsh and irritating to the body, others believed they were worse for the body and more addictive. During a ranking exercise conducted with several of the groups, one group ranked menthol cigarettes as less harsh than nonmenthol cigarettes. Additionally, during these group exercises participants reported taste as the primary driver behind their preference for menthol cigarettes and talked about the perceived "cool factor" they believed was promoting use among African Americans and youth. While focus groups provide useful formative and illustrative information, the qualitative nature of the data makes it impossible to draw causal conclusions or to generalize to a larger population.

Unlike Richter et al. (2006), Wackowski et al. (2010) found that African Americans surveyed in New Jersey were twice as likely as Whites to report menthol cigarettes as more risky than nonmenthol cigarettes, with young adults being three times as likely as adults to think menthol cigarettes were more risky. Among smokers and non-smokers surveyed, 70 percent reported menthol cigarettes were just as risky as nonmenthol cigarettes. Only 4 percent of all respondents and 2.4 percent of menthol smokers believed menthol cigarettes were less risky than nonmenthol cigarettes. Almost one-third of menthol smokers surveyed reported menthol cigarettes were more risky than nonmenthol cigarettes. Davis et al. (2010) found similar results from an analysis of the 2009 HealthStyles survey (n=4,556).

Allen et al. (2010) developed a scale to measure attitudes and beliefs about menthol cigarettes among African American smokers. Researchers identified five factors for the scale: medicinal effects, image, less harmful, tradition, and menthol taste or sensation. They piloted the scale on 720 African American smokers (57% menthol only, 15% nonmenthol only). Findings were mixed based on age, gender, and education. Older respondents had higher scores on medical effects, image, and less harmful. Men had higher scores on medical effects, image, and tradition, while women had higher scores on taste. Education was inversely associated with scores on the medicinal effects, image, less harmful, and tradition factors, with less educated subjects having higher scores.

Lee and Glantz (2011) suggest differences in consumer perception by age may be a related to exposure to early industry advertisements that promoted the health benefits of menthol. This would suggest that older smokers who were exposed to these messages may perceive menthol as less harmful than younger smokers were not exposed to such messages do. Additional research is needed to test this hypothesis.

Conclusion

Many of the studies on the marketing of menthol cigarettes and consumer perceptions of menthol cigarettes were cross-sectional or qualitative in nature and therefore a clear relationship cannot be drawn.

As seen in nonmenthol cigarettes and other consumer goods, marketing has a strong influence on consumer brand preference and use. The relationship between advertising expenditures and brand preference and the research supporting teen sensitivity to advertising illustrates this reality. Based on numerous studies (including American Legacy Foundation, 2007; Arnett et al., 1998; Altman et al., 1991; Balback et al., 2003; Boly et al., 2010; Connolly et al., 2011; Cummings et al., 1987; Cummings et al., 1997; Glantz et al., 2006; Johnston et al., 1999; Landrine et al., 2005; Laws et al., 2002; O'Connor, 2005; Pollay, 1996; Samaji, 2008; Sutton et al., 2004; White et al., 2006), it appears that a targeted marketing mix of price, promotion, product, and place promotes menthol cigarette use among youth and among African Americans in urban communities. It is likely, however, that factors in addition to marketing contribute to the preference and use of menthol cigarettes among consumers. From the available studies, the weight of evidence supports the conclusion that, like nonmenthol cigarettes, the marketing of menthol cigarettes is likely associated with brand preference. The marketing of menthol cigarettes is associated with menthol brand preference among adolescents and the African American community.

Overall, the results appear to be mixed in the perceived risk of menthol cigarettes. While the reviewed studies suggest that people may be more likely to report menthol cigarettes as less risky or just as risky as nonmenthol cigarettes, design limitations prevent researchers from drawing solid conclusions. Additionally, limited use of validated forms of measuring risk perceptions of menthol cigarettes suggests participants may vary in their ways of defining "risk" and "harm." None of the reviewed articles examined risk perceptions of menthol cigarettes among youth. Given the limited data reviewed and mixed results reported, the weight of evidence is not sufficient to support a conclusion that consumer perceptions are associated with the use of menthol cigarettes.

Marketing and Consumer Perception of Risk: Table of Referenced

Author Name(s)	Article Title	Year Pub.	Funded By	Type of Study	Subject Description (Including Special population(s))	Sample Size (N)	Authors' Results/Conclusion(s) related to Menthol* (excerpted directly from article)
Allen B Jr, Unger JB.	Sociocultural correlates of menthol cigarette smoking among adult African Americans in Los Angeles.	2007	The California Tobacco-Related Disease Research Program	Cross-sectional survey	Adult African Americans in Los Angeles, CA at least 18 years old, smoked at least 5 cigarettes/day for the past year	N=432	Menthol smoking was most prevalent among women, 18–30-year-olds, and employed respondents.
Altman DG, Schooler C, Basil MD.	Alcohol and cigarette advertising on billboards.	1991	The Henry J. Kaiser Family Foundation	Neighborhood Census data	901 billboards in San Francisco, CA	Not Applicable	Blacks and Hispanics were the target of the largest proportion of alcohol and cigarette billboard advertising; more tobacco advertisements per 1000 population in black neighborhoods than in other neighborhoods. [Not menthol specific]
American Legacy Foundation	Cigarette preferences among youth—Results from the 2006 Legacy Media Tracking Online.	2007	American Legacy Foundation	Survey	13-18 year olds	N=3,567	The role of mentholated cigarettes may also change if the court's order prohibiting the use of light and related descriptors is upheld. If light cigarettes are no longer sold, more youth may turn to mentholated cigarettes since menthol makes these cigarettes easier to smoke than regular cigarettes. Currently, 37% of youth smokers (and 81% of African-Americans) report usually smoking menthol cigarettes. Currently, 40% of youth smokers report usually smoking menthol cigarettes. Clearly, this type of cigarette has appeal among youth and may increase smoking uptake.

Marketing and Consumer Perception of Risk: Table of Referenced (Continued)

Author Name(s)	Article Title	Year Pub.	Funded By	Type of Study	Subject Description (Including Special population(s))	Sample Size (N)	Authors' Results/Conclusion(s) related to Menthol* (excerpted directly from article)
Anderson S	Marketing of menthol cigarettes and consumer perceptions: a review of tobacco industry documents.	2011	U.S. Department of Health and Human Services	Industry document review	Menthol smokers, including special populations	Not applicable	The tobacco industry knew consumers perceived menthol as healthier than non-menthol cigarettes, and this was the intent behind marketing. Marketing emphasizing menthol attracts consumers who may not otherwise progress to regular smoking, including young, inexperienced users and those who find 'regular' cigarettes undesirable. Such marketing may also appeal to health-concerned smokers who might otherwise quit.
Arnett JJ, Terhanian G.	Adolescents' responses to cigarette advertisements: links between exposure, liking, and the appeal of smoking.	1998	Funding source(s) not provided. Authors affiliated with the University of Missouri and the University of Pennsylvania	Questionnaire/ survey	Adolescents; grades 6-12 (ages 11-18 years) from seven schools in four states, 54% female, 76% white	N=534	The results of the study are consistent with the view that certain cigarette advertisements enhance the appeal of smoking to many adolescents. [not menthol specific]
Balbach ED, Gasior RJ, Barbeau EM.	R.J. Reynolds' targeting of African Americans: 1988-2000.	2003	American Cancer Society	2 phases: systematic search of tobacco co. and documents and content analysis of the company's cigarette magazine	African Americans	Not Specified	Identified escape/fantasy and nightlife fun as two of the three primary images featured in the advertisements of menthol cigarettes to the Black/African American population.

Author Name(s)	Article Title	Year Pub.	Funded By	Type of Study	Subject Description (Including Special population(s))	Sample Size (N)	Authors' Results/Conclusion(s) related to Menthol* (excerpted directly from article)
				advertising.			
Centers for Disease Control and Prevention	Comparison of the cigarette brand preferences of adult and teenaged smokers—United States, 1989, and 10 US communities, 1988 and 1990.	1992	Centers for Disease Control and Prevention	2 surveys: Teenage Attitudes and Practices Survey (TAPS) and survey of selected COMMIT evaluation participations	TAPS: 12-18 year olds nationwide COMMIT: adult smokers and 13-16 year olds from the 10 COMMIT communities	TAPS: 9,135 adolescents COMMIT: 15,415 adults; 9,129 students	TAPS: Although Marlboro was the most popular brand among white and Hispanic adolescents, black adolescents preferred the mentholated brands of Newport, Kool, and Salem. Among 9th-grade students, Marlboro, Newport , and Camel were the most commonly purchased brands. In all regions, Marlboro was the most popular brand. Newport was second in the Northeast, and Camel was second in the West. Among white adolescents, Newport was more popular in the Northeast and the Midwest than in the South and the West. COMMIT: Among 9th-grade smokers across all 10 communities, three cigarette brands -- Marlboro, Camel, and Newport -- were consistently preferred. Camel cigarettes were
							most popular among teenaged smokers in western and midwestern communities. Newport cigarettes were most popular among teenaged smokers from communities in the Northeast. Newport was the most popular brand among black 9th-grade students and third most popular among white 9th-grade students.

Marketing and Consumer Perception of Risk: Table of Referenced (Continued)

Author Name(s)	Article Title	Year Pub.	Funded By	Type of Study	Subject Description (Including Special population(s))	Sample Size (N)	Authors' Results/Conclusion(s) related to Menthol* (excerpted directly from article)
Centers for Disease Control and Prevention	Changes in the cigarette brand preferences of adolescent smokersí United States, 1989-1993.	1994	Centers for Disease Control and Prevention	2 Surveys: 1989 TAPS and 1993 TAPS	12-18 year olds	1989 TAPS: 9,135 1993 TAPS: 7,311	Marlboro, Camel, and Newport were the most frequently purchased brands for 86% of the adolescents. Marlboro was the most commonly purchased brand for both male and female adolescents; the second most commonly purchased brand among males was Camel and among females was Newport. Marlboro was the most commonly purchased brand among white and Hispanic adolescents; black adolescents most frequently purchased Newport. Younger smokers (aged 12-15 years) were more likely than older smokers (aged 16-18 years) to buy Newport and less likely to buy Marlboro; purchasing frequency for Camel cigarettes was similar among all adolescents. Among adolescents nationwide, Marlboro was the most commonly purchased brand. However, by region, Camel was most commonly purchased in the West, and Newport, in the Northeast. From 1989 to 1993, substantial changes in brand preference occurred among adolescents. The percentage of adolescents purchasing Marlboro cigarettes decreased 8.7 percentage points (13% decrease), the percentage of adolescents purchasing Camel cigarettes increased 5.2 percentage points

Author Name(s)	Article Title	Year Pub.	Funded By	Type of Study	Subject Description (Including Special population(s))	Sample Size (N)	Authors' Results/Conclusion(s) related to Menthol* (excerpted directly from article)
							(64% increase), and the percentage purchasing Newport cigarettes increased 4.5 percentage points (55% increase). These changes did not completely correlate with changes in overall cigarette market share during 1989-1993. Increases in brand preference for Camel cigarettes were greatest among white adolescents and adolescents residing in the Midwest and West, and increases for Newport cigarettes were greatest among younger smokers and adolescents residing in the Northeast.
Centers for	Cigarette brand	2009	Centers for Disease	2 Surveys:	Adolescents in grades	2004:	Marlboro was the preferred brand (43.3% and52.3%, respectively), followed by Newport (26.4% and 21.4%, respectively). The use of Newport was significantly higher among blacks in middle school (59.7%) and high school (78.6%) compared with other racial/ethnic groups. Information on brand preferences and tobacco marketing strategies that are attractive to students can be used by tobacco control programs and community initiatives in the design of tobacco countermarketing campaigns. These countermarketing campaigns have been shown to be effective as part of a comprehensive tobacco control program to decrease the initiation of tobacco use among youths and young adults. [Not menthol specific]

Marketing and Consumer Perception of Risk: Table of Referenced (Continued)

Author Name(s)	Article Title	Year Pub.	Funded By	Type of Study	Subject Description (Including Special population(s))	Sample Size (N)	Authors' Results/Conclusion(s) related to Menthol* (excerpted directly from article)
Disease Control and Prevention	preference among middle and high school students who are established smokers—United States, 2004 and 2006.		Control and Prevention	2004 and 2006 National Youth Tobacco Surveys	6-12	N=27,933 2006: N=27,038	
Chen X, Cruz	Receptivity to	2002	Partially by funds from the	Cross-sectional	Ethnic Minority youth	N=20,332	Results indicate that receptivity to protobacco
TB, Schuster DV, Unger JB, Johnson CA.	protobacco media and its impact on cigarette smoking among ethnic minority youth in		University of California Tobacco-Related Disease Research Program, award number 6KT-0191		(boys and girls), 12–17 years of age, in CA		media was lower among African Americans, Asian Americans, and Hispanics than among White youth. There was a consistent dose- response relationship between receptivity to protobacco media and 30-day cigarette smoking
	California.						across ethnic groups. Having a cigarette brand preference was associated with the highest risk for cigarette smoking, having a favorite tobacco ad showed the lowest risk, while having received or being willing to use tobacco promotional items was associated with a moderate risk. [Not menthol specific]
Choi WS, Ahluwalia JS, Harris KJ, Okuyemi K.	Progression to established smoking: the influence of	2002	Robert Wood Johnson Foundation, American Cancer Society, the Tobacco-Related	Data taken from longitudinal survey	Adolescents (12-17 years) in California.	N=965	This study provides evidence that receptivity to tobacco advertising and promotions is an important factor in progressing from experimentation to

Author Name(s)	Article Title	Year Pub.	Funded By	Type of Study	Subject Description (Including Special population(s))	Sample Size (N)	Authors' Results/Conclusion(s) related to Menthol* (excerpted directly from article)
	tobacco marketing.		Disease Research Program at the University of California, the National Cancer Institute				established smoking among adolescents. [Not menthol specific]
Connolly GN, Behm I, Osaki Y, et al.	The impact of menthol cigarettes on smoking initiation among non-smoking young females in Japan	2011	No funding source(s) provided. Authors affiliated with the Center for Global Tobacco Control, Harvard School of Public Health; Tottori University	Industry document review Cross-sectional survey of Japanese adolescents Japanese National Health and Nutrition Survey	Japanese females, including adolescents	Not reported	Japan provides an excellent case-study on the impact of the introduction and marketing of menthol brands to young women and initiation into smoking. Smoking prevalence in Japan has been declining among men for decades, but rates of smoking among women have recently increased. The internal tobacco documents demonstrate the intent of tobacco manufacturers to increase initiation among young females through development and marketing of menthol brands. Adolescent survey data provides evidence that the uptake of smoking among high school aged girls in Japan is largely via menthol brands. Adult survey data, though not segmented by brand type (e.g., menthol), indicates that the increased uptake of smoking among young girls has translated to rising smoking rates among young women as these cohorts age. The Japan experience suggests the importance of brand targeting as a vehicle to capitalize on social changes and encourage initiation and use among a historically non- smoking population.

Marketing and Consumer Perception of Risk: Table of Referenced (Continued)

Author Name(s)	Article Title	Year Pub.	Funded By	Type of Study	Subject Description (Including Special population(s))	Sample Size (N)	Authors' Results/Conclusion(s) related to Menthol* (excerpted directly from article)
Cruz TB, Wright LT, Crawford G.	The menthol marketing mix: targeted promotions for focus communities in the United States.	2010	No funding source(s) provided. Authors affiliated with University of Southern California, National African American Tobacco Prevention Network, Georgia Division of Public Health. Data were partially gathered while an author (Wright) was employed by Brown & Williamson Tobacco Corporation	Interview Review of industry documents	Interview with former Brown and Williamson trade marketing manager Industry review focused on menthol marketing strategies in urban communities	Not applicable	Tobacco companies recognize the growth potential for the menthol segment in these urban communities. They have higher levels of price discounts and signage, exert tight controls over the retail environment, and use hip-hop lifestyle to associate menthol products with urban nightlife, music, fame, and cultural edginess among younger smokers.
Cummings KM, Giovino G, Mendicino AJ.	Cigarette advertising and black-white differences in brand preference.	1987	The National Cancer Institute	Not Applicable	Two Populations: (1) patients seen at the Deaconness Family Medicine Center (FMC) located in Buffalo, NY. During the 4-month period of February to May 1984 (2) white and black smokers who called the Stop Smoking Hotline between August 1984 and June 1985	FMC N=440 Hotline N=1199	Magazines directed to blacks include a much greater proportion of ads for menthol cigarettes compared with magazines similar in content but directed to white readers.

Author Name(s)	Article Title	Year Pub.	Funded By	Type of Study	Subject Description (Including Special population(s))	Sample Size (N)	Authors' Results/Conclusion(s) related to Menthol* (excerpted directly from article)
Cummings KM, Hyland A, Pechacek TF, Orlandi M, Lynn WR.	Comparison of recent trends in adolescent and adult cigarette smoking behavior and brand preferences.	1997	National Cancer Institute; Robert Wood Johnson Foundation	2 cross-sectional phone surveys (adults); and 2 surveys conducted at schools (adolescents)	Adolescent and adult smokers in 18 communities	Jan-May 1988 N=99348; Aug 1993-Jan 1994 N=79890;	No gender difference between males and females who smoked the menthol brand NewportTM or reported smoking menthol cigarettes in general. Cigarette brand use was more tightly concentrated among adolescents compared to adults, with young smokers most likely to use the most heavily marketed cigarette brands.
Davis SP, McClave-	Perceptions of menthol cigarette	2010	Centers for Disease Control and Prevention	Survey	U.S. adults and current smokers	N=4,556	Close to half of adults (45.8%) believed that menthol cigarettes are just as harmful as
Regan AK, Rock VJ, et al.	use among U.S. adults and adult smokers: Findings from the 2009 HealthStyles survey.						nonmenthol cigarettes, and 40.9% of adults did not know whether menthol cigarettes are more or less harmful than nonmenthol cigarettes. Few adults (0.6%), including smokers, perceived menthol cigarettes to be less harmful than nonmenthol cigarettes. Blacks were more likely to believe that menthol cigarettes have health benefits when compared with Whites. Almost half of current smokers believed menthol cigarettes are equally addictive as nonmenthol cigarettes and 74.9% believed menthol and nonmenthol cigarettes are equally hard to quit.
Evans N, Farkas A, Gilipin E, Berry C, Pierce JP.	Influence of tobacco marketing and exposure to smokers on adolescent susceptibility to smoking.	1995	The California Department of Health Services; Robert Wood Johnson Foundation; the American Heart Association.	Survey	1993 California Tobacco Survey of adolescent non-smokers	N=3536	Tobacco marketing may be a stronger current influence in encouraging adolescents to initiate smoking than demographics, school performance, or exposure to other smokers in peers or family network. [Not menthol specific]

Marketing and Consumer Perception of Risk: Table of Referenced (Continued)

Author Name(s)	Article Title	Year Pub.	Funded By	Type of Study	Subject Description (Including Special population(s))	Sample Size (N)	Authors' Results/Conclusion(s) related to Menthol* (excerpted directly from article)
Gardiner PS.	The African Americanization of menthol cigarette use in the United States.	2004	Tobacco Related Disease Research Program at the University of California	Literature Review	African American Population	Not Applicable	Menthol targeting has changed little since the 1960s: African Americans continue to be bombarded with menthol slogans and advertisements.
Glanz K, Sutton NM, Jacob Arriola KR.	Operation storefront Hawaii: tobacco advertising and promotion in Hawaii stores.	2006	Master Tobacco Settlement through the Hawaii State Department of Health, Georgia Cancer Coalition Distinguished Scholar Award	Cross-sectional study of tobacco product store-based advertisements, including the number, location (indoor/outdoor;	Advertisements and promotions among 184 stores	N=3151	Among just 184 stores, more than 3,000 ads and promotions were identified. Kool, which is a mentholated brand, was the most heavily advertised brand, consistent with earlier research that found this brand to be the most heavily smoked by middle school youth in Hawaii
				proximity to candy, toys, school), size, and brand of the ads. Trained youth (ages 12–19 years).			
Henriksen, L, Schleicher, NC, Dauphinee, AL, Fortmann, SP.	Targeted advertising, promotion, and price for menthol cigarettes in California high school	2011 (e-pub ahead of print)	California's Tobacco-Related Disease Research Program, Grant #14RT- 0103	Observational	Tobacco retailers within .5 miles of schools who participated in the California Tobacco Survey	N=726	In high school neighborhoods, targeted advertising exposes Blacks to more promotions and lower prices for the leading brand of menthol cigarettes. This evidence contradicts the manufacturer's claims that the availability of its promotions is not based on race/ethnicity. It also highlights

Author Name(s)	Article Title	Year Pub.	Funded By	Type of Study	Subject Description (Including Special population(s))	Sample Size (N)	Authors' Results/Conclusion(s) related to Menthol* (excerpted directly from article)
	neighborhoods.						the need for tobacco control policies that would limit disparities in exposure to retail marketing for cigarettes.
Johnson DM, Wine LA, Zack S, Zimmer E, Wang JH, Weitzel-O'Neill PA, Claflin V, Tercyak KP	Designing a tobacco counter-marketing campaign for African American youth.	2008	National Institutes of Health/National Cancer Institute grants U56CA101429, U56CA101563, and K07CA091831	Qualitative	African American middle school-aged youth.	N=28	High degree of industry commitment to recruiting and retaining young African American smokers and their preference for mentholated brands.
Johnston LD, O'Malley PM, Bachman JG, Schulenberg JE.	Cigarette brand preferences among adolescents.	1999	National Institute on Drug Abuse	Survey	American students in 8th, 10th, or 12th grade attending public or private secondary schools in the coterminous 48 states.	N=2,048 eighth graders, 2,708 tenth graders, and 2,335 twelfth graders	There are dramatic racial/ethnic differences in brand preferences among those who do smoke. Newport, a mentholated cigarette, predominates among African American teenage smokers to an even greater extent than Marlboro predominates among white teenage smokers.
Kaufman NJ, Castrucci BC, Mowery P, Gerlach KK, Emont S,	Changes in adolescent cigarette-brand preference, 1989 to 1996.	2004	No funding source(s) provided. Authors affiliated with the Robert Wood Johnson, Research Triangle Institute, White	Survey	3 national samples of adolescents collected in 1989, 1993, and 1996.	N=17,287	Brand preference among adolescents has been steadily concentrated among 3 brands. More attention may need to be focused on mentholated brands given the increase in Newport's market share.
Orleans CT.			Mountain Research Associates				

Marketing and Consumer Perception of Risk: Table of Referenced (Continued)

Author Name(s)	Article Title	Year Pub.	Funded By	Type of Study	Subject Description (Including Special population(s))	Sample Size (N)	Authors' Results/Conclusion(s) related to Menthol* (excerpted directly from article)
Klausner, K.	Menthol cigarettes and smoking initiation: a tobacco industry perspective.	2011	No funding source(s) provided. Author affiliated with University of California, San Francisco	Industry document review	Not applicable	N=128 documents	The documents show that menthol is added to cigarettes in part because it is known to be an attractive feature to inexperienced smokers who perceive menthol cigarettes as less harsh and easier to smoke and because of their availability from friends and family. Second, the tobacco industry found that some youths smoke menthols because they perceive them to be less harmful than non-menthol cigarettes. A key product design issue concerns whether to increase brand menthol levels to appeal to the taste preferences of long-term menthol smokers or keep menthol levels lower to appeal to inexperienced smokers. Marketing studies showed that the companies carefully researched the menthol segment of the market in order to recruit younger smokers to their brands. The industry tracked menthol cigarette usage by age, gender and race to inform product development and marketing decisions.
Landrine H, Klonoff EA, Fernandez S, Hickman N, Kashima K, Parekh B, Thomas K,	Cigarette advertising in Black, Latino, and White magazines, 1998-2002: an exploratory	2005	National Cancer Institute, Tobacco Related Disease Research Program at the University of California, the California Department of Health	Review	Analysis of digital photographs of cigarette ads appearing in Ebony (Black), People (White), and People in Spanish (Latino) for	N=274 advertisements	Black magazines were 9.8 times and Latino magazines 2.6 times more likely than White magazines to contain ads for menthol cigarettes...

Author Name(s)	Article Title	Year Pub.	Funded By	Type of Study	Subject Description (Including Special population(s))	Sample Size (N)	Authors' Results/Conclusion(s) related to Menthol* (excerpted directly from article)
Brouillard CR, Zolezzi M, Jensen JA, Weslowski Z.	investigation.		Services		the 4.5-year period of January 1998 to August 2002.		
Laws MB, Whitman J,	Tobacco availability and	2002	No funding source(s) provided. Authors	Survey	Retail businesses in the Boston area that sell	N=1676	Mentholated brands were marketed most heavily in the predominantly African American
Bowser DM, Krech L.	point of sale marketing in demographically contrasting districts of Massachusetts.		affiliated with the Latin American Health Institute, Arias Foundation, Harvard School of Public Health		tobacco products		neighborhood, and disproportionately in the Latino neighborhoods.
Lee, YO, Glantz, SA.	Menthol: putting the pieces together.	2011	The National Cancer Institute grants CA-113710 and CA-87472	Review	Not applicable	Not applicable	Tobacco companies shaped consumer perceptions of menthol cigarettes. Menthol is not just a flavouring agent. Cigarette companies use menthol's ability to mask irritation and provide sensory effects to make menthol cigarettes appeal to youth and health-concerned smokers, in part because menthol makes low-tar cigarettes more palatable. Consistent with targeted marketing, youths, women and African Americans disproportionately smoke menthols. There appear to be complex interactions with addictive effects of nicotine. The ubiquitous addition of menthol by tobacco companies to over 90% of all tobacco products, whether labelled 'menthol' or not, demonstrates that menthol is not simply a flavour or brand. Menthol

Marketing and Consumer Perception of Risk: Table of Referenced (Continued)

Author Name(s)	Article Title	Year Pub.	Funded By	Type of Study	Subject Description (Including Special population(s))	Sample Size (N)	Authors' Results/Conclusion(s) related to Menthol* (excerpted directly from article)
							imparts sensory characteristics to cigarettes and has a complex interaction with nicotine that affects smoking behaviour whether it is perceived or not, or whether cigarettes containing menthol are marketed as 'menthol' or not. Adding menthol increases fine particles in cigarette smoke, which have immediate adverse effects on the risk of heart attack.
Lovato C, Linn G, Stead LF, Best A.	Impact of tobacco advertising and promotion on increasing adolescent	2003	National Cancer Institute of Canada, Canada; Canadian Cancer Society, Canada; Centre for Behavioural Research and	Review	9 Longitudinal studies that assessed individuals' smoking behaviour and exposure to advertising,	N=12,000 baseline nonsmokers.	Tobacco advertising and promotion increases the likelihood that adolescents will start to smoke. [Not menthol specific]
	smoking behaviours.		Program Evaluation, Canada		receptivity or attitudes to tobacco advertising, or brand awareness at baseline, and assessed smoking behaviour at follow-ups. Participants were adolescents aged 18 or younger who were not regular smokers at baseline.		
Mazis MB, Ringold DJ, Perry ES,	Perceived age and attractiveness of models in	1992	The Center for Marketing Policy Research, American	Sample Survey	Two quota samples of 280 and 281 people were recruited in a	N=561	Cigarette ads with young persons were found to appear more often in magazines with younger audiences and for menthol

Author Name(s)	Article Title	Year Pub.	Funded By	Type of Study	Subject Description (Including Special population(s))	Sample Size (N)	Authors' Results/Conclusion(s) related to Menthol* (excerpted directly from article)
Denman DW.	cigarette advertisements.		University, University of Baltimore		racially and economically diverse shopping mall in a suburban area of a large east-coast city.		brands.
O'Connor RJ.	What brands are US smokers under 25 choosing?	2005	No funding source(s) provided. Author affiliated with the Roswell Park Cancer Center	Online Analysis	Data on the cigarette brand preferences of smokers in the 2002 US National Survey on Drug Use and Health from three age groups: 12–17, 18–25 years, and 26+ years.	12–17 years (n = 2290), 18–25 years (n = 7321), 26+ years (n = 5238).	The youth market in the USA appears dominated by varieties of the major advertised brands; other products make up a more modest percentage of the market. Conversely, the adult market is much more diffuse, with the major varieties commanding smaller overall percentages of the market. Light varieties appear to be popular choices for younger smokers. Similar investigations in other countries could shed further light on younger smokers' brand choices, particularly in those countries that have banned descriptors such as "Light'' and "Mild". [Not menthol specific]
Office of Applied Studies.	Results from the 2005 National Survey on Drug Use and Health: National findings	2006	Department of Health and Human Services	Survey	Nationally representative sample of U.S. population ages 12 and older	N=68,308	Marlboro was the cigarette brand used most often by past month cigarette smokers in all four geographic regions. Newport was second in prevalence in the Northeast, Midwest, and South, while Camel was second in the West
Pollay RW, Siddarth S, Siegel M, Haddix A,	The last straw? Cigarette advertising and realized market	1996	The Social Science and Humanities Research Council of Canada	Analysis	Market shares among adults and teenagers for five years between 1979 and 1993 (1979,	Based on information of 9 brands	Cigarette brand shares of advertising voice are found to be significantly related to realized market shares, with advertising sensitivity being about three times larger

Marketing and Consumer Perception of Risk: Table of Referenced (Continued)

Author Name(s)	Article Title	Year Pub.	Funded By	Type of Study	Subject Description (Including Special population(s))	Sample Size (N)	Authors' Results/Conclusion(s) related to Menthol* (excerpted directly from article)
Merritt RK, Giovino GA, Eriksen MR.	shares among youths and adults, 1979–1993.				1986, 1989, 1992, 1993).		among teenagers than among adults. [Not menthol specific]
Richter P, Beistle D, Pederson L, O'Hegarty M.	Small-group discussions on menthol cigarettes: listening to adult African American smokers in Atlanta, Georgia.	2008	Centers for Disease Control and Prevention	Focus Groups	Explored health risk perceptions in two studies using focus groups. In the first, Black/African American men and women (ages 45–64 years) who smoked menthol cigarettes participated in small-group discussions	N=54	The majority of the participants agreed that menthol cigarettes were predominantly featured in Black publications, and that most cigarette advertising and marketing in their communities were for menthol brands, with minimal advertising of non-menthol brands. Some participants thought that tobacco companies targeted menthol cigarettes to Black/African American communities (and non-menthol cigarettes to White communities) and believed that advertising played a role in what brands were sold in an area
Richter PA, Pederson LL, O'Hegarty MM.	Young adult smoker risk perceptions of traditional cigarettes and nontraditional tobacco products.	2006	U.S. Department of Health and Human Services	Focus Groups	African American, non- Hispanic white, and Hispanic young adult current smokers between the ages of 18 and 22 years who had tried or who currently used NTPs (nontraditional tobacco products).	N=137	In comparisons with menthol and regular cigarettes, most college and not-in-college participants chose the same risk or more harmful ratings, regardless of the order of presentation of the products.
Sargent JD, Gibson J,	Comparing the effects of	2009	National Cancer Institute and The	Comparative, Multicenter	Northern New England adolescents	N=4524	Separate roles for entertainment media and tobacco marketing on adolescent smoking.

Author Name(s)	Article Title	Year Pub.	Funded By	Type of Study	Subject Description (Including Special population(s))	Sample Size (N)	Authors' Results/Conclusion(s) related to Menthol* (excerpted directly from article)
Heatherton TF.	entertainment		American Legacy Foundation		aged 10-14 in 1999		Both exposures deserve equal emphasis from a policy
	media and tobacco marketing on youth smoking.						standpoint. [Not menthol specific]
Seidenberg, AB, Caughey, RW, Rees, VW, Connolly, GN.	Storefront cigarette advertising differs by community demographic profile.	2010	American Legacy Foundation grant 6212 and National Cancer Institute grant 5 U01 CA114644	Observational	Tobacco retailers in Brookline, MA (primarily Caucasian) and Dorchester, MA (primarily African American)	N=102	The low-income/minority community had more tobacco retailers, and advertisements were more likely to be larger, promote menthol products, have a lower mean advertised price, and occur within 1000 feet of a school.
Sutton CD, Robinson RG.	The marketing of menthol cigarettes in the United States: populations, messages, and channels.	2004	No funding source(s) provided. Authors affiliated with the Onyx Group, the Centers for Disease Control and Prevention	Commentary	Tobacco industry documents related to specific populations including women, middle school youth, Asian/Pacific Islander immigrants, and African Americans	Not Applicable	Learning more about the messages and media used to promote menthol cigarette brands to target markets such as women, Blacks, and youth can be an invaluable aid in helping to decrease the uptake of menthol brands and in creating improved prevention and cessation strategies for at-risk communities and populations. [Not menthol specific]
Wackowski O, Delnevo CD, Lewis, MJ	Risk perceptions of menthol cigarettes compared with nonmethol cigarettes among New Jersey adults.	2010	New Jersey Department of Health and Senior Services	Statewide random-digit-dial telephone survey	Data from the 2005 New Jersey Adult Tobacco Survey, oversampling young adults aged 18–24 years, smokers, and recent quitters	N=3062	Overall, 70.1% (±2.4) of all survey respondents (including nonsmokers) reported that they perceived menthol cigarettes to have about the same risk as nonmenthol cigarettes. Current smokers overall were significantly more likely than nonsmokers to believe menthol cigarettes were riskier than

Marketing and Consumer Perception of Risk: Table of Referenced (Continued)

Author Name(s)	Article Title	Year Pub.	Funded By	Type of Study	Subject Description (Including Special population(s))	Sample Size (N)	Authors' Results/Conclusion(s) related to Menthol* (excerpted directly from article)
							nonmenthol cigarettes
West JH, Romero RA, Trinidad DR.	Adolescent receptivity to tobacco marketing by racial/ethnic groups in California.	2007	the Tobacco Related Disease Research Program of the University of California, the National Cancer Institute, the California Department of Health Services	Survey	Adolescents	5857 adolescents ages 12-17 years	There may be features of the American and Asian/Pacific cultures that are protective for receptivity to tobacco smoking among those who are susceptible smokers. Prevention strategies emphasizing such features for adolescents of other ethnicities may be beneficial in reducing smoking disparities. [Not menthol specific]
White VM, White MM, Freeman K, Gilpin EA, Pierce JP	Cigarette promotional offers: who takes advantage?	2006	the Tobacco Related Disease Research Program of the University of California, California Department of Health Services	Population	Current smokers	N=4618	With the exception of smokers intending to quit, cigarette promotional offers are effectively reaching most industry-targeted groups. Importantly, young adults, who have the greatest long-term customer potential, are responding. [Not menthol specific]
Yerger VB, Przewoznik J, Malone RE.	Racialized geography, corporate activity, and health disparities: tobacco industry targeting of inner cities.	2007	No funding source(s) provided. Authors affiliated with the University of California, San Fancisco and the University of Pennsylvania	Review	Inner cities containing predominately low-income African American residents	400 internal tobacco industry documents	Tobacco industry's activities contributed to the racialized geography of today's tobacco-related health disparities. [Not menthol specific]

* Note: these statements are taken directly from articles and may not include all relevant results/conclusions. [Bracketed notes added by FDA]

References

Allen B., Cruz TB, Leonard E, et al. (2010) Development and validation of a scale to assess attitudes and beliefs about menthol cigarettes among African-American smokers. Evaluation and the Health Professions 33(4):414-436. [Funded by the Tobacco Related Disease Research Program at the University of California]

Altman DG, Schooler C, Basil MD (1991) Alcohol and cigarette advertising on billboards. Health Education Research 6(4):487–490. [Funded in part by Henry J. Kaiser Family Foundation]

American Legacy Foundation (2007). Cigarette preferences among youth—Results from the 2006 Legacy Media Tracking Online. First Look Report 17. http://www.legacy forhealth.org/4206.aspx

Anderson S (2011) Marketing of menthol cigarettes and consumer perceptions: a review of tobacco industry documents. Tobacco Control 20(suppl.2):ii20-ii28. [Funded by U.S. Department of Health and Human Services]

Arnett JJ, Terhanian G (1998) Adolescents' responses to cigarette advertisements: links between exposure, liking, and the appeal of smoking. Tobacco Control 7(2):129–133. [Funding source(s) not provided. Authors affiliated with the University of Missouri and the University of Pennsylvania]

Balbach ED, Gasior RJ, Barbeau EM (2003) R.J. Reynold's targeting of African Americans: 1988–2000. American Journal of Public Health 93:822–827. [Funded by the American Cancer Society]

Centers for Disease Control and Prevention (1992) Comparison of the cigarette brand preferences of adult and teenaged smokers—United States, 1989, and 10 US communities, 1988 and 1990. Morbidity and Mortality Weekly Report 41(10):169–73,179–81. http://www.cdc.gov/mmwr/preview/mmwrhtml/00016275.htm [Funded by the Centers for Disease Control and Prevention]

Centers for Disease Control and Prevention (1994) Changes in the cigarette brand preferences of adolescent smokersí United States, 1989-1993. Morbidity and Mortality Weekly Report 43:577-581. http://www.cdc.gov/mmwr/preview/mmwrhtml/ 00032326. htm [Funded by the Centers for Disease Control and Prevention]

Centers for Disease Control and Prevention (2009). Cigarette brand preference among middle and high school students who are established smokers—United States, 2004 and 2006. Morbidity and Mortality Weekly Report, 58(05): 112-115.

Chen X, Cruz TB, Schuster DV, et al. (2002) Receptivity to protobacco media and its impact on cigarette smoking among ethnic minority youth in California. Journal of Health Communication 7(2):95–111. [Funded in part by the Tobacco-Related Disease Research Program at the University of California]

Choi WS, Ahluwalia JS, Harris KJ, Okuyemi K (2002) Progression to established smoking: the influence of tobacco marketing. American Journal of Preventive Medicine 22(4):228–233. [Funded by the Robert Wood Johnson Foundation, American Cancer Society, the Tobacco-Related Disease Research Program at the University of California, the National Cancer Institute]

Connolly GN, Behm I, Osaki Y, et al. (2011) The impact of menthol cigarettes on smoking initiation among non-smoking young females in Japan. International Journal of Environmental Research and Public Health 8(1):1-14 [No funding source(s) provided.

Authors affiliated with the Center for Global Tobacco Control, Harvard School of Public Health; Tottori University]

Cruz TB, Wright LT, Crawford G (2010) The menthol marketing mix: targeted promotions for focus communities in the United States. Nicotine and Tobacco Research 2(suppl 2):S147-S153. [No funding source(s) provided. Authors affiliated with University of Southern California, National African American Tobacco Prevention Network, Georgia Division of Public Health. Data were partially gathered while an author (Wright) was employed by Brown & Williamson Tobacco Corporation]

Cummings KM, Hyland A, Pechacek TF, Orlandi M, Lynn WR (1997) Comparison of recent trends in adolescent and adult cigarette smoking behaviour and brand preferences. Tobacco Control 6(Suppl 2):S31-7. [Funded by the National Cancer Institute, Robert Wood Johnson Foundation]

Cummings KM, Giovino G, Mendicino AJ (1987) Cigarette advertising and Black-White differences in brand preference. Public Health Report 102(6):698–701. [Funded by the National Cancer Institute]

Davis SP, McClave-Regan AK, Rock VJ, et al.(2010) Perceptions of menthol cigarette use among U.S. adults and adult smokers: Findings from the 2009 HealthStyles survey. Nicotine and Tobacco Research 12(suppl 2);S125-35. [Funded by the Centers for Disease Control and Prevention]

Evans N, Farkas A, Gilpin E, et al. (1995) Influence of tobacco marketing and exposure to smokers on adolescent susceptibility to smoking. Journal of the National Cancer Institute 87(20):1538–1545. [Funded in part by the California Department of Health Services, Robert Wood Johnson Foundation, American Heart Association]

Gardiner PS (2004) The African Americanization of menthol cigarette use in the United States. Nicotine and Tobacco Research 6(suppl 1):S55–S65. [Funded by Tobacco Related Disease Research Program at the University of California]

Glanz K, Sutton NM, Arriola KRJ (2006) Operation storefront Hawaii: tobacco advertising and promotion in Hawaii stores. Journal of Health Communication 11(7):699–707. [Funded in part by Master Tobacco Settlement through the Hawaii State Department of Health, Georgia Cancer Coalition Distinguished Scholar Award]

Henriksen, L, Schleicher, NC, Dauphinee, AL, Fortmann, SP (2011). Targeted advertising, promotion, and price for menthol cigarettes in California high school neighborhoods. Nicotine and Tobacco Research. epub ahead of print. [Funded by California's Tobacco-Related Disease Research Program, Grant #14RT-0103]

Johnson DM, Wine LA, Zack S, et al. (2008) Designing a tobacco counter-marketing campaign for African American youth. Tobacco Induced Diseases 4(1):7. [Funded in part by National Cancer Institute, Lombardi Comprehensive Cancer Center at Georgetown University, University of the District of Columbia]

Johnston LD, O'Malley PM, Bachman JG, Schulenberg JE (1999) Cigarette brand preferences among adolescents. Monitoring the Future Occasional Paper No. 45, Ann Arbor, MI: Institute for Social Research. http://www.monitoringthefuture.org/pubs/occpapers/occ45.pdf [Funded by the National Institute on Drug Abuse]

Kaufman NJ, Castrucci BC, Mowery P, Gerlach KK, Emont S, Orleans TC (2004) Changes in adolescent cigarette-brand preference, 1989 to 1996. American Journal of Health Behavior 28(1):54-62. [No funding source(s) provided. Authors affiliated with the Robert Wood Johnson, Research Triangle Institute, White Mountain Research Associates]

Klausner, K (2011). Menthol cigarettes and smoking initiation: a tobacco industry perspective. Tobacco Control 20(suppl 2): ii12-ii19. [No funding source(s) provided. Author affiliated with University of California, San Francisco]

Landrine H, Klonoff EA, Fernandez S, et al. (2005) Cigarette advertising in Black, Latino, and White magazines, 1998–2002: an exploratory investigation. Ethnicity and Disease 15(1):63–67. [Funded by the National Cancer Institute, Tobacco Related Disease Research Program at the University of California, the California Department of Health Services]

Laws MB, Whitman J, Bowser DM, et al. (2002) Tobacco availability and point of sale marketing in demographically contrasting districts of Massachusetts. Tobacco Control 11(suppl 2):S71–S73. [No funding source(s) provided. Authors affiliated with the Latin American Health Institute, Arias Foundation, Harvard School of Public Health]

Lee, YO, Glantz, SA (2011). Menthol: putting the pieces together. Tobacco Control 20(suppl 2): ii1-ii7. [Funding provided by The National Cancer Institute grants CA- 113710 and CA-87472]

Lovato C, Linn G, Stead LF, Best A (2003) Impact of tobacco advertising and promotion on increasing adolescent smoking behaviours. Cochrane Database of Systematic Review (4):CD003439. [Funded by National Cancer Institute of Canada, Canada; Canadian Cancer Society, Canada; Centre for Behavioural Research and Program Evaluation, Canada]

Mazis MB, Ringold DJ, Perry ES, Denman DW (1992) Perceived age and attractiveness of models in cigarette advertisements. Journal of Financial Markets 56(1):22–37.

[Funded in part by the Center for Marketing Policy Research, American University, University of Baltimore]

O'Connor RJ (2005) What brands are US smokers under 25 choosing? Tobacco Control 14:213-218. [No funding source(s) provided. Author affiliated with the Roswell Park Cancer Center]

Office of Applied Studies. (2002). Results from the 2001 National Household Survey on Drug Abuse: Volume I. Summary of national findings (DHHS Publication No. SMA 02–3758, NHSDA Series H–17). Rockville, MD: Substance Abuse and Mental Health Services Administration. [Funding provided by the Department of Health and Human Services]

Pollay RW, Siddarth S, Siegel M, et al. (1996) The last straw? Cigarette advertising and realized market shares among youths and adults, 1979–1993. Journal of Financial Markets 60:1–16. [Funded by the Social Science and Humanities Research Council of Canada]

Richter P, Beistel D, Pederson L, O'Hegarty M (2008) Small-group discussions on menthol cigarettes: listening to adult African American smokers in Atlanta, Georgia. Ethnicity and Health 13(2):171–182. [Funded by the Centers for Disease Control and Prevention]

Richter PA, Pederson LL, O'Hegarty MM (2006) Young adult smoker risk perceptions of traditional cigarettes and nontraditional tobacco products. American Journal of Health Behavior 30(3):302-12. [Funded by the Centers for Disease Control and Prevention]

Sargent JD, Gibson J, Heatherton TF (2009) Comparing the effects of entertainment media and tobacco marketing on youth smoking. Tobacco Control 18(1):47–53. [Funded by the National Cancer Institute, American Legacy Foundation]

Seidenberg, AB, Caughey, RW, Rees, VW, Connolly, GN (2010). Storefront cigarette advertising differs by community demographic profile. American Journal of Health Promotion 24(6): e26-e31. [Funded by American Legacy Foundation grant 6212 and National Cancer Institute grant 5 U01 CA114644]

Sutton D, Robinson RG (2004) The marketing of menthol cigarettes in the United States: populations, messages, and channels. Nicotine and Tobacco Research, 6 (suppl 1):S83–S91. [No funding source(s) provided. Authors affiliated with the Onyx Group, the Centers for Disease Control and Prevention]

Wackowski O, Delnevo CD, Lewis, MJ (2010) Risk perceptions of menthol cigarettes compared with nonmethol cigarettes among New Jersey adults. Nicotine and Tobacco Research 12(7): 786-790. [Funded by the New Jersey Department of Health and Senior Services]

West JH, Romero RA, Trinidad DR (2007) Adolescent receptivity to tobacco marketing by racial or ethnic groups in California. American Journal of Preventive Medicine 33(2):121–123. [Funded by the Tobacco Related Disease Research Program of the University of California, the National Cancer Institute, the California Department of Health Services]

White VM, White MM, Freeman K, et al. (2006) Cigarette promotional offers: who takes advantage? American Journal of Preventive Medicine 30(3):225–231. [Funded by the Tobacco Related Disease Research Program of the University of California, California Department of Health Services]

Yerger VB, Przewoznik J, Malone RE (2007) Racialized geography, corporate activity, and health disparities: tobacco industry targeting of inner cities. Journal of Health Care for the Poor and Underserved 18(suppl 4):S10–S38. [No funding source(s) provided. Authors affiliated with the University of California, San Fancisco and the University of Pennsylvania]

F. Initiation and Progression to Regular Use

Close to 90 percent of adult smokers in the United States started to smoke before age 18 (Substance Abuse and Mental Health Services Administration, 2009; U.S. Department of Health and Human Services, 2012). Thus, youth and young adulthood appear to be critical developmental periods for initiation of cigarette smoking. Menthol cigarettes may have an impact on initiation rates and progression to regular use that differ from nonmenthol cigarettes. Since even a small increase in the rate of initiation of cigarette smoking may have a large impact on public health, assessing this possible impact is important. Although some assessments of initiation have included data on switching behavior (i.e., switching between menthol and nonmenthol preferences), this is not included in the current assessment due to difficulties in interpretation. This report assesses the available, though limited, data on the possible impact of menthol cigarettes on initiation of cigarette smoking and progression to regular use, and focuses primarily on smoking behavior by youth and young adults. Given that no large scale, carefully designed cohort study has been carried out to clearly delineate initiation dynamics (progression from experimentation to regular smoking), this assessment examines both age and period data estimates from many data sources.

Differences in Preference Rates

Appleyard et al. (2001) analyzed data from the 2000 National Youth Tobacco Survey (NYTS), using data from 35,828 middle and high school students from across the country for a cross- sectional survey of school-age children. They found that, among those surveyed who reported smoking in the past 30 days, 32 percent of White middle and high school students said their usual brand of cigarette was a menthol brand, as compared to higher values of Asian American (58%), Hawaiian/Pacific Islander (46%), African American (74%) and Hispanic (51%) middle and high school students who reported that they usually smoke menthol cigarettes. An overall number of youth who regularly smoke nonmenthol cigarettes was not provided. This study included a nationally representative population with a high response rate and adequate representation from most racial or ethnic groups. Participating students were from both public and private schools; however results may not generalize to students in non-traditional schools.

Hersey et al. (2006) analyzed data from over 1700 participants of the National Youth Tobacco Survey and found that, after adjusting for demographic differences, menthol use was more common among newer, younger smokers. Younger adolescents were more likely to smoke menthol cigarettes as compared to older adolescents, with both age groups increasing in menthol cigarette use from 2000 to 2002. In 2000, 52 percent of middle school smokers and 37 percent of high school smokers reported menthol cigarette use. In 2002, this percentage increased for both age groups (60% of middle school youth, 44% of high school youth). Rock et al. (2010) found similar results, and addressed the issue of misclassification of the kind of cigarettes smoked through a modification of the response options.

Lawrence et al. (2010), in a cross-sectional study of adults, analyzed data from the 2003 and 2006/2007 CPS-TUS. As with Appleyard et al. (2001), this study found that the prevalence of smoking menthol cigarettes was highest in participants 18-24 years old. Smokers in the 18-24 and 45-64 year old age groups were approximately 1.4 and 1.3 times as likely, respectively, to be menthol smokers as compared to smokers in the 65 years old or over age group. There was no significant difference between the 25-44-year age group and the 65 years age group (CI 1.07; 0.89-1.28). This suggested that smokers 65 years old or over tend to smoke menthol cigarettes at a lower rate than other age groups (Lawrence et al., 2010).

Hersey et al. (2010) analyzed data from the cross-sectional 2006 National Youth Tobacco Survey, a survey of over 27,000 students in grades 6-12. They found that youth (n=3281) who smoked in the past month were more likely to report smoking menthol cigarettes at rates inversely proportional to age. Of middle school students who reported smoking in the past month, over 50 percent reported smoking menthol cigarettes, whereas of high school students who reported smoking in the past month, 43 percent reported smoking menthol cigarettes. Differences exist in prevalence of menthol smoking depending on race and ethnicity, with African American youth reporting the highest prevalence (80.6% middle school smokers and 84.8% high school smokers), followed by both Hispanics (57.9% and 56.4% for middle and high school smokers) and Asian Americans (57.4% middle school smokers and 43.6% high school smokers). White youth smokers reported the lowest levels, but still higher than that seen in adults. Among current non-Hispanic White smokers who smoked in the past month, 43.1 percent and 37.6 percent for middle and high school smokers smoked menthol cigarettes. This study included a large nationally representative population with a high response rate (80.2%) and weighted estimates, used three menthol smoking status definitions to model the relationship between menthol cigarette use, and included a nicotine dependence measure to assess the robustness of the association.

Rock et al. (2010) analyzed data from the 2004-2008 NSDUH (n=71,605) and found that 35.7 percent of current smokers 12 years old or over smoked menthol cigarettes. Among smokers age 12-17, 71.9 percent of African American youth reported smoking menthol cigarettes, followed by 51.5 percent of Asian Americans, 47.0 percent of Hispanics, 41.0 percent of Whites, and 34.7 percent of American Indian/Alaska Natives. This pattern remained relatively consistent among 18-25 year olds, with a slight increase for African American smokers (85%). Among adult smokers 26 years old or over in the survey, the prevalence of current menthol use was only modestly lower (and still high) for African American smokers (82.2%), however rates were much lower for Hispanics (29.5%), Asian Americans (28.6%), American Indian/Alaska Natives (23%), and Whites (21.9%). From 2004 to 2008, menthol cigarette smoking among White smokers 12-17 years old increased from 40.3 percent to 46.0 percent. In addition, menthol cigarette use among individuals 18-25 years old increased for Hispanic (from 33.9% to 42.4%) and White (from 26.7% to 32.5%) smokers. Thus, not only were younger smokers more likely to be menthol smokers, but prevalence may be increasing.

Fernander et al. (2010) analyzed data from the 2003 and 2006/2007 CPS-TUS. They found that current smokers 18-24 years old were more likely to smoke menthol cigarettes. Odds ratios indicated that, relative to the 65+ year group, smokers who were 18-24 years old, 25-44 years old, and 45-65 years old were significantly more likely to be menthol smokers (66%, 20%, and 22%, respectively).

First Smoking Experience

Pletcher et al. (2006) analyzed data collected during the CARDIA study, which included data from 972 menthol and 563 nonmenthol smokers (18-30 years old). They found that there was no difference in age of first cigarette use when comparing menthol and nonmenthol smokers; both groups smoked their first cigarette at an average age of 16. This was a cohort study with a long follow up period. Although not nationally representative, there was a diverse group of participants. Participants were limited to adults 30 years old and younger, which was appropriate to assess smoking initiation.

Okuyemi et al. (2004) analyzed data from a cross-sectional survey of 480 African American smokers and asked about age of first cigarette use as part of the subjects' demographic and smoking characteristics. No significant differences were found; menthol smokers smoked their first cigarette on average at 15 years old, nonmenthol smokers at around 16 years old. Although there were more menthol smokers (n=407) than nonmenthol smokers (n=73), there was sufficient power to make statistically comparisons between these two groups.

Gandhi et al. (2009) analyzed data from 1,688 patients of a specialist smoking cessation service. No differences were found in the age at which menthol and nonmenthol smokers reported first using tobacco. For menthol smokers, "age first used tobacco" was an average of 14.87 years old; for nonmenthol smokers, "age first used tobacco" was an average of 15.21 years old. The study included comparable numbers of menthol (n=778) and nonmenthol (n=910) smokers, however generalizability may be limited because of the use of a non-nationally representative community sample and the inclusion of only those who were seeking smoking cessation treatment.

Progression to Regular Smoking

Hyland et al. (2002) analyzed data (n=13,268) from the Community Intervention Trial for Smoking Cessation (COMMIT), a telephone tobacco use survey in 1988 with re-interviews in 1993. When "age started smoking" of menthol smokers was compared with nonmenthol smokers, there were no significant differences. This study used 11 matched pairs of communities (10 in the United States and one in Canada), which decreased confounding by pairing controls with similar groups, and had a large sample size. However, there was a lack of definition of "age started smoking", so it is unknown if this refers to first experience or to onset of regular smoking. Generalizability may be limited due to the use of a community based sample that was not nationally representative.

Okuyemi et al. (2004) surveyed a cross-section of 480 inner-city African American smokers and examined the relationship between menthol smoking and smoking cessation. This survey examined sociodemographics, smoking characteristics, and smoking cessation experiences of participants and compared menthol smokers (n=407) to nonmenthol smokers (n=73). No differences were seen in age of onset of regular smoking. The inclusion of only African American smokers is both a strength and a limitation of the study. It limits generalizability but also eliminates the effect of disproportionate subgroup size (see Fagan et al., 2010 and Fernander et al., 2010). Although the sample sizes were small, there was sufficient power to make comparisons.

Okuyemi et al. (2007) conducted a randomized, double-blind, placebo-controlled clinical trial looking at African American "light" smokers (n=755). "Light" refers to a low number of cpd smoked, and does not refer to the cigarettes themselves. In this case, a light smoker is defined as one who smoked 10 or fewer cpd. No differences were found in "age started smoking regularly" between menthol and nonmenthol smokers. The study included a large number of participants, however, the majority (81.7%) was self-identified menthol smokers. Despite this uneven distribution, there appears to be sufficient statistical power to compare these groups. The inclusion of only African American smokers of 10 or fewer cpd limits the generalizability of the findings (see Fagan et al., 2010 and Fernander et al., 2010).

Fagan et al. (2010) analyzed data from the 2003 and 2006/2007 CPS-TUS to study progression to regular smoking. The study compared the age of onset of "fairly regular smoking" of menthol and nonmenthol smokers. Smokers were defined as those who had smoked at least 100 cigarettes, however no formal definition for "smoking fairly regularly" was given. Covariates included age, race or ethnicity, marital status, and socioeconomic variables, as well as total years smoked daily and smoking status 12 months ago. Since African Americans typically initiate smoking at later ages (Finkenauer et al., 2009), it was important to include race or ethnicity as a covariate. Menthol smokers started smoking regularly at a later age. When investigating the age of onset to regular smoking, menthol smokers were less likely to start before 15 years old as compared to nonmenthol smokers or smokers with no usual type. Although there were no significant differences in the 15-17 year old groups, menthol smokers were more likely to report 18 years old or more as the age of onset of regular smoking. The tabular data had uneven racial or ethnic representations with more White smokers identifying as nonmenthol smokers and more African Americans identifying as menthol smokers. The study had a large sample size with nationally representative data.

Like Fagan et al. (2010), Fernander et al. (2010) analyzed data from the 2003 and 2006/2007 CPS-TUS to study progression to regular smoking. They also assessed the age of onset of regular smoking by asking respondents, who had smoked at least 100 cigarettes, at what age they first started "smoking fairly regularly." Like the results from Fagan et al. (2010), menthol smokers started smoking regularly at a later age. The CPS-TUS data set contains an uneven distribution of racial or ethnic subpopulations in the cell sizes, with more White smokers identifying as nonmenthol smokers and more African Americans identifying as menthol smokers.

Hispanics and other minorities were more likely to smoke menthols, and African Americans tend to start smoking later, which can complicate the interpretation of what drives a later onset of progression to regular smoking in menthol smokers (see Okuyemi et al., 2004 and 2007).

Like Fagan et al. (2010) and Fernander et al. (2010), Lawrence et al. (2010) analyzed data from the 2003 and 2006/2007 CPS-TUS. A significant association exists between use of menthol cigarettes and the age of onset of regular smoking among women, but not among men.

That is, women who reported smoking menthol cigarettes were more likely to report having an earlier onset of regular smoking. Importantly, however, this was limited to smokers in the 45-64 year old age group as compared to the 65 and over age group.

Cubbin et al. (2010) analyzed cross-sectional, nationally representative data in the United States from the 2005 NHIS – CCS (n = 31,428 18 years old and over). Among current smokers (identified as having smoked at least 100 cigarettes and currently smoking some days or everyday), Cubbin et al. compared the "age of initiation" of menthol and nonmenthol smokers and found no significant differences between menthol and nonmenthol smokers on this measure.

All analyses were adjusted for age, income, and education levels, and stratified by gender and race or ethnicity. Readers likely assume that the researchers are using data from the "How old were you when you FIRST started to smoke fairly regularly?" question because there is no question that uses 'age of initiation' language. In addition, no indication of whether someone started out as a menthol or nonmenthol smoker is provided. Among both menthol and nonmenthol smokers, White smokers have been shown to initiate regular smoking one and a half to three years earlier than non-Whites (Cubbins et al., 2010).

Stahre et al. (2010) also analyzed data from the 2005 NHIS – CCS, which examined current smokers (n=6511) and former smokers (n=6774). No significant difference existed in the average age of first smoking regularly. Menthol smokers reported an average age of 19.6 and nonmenthol smokers reported an average age of 19.7.

Among a set of secondary data analyses conducted in 2010 that have not been peer-reviewed, one study included an analyis related to initiation. The Nonnemaker secondary data analysis used a measure of progression that was based on several measures, including a transition from smoking less than 100 cigarettes to smoking more than 100 cigarettes, a transition from smoking on less than 20 days per month to smoking 20 or more days per month, and a transition from nondaily smoking to daily smoking. Survey data were collected over three consecutive school years (2000-2001, 2001-2002, 2002-2003). Middle and high school students who initiated to menthol cigarettes during the first or second year of data collection were more likely to report being daily smokers at the third year of data collection. Racial or ethnic subpopulations were unevenly distributed, but the analysis accounted for baseline characteristics. Although this analysis pulled from a large sample, this study lacked appropriate controls for socioeconomic status, and the point estimates for other (non-progression) covariates were somewhat implausible due to small sample size.

Industry Documents Research

Two studies examined publicly available tobacco industry documents. Although utility of these kinds of studies may be limited due to unknown details related to the original data, they can be useful in providing some insight into tobacco industry communications, plans, and research. Kreslake et al. published two articles that reviewed such documents on the topic of initiation of smoking behavior.

The documents mainly focused on the possible palliative effect of menthol on smoking; menthol appears to moderate or alleviate negative sensory experiences that often accompany a first-smoking experience (Kreslake et al., 2008a). Indeed, Kreslake et al. (2008b) also found an internal Brown and Williamson memo stating that "Kool's menthol level may be considered too high for new smokers, and that a successful 'starter' cigarette would need to include a low tobacco taste, low impact and irritation, low tobacco aftertaste and low menthol content." Although these are single examples, they indicate tobacco industry knowledge and acceptance that menthol provides a mechanism through which new smokers are able to more successfully initiate smoking.

Conclusion

In all peer-reviewed articles, data were collected through self-report. Although this could be associated with recall bias or misclassification, self-report is the standard of this research field and not considered detrimental to the study results. The data do not support the claim that a substantial number of adult respondents intentionally under-report tobacco use (Everhart et al., 2009; Yeager & Krosnick, 2010). Furthermore, as noted by Caraballo et al. (2011), while evidence exists of some self-report bias in reporting menthol or nonmenthol cigarette use, especially among adolescents, this is not necessarily problematic since it is likely that this type of bias is fairly constant over time.

There is no indication that menthol smokers first experience cigarette smoking any earlier or later than nonmenthol smokers (Pletcher et al., 2006; Okuyemi et al., 2004; Gandhi et al., 2009). However, data regarding age of onset of regular smoking are mixed. Six studies found no difference (Hyland et al., 2002; Okuyemi et al., 2004; Okuyemi et al., 2007; Cubbin et al., 2010; Stahre et al., 2010; Lawrence et al., 2010 – males only), two found that menthol smokers began regular smoking at a later age (Fagan et al., 2010; Fernander et al., 2010), and two found that menthol smokers began regular smoking at an earlier age (Lawrence et al., 2010 – females only; Nonnemaker secondary data analysis).

Data that appear to indicate that menthol smokers start smoking later than nonmenthol smokers are difficult to interpret because differences may be driven by racial or ethnic differences. Evidence exists of significant racial or ethnic differences in early experiences with smoking and transitioning to regular smoking, with African Americans experimenting and transitioning later than White smokers (Finkenauer et al., 2009). Age of smoking initiation may also be dependent on the ethnic background in which the smokers grow up (Baron-Epel & Haviv-Messika, 2004).

Although there were no consistent differences in the onset of regular smoking, the non-peer-reviewed Nonnemaker secondary data analysis indicated that those who start smoking with menthol cigarettes were more likely to progress to regular smoking.

Prevalence data from cross sectional studies make a case for the involvement of menthol in the initiation process; all six studies found that youth/younger smokers were more likely to smoke menthol cigarettes as compared to older smokers (Appleyard et al., 2001; Hersey et al., 2006; Lawrence et al., 2010; Hersey et al., 2010; Rock et al., 2010; Fernander et al., 2010). Although cohort effects could be a factor in these differences, the consistency of findings across datasets gathered from different years suggests that this is not the case. When the logical connections between and among cohorts are considered in several articles, the suggestion of greater influence on initiation dynamics grows. Younger, newer smokers prefer menthol at levels far above that of the general population, a finding that is generally consistent across racial or ethnic groups.

The data that support the finding that those of younger age have greater menthol preference are consistent. This suggests that as smokers grow older, menthol preferences change. Additionally, while this is not a direct measure of individual initiation, it tracks very well to the ages that initiation typically occurs.

Given that the general adult smoking population smokes menthol cigarettes at rates lower than the younger age groups, the type of cigarette chosen does not appear to be purely based on availability through parents or other adults, which suggests that younger smokers may intentionally seek out menthol cigarettes. This could be for a variety of reasons, some of which have been discussed in publicly available internal tobacco industry documents, including effects directly related to menthol (e.g., soothing or cooling effects) or for social reasons and marketing. However, as stated previously, since the studies addressing differences in menthol or nonmenthol in prevalence are all fairly recent (within the past 10 years), it is possible that these differences may be due to cohort effects. Despite this caveat, from the available studies, the weight of evidence supports the conclusion that menthol in cigarettes is likely associated with increased initiation and progression to regular use of cigarette smoking.

References

Appleyard J, Messeri P, Haviland ML (2001) Smoking among Asian American and Hawaiian/Pacific Islander youth: data from the 2000 National Youth Tobacco Survey. Asian American & Pacific Islander Journal of Health 9(1):5-14. [Funded by the American Legacy Foundation]

Baron-Epel O, Haviv-Messika A. (2004) Factors associated with age of smoking initiation in adult populations from different ethnic backgrounds. European Journal of Public Health 14(3):301-5. [No funding source(s) provided. Authors affiliated with the University of Haifa and the Israel Center for Disease Control]

Caraballo, RS & Asman, K (2011). Epidemiology of menthol cigarette use in the United States. Tobacco Induced Diseases, 9 (Suppl 1): S1. [No funding source(s) provided. Authors affiliated with the Centers for Disease Control and Prevention]

Smoking Initiation: Table of Referenced Sources

Author Name(s)	Article Title	Year Pub.	Funded By	Type of Study	Subject Description (Including Special population(s))	Sample Size (N)	Authors' Results/Conclusion(s) related to Menthol* (excerpted directly from article)
Appleyard J, Messeri P, Haviland ML.	Smoking among Asian American and Hawaiian/Pacific Islander youth: data from the 2000 National Youth Tobacco Survey.	2001	American Legacy Foundation)	National Youth Tobacco Survey	Asian American and Hawaiian/ Pacific Islander youth	N=35,828.The schools response Rate was 90% and the student response rate was 93%, resulting in an overall response rate of 84%.	While many studies have documented the high prevalence of Menthol cigarette use among African Americans, NYTS 2000 data reveal that smoking mentholated cigarettes is also common among Asian American youth. Overall, 74% of African Americans and 58% of Asian Americans reported that their usual brand of cigarette is menthol brand.
Baron-Epel O, Haviv-Messika A.	Factors associated with age of smoking initiation in adult populations from different ethnic backgrounds.	2004	No funding source(s) provided. Authors affiliated with the University of Haifa and the Israel Center for Disease Control	Cross-sectional National (Israel) survey	Households with at least one resident 21+ years old	4248 Jews, 858 Arabs and 915 Immigrants (856 from the former Soviet)	Age of smoking initiation is dependent on the ethnic background in which the smokers grow up, however, the influence of the father smoking seems to be similar in all population groups. [Not menthol specific]
Caraballo, RS & Asman, K	Epidemiology of menthol cigarette use in the United States.	2011	No funding source(s) provided. Authors affiliated with the Centers for Disease Control and Prevention	Review and secondary analyses of national surveys	NSDUH: adolescents aged 12-17 years old who smoked in the past month and adult smokers (aged 18 years or older) who smoked in the past month NYTS: middle school (MS) and high school (HS) students with school year, past	NSDUH: 9,595 adolescents; 62,010 adults NYTS: 1,978 MS students and 6,163 HS students MTF:	Menthol cigarettes are disproportionately smoked by adolescents, blacks/African Americans, adult females, those living in the Northeast of the United States and those with family incomes lower than $50,000. Based on self-reports of menthol cigarette use, menthol cigarette use among smokers have increased from 2004 to 2008.

Author Name(s)	Article Title	Year Pub.	Funded By	Type of Study	Subject Description (Including Special population(s))	Sample Size (N)	Authors' Results/Conclusion(s) related to Menthol* (excerpted directly from article)
					30 day smoking, brand use, and menthol information. MTF: current smokers in 8t^{h}, 10t^{h} and 12th	20,863 8th graders; 30,722 10th graders; 40,914 12th Graders	
					Grade NHANES: 20 years and older who had Smoked and were non- Hispanic white, non- Hispanic black/African American, or Mexican American	NHANES: 1571 individuals with UPC information	
Cubbin C, Soobader M-J, LeClere FB.	The intersection of gender and race/ethnicity in smoking behaviors among menthol and non-menthol smokers in the United States.	2010	Research Network on Disparities	Cross-sectional national survey (2005 National Health Interview Survey and Cancer Control Supplement)	Black, Hispanic and white men and women, 25-64 years old	N= 7688	After adjusting for age, income and education, black (compared with Hispanic and white) and female (compared with male) smokers were more likely to choose menthol cigarettes. There was only one statistically significant difference in age of initiation, cigarettes smoked per day, quit attempts or time since quitting between menthol and non-menthol smokers: white women who smoked menthol cigarettes reported longer cessation compared with those who smoked non-menthol cigarettes.
Everhart J, Ferketich AK,	Acculturation and misclassification	2009	Summer Research Opportunities Program	Survey (1999 – 2002 National	Self-identified "Mexican American"	N=9965 (wave 1999-	A gender-specific association between misclassification and acculturation was

Author Name(s)	Article Title	Year Pub.	Funded By	Type of Study	Subject Description (Including Special population(s))	Sample Size (N)	Authors' Results/Conclusion(s) related to Menthol* (excerpted directly from article)
Browning K et al.	of tobacco use status amont Hispanic men and women in the United States.		at the Ohio State University	Health and Nutrition Examination Surveys)	or "other Hispanic" and were at least 20 years old.	2000) N=11,039 (wave 2001-2002)	found. Among males (n=1,175), the prevalence estimates of misclassification were 4.8%, 1.8%, and 2.2% for low, medium, and highly acculturated males, respectively ($p < .02$). Among females (n=1,345), the prevalence estimates of misclassification were 0.8%, 2.0%, and 4.9% for low, medium, and highly acculturated females, respectively ($p < .03$). [not menthol specific]
Fagan P, Moolchan ET et al.	Nicotine dependence and quitting behaviors among menthol and non-menthol smokers with similar consumptive patterns.	2010	The National Cancer Institute, Virginia Commonwealth University and the Massey Cancer Center	Cross-sectional survey (2003 and 2006/07 Tobacco Use Supplements to the Current Population Surveys)	Civilian non-institutionalized daily smokers aged 18 years and above.	N=11,671 (menthol smokers) N=33,644 (nonmenthol smokers) N=958 (no usual type)	...among adults, daily menthol smokers consuming six to 10 cigarettes per day were more likely than non-menthol smokers consuming six to 10 cigarettes per day to smoke their cigarette within the first 5 minutes after waking.
Fernander A, Rayens ML et al.	Are age of smoking initiation and purchasing patterns association with menthol smoking?	2010	No funding source(s) provided. Authors affiliated with the University of Kentucky	Cross-sectional survey (2003 and 2006/07 Tobacco Use Supplement to the Current Population Survey)	Civilian non-institutionalized individuals aged 18 years and above.	N= 16,294 (menthol smokers) N= 46,899 (non-menthol smokers)	The multivariate logistic model only marginally revealed that age of smoking initiation predicted menthol smoking: findings are suggestive that the longer the delay of initiation the more likely that an individual smoked menthol cigarettes [odds ratio (OR) = 1.01; 95% confidence interval (CI): 1.00–1.01]. Menthol smokers in the United States are more likely to be female, younger, from ethnic minority groups, and to have a high school education

Smoking Initiation: Table of Referenced Sources (Continued)

Author Name(s)	Article Title	Year Pub.	Funded By	Type of Study	Subject Description (Including Special population(s))	Sample Size (N)	Authors' Results/Conclusion(s) related to Menthol* (excerpted directly from article)
Finkenauer R, Pomerleau CS, Snedecor SM, Pomerleau OF.	Differences in factors relating to smoking initiation.	2009	NIH grants DA017640 and R01 DA006529	Research study	Regular daily smokers (• 5 cpd for at least 5 years) between 25 and 65 years old	N=203	Ninety percent of African American smokers consumed menthol cigarettes, as opposed to 25% of Caucasian smokers.
Gandhi KK, Foulds J, Steinberg MB, Lu SE, Williams JM.	Lower quit rates among African American and Latino menthol cigarette smokers at a tobacco treatment clinic.	2009	The New Jersey Department of Health and Senior Services, the Cancer Institute of New Jersey, the Robert Wood Johnson Foundation, National Institute on Drug Abuse, the American Legacy Foundation and the National Institute on Mental Health]	Retrospective Cohort/ Population Studies	Specialized smoking cessation outpatient clinic in New Jersey: patients who set a quit date and attempted to quit smoking, between 1 January 2001 and 30 June 2005; African American, Latinos, Whites	N=1688 (787 Menthol, 910 Nonmenthol)	This study found lower short-term (4-week followup) quit rates among AA and Latino menthol smokers as compared with non-menthol smokers within the same racial/ ethnic subgroups.
Hersey JC, Ng SW, Nonnemaker JM, Mowery P, Thomas KY, Vilsaint MC,	Are menthol cigarettes a starter product for youth?		American Legacy Foundation	2000 and 2002 NYTS, School-based, national survey	Data from the 2000 NYTS and from the 2002 NYTS.The survey used a three-stage cluster sample design that oversampled	N=5,512 youth (2000 NYTS) and 3,202 youth (2002 NYTS)	Additionally, youth who smoked menthol cigarettes had significantly higher scores on a scale of nicotine dependence compared with nonmenthol smokers, controlling for demographic background and the length, frequency, and level of smoking.
Allen JA, Haviland ML.					African American, Hispanic, and Asian students. The NYTS was administered to 35,828 students in		

Author Name(s)	Article Title	Year Pub.	Funded By	Type of Study	Subject Description (Including Special population(s))	Sample Size (N)	Authors' Results/Conclusion(s) related to Menthol* (excerpted directly from article)
					grades 6 through 12 in spring 2000 and to 26,149 students in spring 2002. The		
Hersey JC, Nonnemaker JM, Homsi G.	Menthol cigarettes contribute to the appeal and addiction potential of smoking for youth.	2010	American Legacy Foundation and RTI International	Survey (2006 National Youth Tobacco Survey)	Middle and high school students who smoked in the past 30 days who reported that they had a usual brand of cigarette and who could identify whether the usual brand was menthol or nonmenthol.	N=1458 (menthol smokers) N=1710 (nonmenthol smokers)	A logistic regression model of dependence, controlling for background (i.e., school level, gender, and race/ethnicity) and smoking level (i.e., years, frequency, and level of smoking) found that smoking menthol cigarettes was significantly associated with reduced time to needing a cigarette among smokers with a regular brand (odds ratio [OR]: 1.86, $p = .003$) and among established smokers (OR: 2.06, $p = .001$).
Hyland A, Garten S, Giovino GA, Cummings KM.	Mentholated cigarettes and smoking cessation: findings from COMMIT.	2002	The National Cancer Institute grant CA016056- 26	Telephone survey	COMMIT study: Baseline smokers who reported whether their current cigarette brand or not in 1988, and had a known smoking status in 1993.	N=13,268 (3,184 menthol, 10084 non-menthol)	No clear associations were observed between menthol cigarette use and indicators of nicotine dependence, even after controlling for race/ethnicity and other demographics..
Kreslake JM, Wayne GF, Alpert HR, Koh HK, Connolly GN.	Tobacco industry control of menthol in cigarettes and targeting of adolescents and young adults.	2008	American Legacy Foundation grant 6212 and the National Cancer Institute grant RO1 CA87477-07	Review	Tobacco industry documents from 1985-2007, describing menthol product development, results of laboratory testing of US menthol brands, market research	N=580 documents	Tobacco companies manipulate the sensory characteristics of cigarettes, including menthol content, thereby facilitating smoking initiation and nicotine dependence. Menthol brands that have used this strategy have been the most successful in attracting youth and young adult smokers and have grown in popularity.

Smoking Initiation: Table of Referenced Sources (Continued)

Author Name(s)	Article Title	Year Pub.	Funded By	Type of Study	Subject Description (Including Special population(s))	Sample Size (N)	Authors' Results/Conclusion(s) related to Menthol* (excerpted directly from article)
					reports, and the 2006 National Survey on Drug Use and Health Results.		
Kreslake JM, Wayne GF, Connolly GN.	The menthol smoker: tobacco industry research on consumer sensory perception of menthol cigarettes and its role in smoking behavior.	2008	National Cancer Institute Grant R01 CA87477-07 and American Legacy Foundation Grant 6212	Review	Internal tobacco industry documents ranging in date from 1965-2000.	N=440 documents	Two unique types of menthol smoker emerged from this analysis: those who cannot tolerate the harshness and irritation associated with smoking nonmenthol cigarettes, and those who seek out the specific menthol flavor and associated physical sensation.
Lawrence DL, Rose A et al.	National patterns and correlates of menthol cigarette use in the United States.	2010	National Cancer Institute	Cross-sectional survey (2003 and 2006/07 Tobacco Use Supplements to the Current Population Survey)	Smokers at least 18 years old.	N=63,193	Use of mentholated cigarettes was higher among women than among men. Additional significant factors associated with mentholated cigarette smoking included being unmarried (never married: OR: 1.21, 99% CI: 1.09–1.34; divorced/separated: OR: 1.13, 99% CI: 1.03–1.23), being born in a US territory (OR: 2.01, 99% CI: 1.35–3.01), living in a non- metropolitan area (OR: 0.87, 99% CI: 0.80– 0.96), being unemployed (OR: 1.24, 99% CI: 1.06–1.44) and lower levels of education.
Okuyemi KS,	African-	2004	Grants from the National	Cross sectional	African-American	N=480	Based on the consistency of the direction of

Author Name(s)	Article Title	Year Pub.	Funded By	Type of Study	Subject Description (Including Special population(s))	Sample Size (N)	Authors' Results/Conclusion(s) related to Menthol* (excerpted directly from article)
Ebersole-Robinson M, Nazir N, Ahluwalia JS.	American menthol and nonmenthol smokers: differences in smoking and cessation experiences.		Institutes of Health (K08 CA90334) and the Cancer Research Foundation of America	surbey	smokers at an inner-city health center. Menthol smokers (n = 407) were compared to nonmenthol smokers (n = 73) in these characteristics.		the three measures of cessation success, the authors suggested that Black/African American individuals who smoke menthol cigarettes may be less likely to be successful in their quit attempts.
Okuyemi KS, Faseru B, Sanderson Cox L, Bronars CA,	Relationship between menthol cigarettes and smoking cessation	2007	National Cancer Institute at the National Institutes of Health grant R01 CA091912	Randomized Controlled Trial	African American light smokers	N=755	Among African American light smokers, use of menthol cigarettes is associated with lower smoking cessation rates.
Ahluwalia JS.	among African American light smokers.						
Pletcher MJ, Hulley BJ, Houston T, Kiefe CI, Benowitz N, Sidney S.	Menthol cigarettes, Smoking cessation, atherosclerosis, and pulmonary function: the Coronary Artery Risk Development in Young Adults (CARDIA) Study.	2006	Contracts N01-HC-48047, N01-HC-48048, N01-HC- 48049, N01-HC-48050, and N01-HC-95095 from the National Heart, Lung, and Blood Institute	Multi-center U.S.cohort study (CARDIA)	African American and European American smokers aged 18 to 30 years and healthy at the time of enrollment in 1985	1544 (non-menthol smokers (n = 563) and menthol smokers (n = 972))	Menthol and nonmenthol cigarettes seem to be equally harmful per cigarette smoked in terms of atherosclerosis and pulmonary function decline, but menthol cigarettes may be harder to quit smoking.
Rock VJ, Davis SP, Thorne SL,	Menthol cigarette use among racial	2010	No funding source(s) provided. Authors	Cross-sectional survey (2004–	Current smokers age 12 and over	N=71,605	Over half of menthol cigarette smokers were female (52.2%), and approximately

Author Name(s)	Article Title	Year Pub.	Funded By	Type of Study	Subject Description (Including Special population(s))	Sample Size (N)	Authors' Results/Conclusion(s) related to Menthol* (excerpted directly from article)
	and ethnic groups in the United States, 2004-2008.		affiliated with Centers for Disease Control and Prevention and RTI International	2008 National Survey on Drug Use and Health)			29.4% of all menthol smokers were Black, which was almost 10 times the percentage of nonmenthol smokers who were Black (3.0%, $p < .01$). Prevalence of past month menthol cigarette use was highest among current smokers aged 12–17 years (44.7%) and decreased as age group increased.
Stahre et al.M, Okuyemi KS et al.	Racial/ethnic differences in menthol cigarette smoking, population quit ratios and utilization of evidence-based tobacco cessation treatments.	2010	Department of Veterans Affairs, Veterans Health Administration, Office of Research and Development and Health Services Research and Development	Cross-sectional survey (2005 National Health Interview Survey (NHIS) Cancer Control Supplement)	Current or former smokers, age 18 and over	N= 6511 (smoker) N= 6774 (former smoker)	Overall menthol smoking prevalence was significantly different by sex, region of the United States, race, marital status and average number of cigarettes smoked per day for both current and former smokers and age for former smokers only. For current and former smokers, non-menthol smokers reported a higher number Menthol smoking status was not associated with differences in utilization of quit aids.Menthol smoking status was not associated with differences in utilization of quit aids.of cigarettes smoked per day on average than menthol smokers.
U.S. Department of Health and Human Services.	Preventing Tobacco Use Among Young People: A Report of the Surgeon General.	1994	Centers for Disease Control and Prevention	Review	Not applicable	Not applicable	[Not applicable]
U.S.	Preventing	2012	U.S. Department of	Review	Not applicable	Not	[Not applicable]

Author Name(s)	Article Title	Year Pub.	Funded By	Type of Study	Subject Description (Including Special population(s))	Sample Size (N)	Authors' Results/Conclusion(s) related to Menthol* (excerpted directly from article)
Department of Health and Human Services	tobacco use among youth and young adults – A report of the Surgeon General. Rockville, MD.		Health and Human Services			applicable	
Yeager DS & Krosnick JA	The validity of self-reported nicotine product use in the 2001-2008 National Health and Nutrition Examination Survey.	2010	No funding source(s) provided. Authors affiliated with Stanford University	Study based on National Health and Nutrition Examination Survey (multiple waves)	Adult smokers age 20 and over	N=21,414	These analyses of NHANES data collected between 2001 and 2008 suggest that if any nicotine product users under-reported this behavior, the proportion of people who did so was exceedingly small. [Not menthol specific]

* Note: these statements are taken directly from articles and may not include all relevant results/conclusions. [Bracketed notes added by FDA]

Cubbin C, Soobader M-J, LeClere FB (2010) The intersection of gender and race or ethnicity in smoking behaviors among menthol and non-menthol smokers in the United States. Addiction 105(suppl. 1):32–8. [Funded by Research Network on Disparities]

Everhart J, Ferketich AK, Browning K et al. (2009) Acculturation and misclassification of tobacco use status amont Hispanic men and women in the United States. Nicotine and Tobacco Research 11(3): 240-247. [Funding provided by the Summer Research Opportunities Program at the Ohio State University].

Fagan P, Moolchan ET et al. (2010) Nicotine dependence and quitting behaviors among menthol and non-menthol smokers with similar consumptive patterns. Addiction 105(suppl. 1):55–74. [Funded by the National Cancer Institute, Virginia Commonwealth University and the Massey Cancer Center]

Fernander A, Rayens ML et al. (2010) Are age of smoking initiation and purchasing patterns association with menthol smoking? Addiction 105(suppl. 1): 39–45. [No funding source(s) provided. Authors affiliated with the University of Kentucky]

Finkenauer R, Pomerleau CS, Snedecor SM, Pomerleau OF (2009) Differences in factors relating to smoking initiation. Addictive Behaviors 34(12):1056-9. [Funded by NIH grants DA017640 and R01 DA006529]

Gandhi KK, Foulds J, Steinberg MB, et al. (2009) Lower quit rates among African American and Latino menthol smokers at a tobacco treatment clinic. International Journal of Clinical Practice 63:360–367. [Funded by the New Jersey Department of Health and Senior Services, the Cancer Institute of New Jersey, the Robert Wood Johnson Foundation, National Institute on Drug Abuse, the American Legacy Foundation and the National Institute on Mental Health]

Hersey JC, Ng SW, Nonnemaker JM, et al. (2006) Are menthol cigarettes a starter product for youth? Nicotine and Tobacco Research 8:403–13. [Funded by the American Legacy Foundation]

Hersey JC, Nonnemaker JM, Homsi G. (2010) Menthol cigarettes contribute to the appeal and addiction potential of smoking for youth. Nicotine and Tobacco Research 12(suppl 2):S136-46. [Funded by the American Legacy Foundation and RTI International]

Hyland A, Garten S, Cummings KM (2002) Menthol cigarettes and smoking cessation: findings from COMMIT (Community Intervention Trial for Smoking Cessation). Tobacco Control 11(2):135–9. [Funded by the National Cancer Institute Grant CA016056-26]

Kreslake JM, Wayne GF, et al. (2008a) Tobacco industry control of menthol in cigarettes and targeting of adolescents and young adults. American Journal of Public Health 98(9):1685–92. [Funded by National Cancer Institute Grant R01 CA87477-07 and American Legacy Foundation Grant 6212]

Kreslake JM, Wayne GF, Connolly GN (2008b) The menthol smoker: Tobacco industry research on consumer sensory perception of menthol cigarettes and its role in smoking behavior. Nicotine and Tobacco Research, 10(4):705–715. [Funded by National Cancer Institute grant R01 CA87477-07 and American Legacy Foundation Grant 6212]

Lawrence DL, Rose A et al. (2010) National patterns and correlates of menthol cigarette use in the United States. Addiction 105(suppl. 1):13–31. [Funded by the National Cancer Institute]

Okuyemi KS, Ebersole-Robinson M, Nazir N, et al. (2004) African-American menthol and non-menthol smokers: differences in smoking and cessation experiences. Journal of the

National Medical Association, 96(9):1208–11. [Funded by grants from the National Institutes of Health (K07 CA90334) and the Cancer Research Foundation of America]
Okuyemi KS, Faseru B, Cox LS, et al. (2007) Relationship between menthol cigarettes and smoking cessation among African American light smokers. Addiction 102(12):1979–86. [Funded by National Institutes of Health grant R01 CA091912]
Pletcher MJ, Hulley BJ, Houston T, et al. (2006) Menthol cigarettes, smoking cessation, atherosclerosis, and pulmonary function: the Coronary Artery Risk Development in Young Adults (CARDIA) study. Archives of Internal Medicine 166(17):1915–22. [Funded by contracts N01-HC-48047, N01-HC-48048, N01-HC-48049, N01-HC-48050, and N01-HC95095 from the National Heart, Lung, and Blood Institute]
Rock VJ, Davis SP, Thorne SL, et al. (2010) Menthol cigarette use among racial and ethnic groups in the United States, 2004-2008. Nicotine and Tobacco Research 12(suppl 2):S117-24. [No funding source(s) provided. Authors affiliated with Centers for Disease Control and Prevention and RTI International]
Stahre M, Okuyemi KS et al. (2010) Racial or ethnic differences in menthol cigarette smoking, population quit ratios and utilization of evidence-based tobacco cessation treatments. Addiction 105(suppl. 1):75–83. [Funded by Department of Veterans Affairs, Veterans Health Administration, Office of Research and Development and Health Services Research and Development]
Substance Abuse and Mental Health Services Administration. Results from the 2008 National Survey on Drug Use and Health: national findings. Rockville, MD: US Department of Health and Human Services, Substance Abuse and Mental Health Services Administration; 2009. [Funded by the US Department of Health and Human Services]
U.S. Department of Health and Human Services (2012). Preventing tobacco use among youth and young adults – A report of the Surgeon General. Rockville, MD.
Yeager DS & Krosnick JA (2010) The validity of self-reported nicotine product use in the 2001-2008 National Health and Nutrition Examination Survey. Medical Care 48(12): 1128-1132. [No funding source(s) provided. Authors affiliated with Stanford University]

G. Dependence

Nicotine dependence is the primary driver of continued tobacco use and may affect the overall adverse health impact of smoking (e.g., failure of quit attempts). Researchers have used peer-reviewed literature, data from the Altria TES, and menthol secondary data analyses to evaluate the impact of nicotine dependence. This assessment includes primary measures that have historically been used to assess nicotine dependence: time to first cigarette (TTFC), cpd, the Fagerström Test for Nicotine Dependence (FTND; a composite measure), and craving. Night waking to smoke has also emerged as a reliable indicator of strength of dependence and is therefore included in this assessment. This assessment also includes other scales of nicotine dependence and craving if there were direct menthol versus nonmenthol assessments, particularly if they were used to assess dependence in youth. Although relapse to smoking has been used as an indicator of strength of dependence, those studies are included in the assessment of the literature on cessation later in this report.

Time to First Cigarette (TTFC)

Baker et al. (2007) used data from four placebo-controlled smoking cessation trials and one international epidemiologic study to determine the relationships between cessation success and each of the following: FTND (Heatherton et al., 1991), the Heaviness of Smoking Index (Kozlowski et al., 1994), the Nicotine Dependence Syndrome Scale (Shiffman et al., 2004), and the Wisconsin Inventory of Smoking Dependence Motives (Piper et al., 2004). TTFC in the morning had the strongest predictive validity of all of the questions on the FTND and had greater validity than any other single measure. TTFC is therefore considered to be the best single measure of assessing nicotine dependence.

Fagan et al. (2010) analyzed data from the 2003 and 2006/2007 CPS-TUS to examine the relationship between menthol and nicotine dependence, including TTFC. All analyses were adjusted for age, income and education levels, and stratified by gender and race or ethnicity. This large (n= 46,273) cross-sectional survey found that moderate menthol smokers (6-10 cpd) were 22 percent more likely to have less than five minutes TTFC compared to nonmenthol smokers. For light smokers (" 5 cpd) or heavy smokers (11+ cpd), there were no differences associated with menthol in TTFC.

Collins and Moolchan (2006) analyzed data from a telephone survey of 572 adolescent smokers who participated in a treatment study. TTFC reported by menthol smokers was compared with nonmenthol smokers. Statistical analysis revealed a significant difference in TTFC in the five minutes or less groups, with the menthol groups significantly higher than nonmenthol groups (45% versus 29%), but no significant differences between the 6-30 minutes, 31-60 minutes, or 60 or more minuntes groups. The majority of smokers surveyed were menthol smokers (n=531) with no additional racial or ethnic breakdowns by menthol or nonmenthol preference. Since the participants were adolescents recruited from a single urban community and who were seeking treatment to stop smoking, generalizability may be limited to other populations of smokers. Results may not hold true across communities, to adults, or to smokers who are not seeking treatment to stop smoking.

Bover et al. (2008) analyzed data from 2,312 cessation treatment-seeking smokers. They compared TTFC after waking reported by 1,048 menthol smokers with that reported by 1,226 nonmenthol smokers and found that smokers who wake at night to smoke had a significantly shorter time before smoking their first cigarette after waking in the morning. While a direct comparison of menthol to nonmenthol smokers and TTFC was not made, a majority of menthol smokers (57.9%) as compared to nonmenthol smokers (45.4%) woke at night to smoke. This suggests that menthol smokers may also be more likely to have a shorter TTFC. Generalizability may be limited by the use of a local population of smokers seeking treatment to stop smoking.

FDA's independent analysis of Altria TES data showed significantly higher nicotine dependence scores for TTFC (p=0.0374) for menthol smokers using an ordinal response model adjusting for number of cigarettes smoked, number of years smoked, total puff volume, and SES or demographic characteristics. FDA did not include a tar delivery content (TDC) category in its statistical model. FDA did not want to include this in its model because models with TDC assume that a menthol user would necessarily switch to a nonmenthol brand in the same TDC if menthol brands were no longer available.

Hyland et al. (2002) conducted a large, community-based cohort study to evaluate the associations between menthol use and future nicotine dependence using data collected in the COMMIT study. Hyland found no differences in TTFC, however the two shortest intervals that are typically used with TTFC ("5 minutes and 6-10 minutes) were combined. From other studies, the five minutes or less time period appears to be the most sensitive to differences, thus the comparison of the results of this study to others is limited.

Okuyemi et al. (2003) analyzed data from 600 African American smokers enrolled in a clinical trial for smoking cessation. Menthol smokers (n=471) reported smoking their first cigarette within 30 minutes of waking significantly more often than nonmenthol smokers (n= 129) (81.7% compared to 69.8%). This study cannot be directly compared with other TTFC data because the TTFC bins were combined, losing all of the fastest time intervals. Data from this randomized clinical trial were self-reported and may have limited generalizability due to the inclusion of only African Americans and an individual community sample. Furthermore, as with Hyland et al. (2002), the lack of the five minutes or less time period, which appears to be the most sensitive to differences, limits the comparison to other studies.

Muscat et al. (2009) analyzed data from a community-based cross-sectional study of 525 African American and White hospital-based, older smokers. TTFC was separated into only two broad categories. Analysis of data collected from this study found no differences in either the 30 minutes or less or the more than 30 minutes groups. As with Hyland et al. (2002) and Okuyemi et al. (2003), the lack of the five minutes or less time period, which appears to be the most sensitive to differences, limits the interpretation of the results of this study.

Lawrence et al. (2010) analyzed data from the 2003 and 2006/2007 CPS-TUS and compared menthol (n=16,294) and nonmenthol smokers' (n=46,899) responses to a question asking if they had smoked a cigarette within their first 30 minutes of waking. Lawrence et al. (2010) found no significant difference in the responses between the two groups. As with Hyland et al. (2002), Okuyemi et al. (2003), and Muscat et al. (2009), the lack of the five minutes or less time period, which appears to be the most sensitive to differences, limits the comparison of the results of this study to other studies.

Through non-peer-reviewed secondary data analyses using the same dataset that was used previously (Muscat et al., 2009), Muscat categorized TTFC into four categories (<15 minutes, 15-30 minutes, 31-60 minutes and >60 minutes). After adjusting for race, sex and BMI, no significant differences existed between menthol and nonmenthol smokers for TTFC. Since the previous differences have been in the five minutes or less timeframe, caution should be exercised with interpreting these results. This analysis is somewhat limited by its small sample size, and it may be difficult to generalize from its results due to the use of a community sample.

Through secondary data analyses that have not been peer-reviewed, Hyland and Kasza analyzed data from the International Tobacco Control Four Country Survey, with data from the United States, United Kingdom, Canada and Australia. Data were collected from 7,532 individuals in the United States between 2002 and 2008. This study had a large and nationally representative sample population. After adjustment for demographic and smoking behavior variables, menthol smokers reported fewer minutes to first cigarette compared to nonmenthol smokers. Additionally, the strength of this relationship differed between racial or ethnic groups, with

Hispanic respondents (particularly men), experiencing the greatest difference in TTFC. Hispanic nonmenthol smokers had an average TTFC of nearly three hours, while Hispanic menthol smokers had an average time of slightly over one hour. The "minutes to first cigarette" (equivalent to TTFC) was, on average, an hour or more, with a median of about 20 minutes.

This average is well beyond those of the previously discussed studies. This may have been influenced by a liberal definition of a smoker as someone who smokes at least one cpd, with approximately 12 percent of included smokers smoking fewer than five cpd. The authors suggest that the inclusion of these light smokers influenced the distribution, which could also limit this study's generalizability.

Cigarettes per Day (cpd)

Historically, cpd has been used as an indicator of nicotine dependence, however changing policies such as smoke-free workplaces, smoking restrictions in and around public buildings and restaurant and bar smoking restrictions have made this an increasingly problematic and less- reliable indicator. These issues are exaggerated when evaluating youth smokers because adolescents are subject to greater social restrictions on smoking than adults (e.g., school and household rules, age restrictions for legal purchase). Nevertheless, given the historical record of use of cpd as an index of nicotine dependence, it is included in this discussion.

Okuyemi et al. (2003) analyzed data from 600 African American smokers who were enrolled in a clinical trial for smoking cessation. They compared cpd for menthol smokers (n=471) with cpd reported by nonmenthol smokers (n= 129). There was no difference in cpd; both groups smoked an average of 18 cpd. Although helpful in addressing issues of menthol use in this population, results cannot be generalized to menthol smokers from other racial or ethnic groups. Generalizability is also limited due to the use of a single community.

Okuyemi et al. (2004) analyzed data from a cross-sectional survey of 480 African American smokers at an inner-city health center. Menthol smokers (n=407) were compared to nonmenthol smokers (n=73). Both menthol and nonmenthol smokers smoked, on average, 10 cpd. Although there were more menthol smokers than nonmenthol smokers, there was sufficient power to make this comparison. The use of a single racial or ethnic group eliminates race or ethnicity as a possible confounder but limits the conclusions to only smokers who are African American and live in urban communities. Although helpful in addressing issues of menthol use in this population, results cannot be generalized to menthol smokers from other racial or ethnic groups.

Collins and Moolchan (2006) analyzed data from telephone interviews of 572 adolescent menthol and nonmenthol smokers who were recruited to participate in a treatment study. Analysis with independent t-tests revealed no significant difference, with both menthol and nonmenthol smokers smoking 11-12 cpd. The majority of smokers were menthol smokers (n=531) with no additional racial or ethnic breakdowns by menthol or nonmenthol preference. Data were not stratified by race or ethnicity. Generalizability may be limited due to the local sample and use of treatment-seekers. The limit to adolescence increased sensitivity to this group, but findings may not generalize to adults.

Pletcher et al. (2006) analyzed data from the CARDIA study, a longitudinal study of risk factors for coronary artery disease, including 972 menthol smokers and 563 nonmenthol smokers. Menthol smokers smoked significantly fewer cpd as compared to nonmenthol smokers (10 and 15 cpd, respectively). Although there were reasonable numbers of menthol and nonmenthol smokers, the majority of menthol smokers were African American while the majority of nonmenthol smokers were White. Since there was no adjustment for race or ethnicity, this difference could be due to racial/ethnic factors rather than menthol use.

Gandhi et al. (2009) evaluated the relationship between menthol cigarette smoking and short- term and long-term smoking cessation rates among 1,688 patients attending a tobacco treatment clinic. This retrospective clinical trial cohort study found that African American and Latino menthol smokers smoked fewer cpd than nonmenthol smokers, however there were no differences among White smokers.

Fagan et al. (2010) analyzed data from daily current smokers who were at least 18 years old and participated in the 2003 and 2005/2007 CPS-TUS. Covariates included age, race or ethnicity, marital status, and socioeconomic variables, as well as total years smoking daily and smoking status 12 months ago. This large (n= 46,273) cross-sectional, nationally representative survey found that menthol smokers smoked fewer cpd (mean=13.05) compared with nonmenthol smokers (mean = 15.01).

Lawrence et al. (2010) also analyzed data from the 2003 and 2005/2007 CPS-TUS. This large (n= 63,193) cross-sectional, nationally representative survey found that adult current smokers of less than 10 cpd were more likely to be menthol smokers than nonmenthol smokers (52% as compared to 42%), while smokers of 20 or more cpd were more likely to be nonmenthol smokers compared to menthol smokers (44% as compared to 34%).

Stahre et al. (2010) analyzed data from the 2005 NHIS-CCS, a nationally representative household survey. Among current smokers (n=6511), menthol smokers reported smoking significantly fewer cpd as compared to nonmenthol smokers (14.6 and 17.5, respectively). There was no adjustment for race or ethnicity, which limits the conclusions that can be drawn since the majority of menthol smokers were non-White while the majority of nonmenthol smokers were White.

As part of the secondary data analyses conducted in 2010 that were not peer-reviewed, Hyland and Kasza analyzed data from adult smokers who were interviewed in the United States as part of the International Tobacco Control Four Country Survey (ITC-4). Researchers collected data from 7,532 individuals between 2002 and 2008, including cpd data, but did not provide statistical results. Menthol smokers smoked 18.7 cpd and nonmenthol smokers smoked 16.5 cpd. A strength of this data set is that the sample size was generally larger than many of the other post- hoc analyses of similar measures and outcomes.

Scales of Nicotine Dependence (e.g., FTND)

The FTND is an aggregate of several measures of dependence including measures of cigarette craving, as well as the previously discussed time to first cigarette and number of cpd smoked. Use of the FTND score may be limited because cpd accounts for 30 percent of the total FTND score, which, as previously discussed, may not be as reliable a measure of nicotine dependence due to the influence of smoking policies and restrictions.

Okuyemi et al. (2004) analyzed data from 480 African American smokers at an inner-city health center. There was no significant difference in FTND scores. The restriction to African Americans eliminates racial or ethnic variability, however the majority of smokers were menthol smokers (n=407), leaving only a small number of nonmenthol smokers (n=73).

Collins and Moolchan (2006) analyzed data from telephone interviews with 572 White and African American adolescent smokers in a treatment study. There were no differences in the FTND scores of menthol and nonmenthol smokers. The majority of smokers were menthol smokers (n=531), with no additional racial or ethnic breakdowns by menthol or nonmenthol preference. Generalizability may be limited due to the local sample and use of treatment- seekers. The limit to adolescence increases sensitivity to this group, but findings may not generalize to adults.

Muscat et al. (2009) conducted a community-based cross-sectional study (n=525) and compared FTND scores of menthol and nonmenthol smokers. No significant differences existed in either those with a low to medium FTND score or those with a high FTND score. There was good distribution by race or ethnicity across menthol and nonmenthol groups. However, generalizability may be limited due to the community sample.

Hersey et al. (2010) analyzed data from the cross-sectional 2006 NYTS, a survey of over 27,000 students in grades 6-12 in public and private schools. After controlling for demographic background and the length, frequency, and level of smoking, Hersey concluded that young smokers who smoked menthol cigarettes had significantly higher scores on a scale of nicotine dependence compared with nonmenthol smokers. This study included a large nationally representative population with a high response rate (80.2%) and weighted estimates. Three menthol smoking status definitions were used to model the relationship between menthol cigarette use and nicotine dependence measure to test the robustness of the association. Data were not stratified by race or ethnicity.

FDA's independent analysis of the Altria TES data showed significantly higher nicotine dependence scores for FTND (p=0.0437) for menthol smokers using an ordinal response model adjusting for cpd, number of years smoked, total puff volume, and SES or demographic characteristics. In FDA's analysis, tar delivery content (TDC) category was not included in the statistical model. FDA did not want to include this in its model because models with TDC assume that a menthol user would necessarily switch to a nonmenthol brand in the same TDC if menthol brands were no longer available.

As part of the secondary data analyses conducted in 2010 that were not peer-reviewed, two analyses used scales geared toward youth. Nonnemaker analyzed a school-based study of students 12-18 years old that collected longitudinal cohort data once a year for three years. The Nonnemaker secondary data analysis used an aggregate of four measures:

1) The average score for the response to two survey questions: "How soon after you wake up do you usually smoke your first cigarette on weekdays?" and "How soon after you wake up do you usually smoke your first cigarette during the weekend?"
2) The score for responses to the survey question "If you are sick with a bad cold or sore throat, do you smoke cigarettes?"
3) The score for the response to the survey question "How true is this statement for you? When I go without a smoke for a few hours, I experience cravings?"
4) The score for response to the survey question "How true is this statement for you? I sometimes have strong cravings for cigarettes where it feels like I'm in the grip of a force that I can't control?"

Nonnemaker found that middle and high school students who initiated to menthol cigarettes reported higher dependence at the third yearly assessment compared to those who initiated to nonmenthol cigarettes (consistent with students who were more likely to be a daily smoker). Nonnemaker also found that those who switched from menthol to nonmenthol reported a higher level of dependence than those who smoked nonmenthol across the yearly assessments. In this study the majority of menthol smokers were White. Although this analysis pulled from a large sample, this study did not control for socioeconomic status, and point estimates for the other covariates in the model were somewhat implausible due to the small sample size (e.g., the odds ratio for becoming an established smoker for African

Americans was 0.23). In addition, researchers included youth who reported initiation in the final wave in an expanded analysis in order to increase sample size, even though these smokers are not followed for smoking progression or menthol use change over time.

The Hersey analysis is a second non-peer-reviewed secondary data analysis that used a dependence scale geared toward youth. Using data from a Legacy for Health-supported national survey of 5511 youth, which included responses to the Nicotine Dependence Scale for Adolescents, Hersey found that, among youth who smoked for less than one year, smoking menthol cigarettes was associated with significantly higher nicotine dependence. Data did not appear to be stratified by race or ethnicity.

Craving

Wackowski & Delnevo (2007) examined rates of menthol smoking and measures of nicotine dependence among 1,345 current established smokers in grades 9-12 who participated in the 2004 NYTS, a nationally representative survey of public and private school students. Logistic regression was used to generate an adjusted odds ratio for menthol smoking for four measures of nicotine dependence, controlling for demographic characteristics and smoking patterns. Approximately 46 percent of current established cigarette smokers in the study were menthol smokers. Menthol smokers had 2.6 and 1.6 greater odds than nonmenthol smokers for reporting that they could go for less than one hour before feeling like they needed a cigarette and that they experienced cravings after not smoking for a while, respectively. This study found that high school menthol smokers were more likely to report symptoms of dependence compared to high school nonmenthol smokers, even when controlling for race, age, and cigarette consumption. The responses to one question (how long before needing a cigarette) had a strong association with menthol use. Although not specifically TTFC, this question resembles this measure. When considering this NYTS question to be a proxy for the "time to first cigarette" question, the results of this study are consistent with previous studies that found adult menthol smokers were more likely to have their first cigarette within a shorter time period than nonmenthol smokers (Ahijevych & Parsley, 1999; Okuyemi et al., 2003; Collins and Moolchan, 2006).

Hersey et al. (2010) analyzed data from the cross-sectional 2006 NYTS, a survey of over 27,000 students in grades 6-12 in public and private schools that garnered a response rate 80.2 percent in a three stage cluster sample design that oversampled African American, Hispanic, and Asian American students.After controlling for demographic background and the length, frequency, and level of smoking, the odds of needing a cigarette within one hour after smoking was greater in menthol smokers than nonmenthol smokers in new youth smokers and in established youth smokers. The need for a cigarette within one hour after smoking was significantly associated with being a likely menthol smoker in both the youth smoker and established youth smoker groups (86% and 106% more likely, respectively). This large, nationally representative sample used two menthol smoking status definitions (including self-description as a menthol smoker and reporting of brand) to model the relationship between menthol cigarette use and nicotine dependence in order to test the robustness of the association. In addition, data were not stratified by race or ethnicity.

Night Waking to Smoke

Night waking to smoke has emerged as a reliable indicator of nicotine dependence. It is strongly associated with several measures associated with nicotine dependence, including TTFC (Bover et al., 2008) and risk for relapse to smoking (Scharf et al., 2008; Foulds et al., 2006). Bover et al. (2008) examined data from 2,312 cigarette smokers who sought treatment at a specialist tobacco dependence clinic. Waking at night to smoke was reported as a "yes" or "no," with no information about the number of wakings. Significantly more menthol smokers (58%) reported waking at night to smoke as compared to nonmenthol smokers (45%). This was a large study, but generalizability may be limited due to the treatment-seeking sample.

Gandhi et al. (2009) conducted a retrospective cohort analysis of 1,688 patients who attempted to quit smoking. Waking at night to smoke was reported as a "yes" or "no," with no information about the number of wakings. Significantly more menthol smokers (55.3%) reported waking at night to smoke as compared to nonmenthol smokers (44.9%). As above, this was a large study, but generalizability may be limited due to the treatment-seeking sample.

Conclusion

In all peer-reviewed articles, researchers collected data through self-report. Although this could be associated with recall bias or misclassification, self-report is the standard of this research field and not considered detrimental to the study results. The data do not support the claim that a substantial number of adult respondents intentionally under-report tobacco use (Everhart et al., 2009; Yeager & Krosnick, 2010). Furthermore, as noted by Caraballo et al. (2011), although evidence exists that there is some self-report bias in reporting menthol or nonmenthol cigarette use, especially among adolescents, this is not necessarily problematic since it is likely that this type of bias is fairly constant over time.

Cpd and FTND, two measures that have historically been used to assess nicotine dependence, find no consistent effect of menthol. Three studies failed to find any differences in cpd (Okutemi et al., 2003; Okuyemi et al., 2004; Collins and Moolchan, 2006), two studies found that menthol smokers smoked fewer cpd (Pletcher et al., 2006; Fagan et al., 2010), and one study found mixed results that varied by racial/ethnic group (Gandhi et al., 2009). Three studies failed to find any differences in FTND score (Okuyemi et al., 2004; Collins and Moolchan, 2006; Muscat et al., 2009) and one study found that menthol smokers scored higher than nonmenthol smokers (FDA analysis of Atria TES). However, as previously discussed, there are questions concerning the applicability of cpd and FTND measures to the current smoking situation in adults. There is even greater concern when applied to youth, as they smoke fewer cigarettes than established adult smokers and have greater social limitations on when/where they can smoke. In contrast there is consistent evidence that menthol smokers are more likely to smoke their first cigarette within 5 min of waking (Fagan et al., 2010; Collins and Moolchan et al., 2006; Bover et al., 2008; FDA analysis of Altria TES; Okuyemi et al., 2003; Hyland and Kasza secondary data analysis), indicating more severe dependence. Those studies that failed to find a difference in TTFC collapse the fastest timeframes, with either smoking within ten minutes (Hyland et al., 2992) or smoking within 30 minutes (Muscat et al., 2009; Lawrence et al., 2010; Muscat secondary data analysis) as their shortest option. As with TTFC, other measures of dependence consistently indicate that menthol smokers are more dependent as compared to nonmenthol smokers. This includes studies that use non-FTND scales of dependence (Hersey et al., 2010; Nonnemaker secondary data analysis; Hersey secondary data analysis), as well as measures of craving (Wachowski and Delnevo, 2007; Hersey et al., 2010) and waking at night to smoke (Bover et al., 2008; Gandhi et al., 2009). These studies consistently found that menthol smokers were more dependent. Based on the findings of TTFC, non-FTND scales of dependence, craving measures, and waking at night to smoke, the weight of evidence supports the conclusion that menthol in cigarettes is likely associated with increased dependence.

References

Ahijevych K, Parsley LA (1999) Smoke constituent exposure and stage of change in Black and White women cigarette smokers. Addictive Behaviors 24:115-120. [Funding provided by an American Lung Association Research Grant, and General Clinical Research Center M01 RR00034]

Baker TB, Piper ME, McCarthy DE, et al. (2007) Time to first cigarette in the morning as an index of ability to quit smoking: implications for nicotine dependence. Nicotine and Tobacco Research 4:S555-70. [Funding provided by a grant through the National Institutes of Health]

Bover MT, Foulds J, Steinberg MB, et al. (2008) Waking at night to smoke as a marker for tobacco dependence: patient characteristics and relationship to treatment outcome. International Journal of Clinical Practice 62:182-190. [Funding provided by a grant from the New Jersey Department of Health and Senior Services as part of New Jersey's Comprehensive Tobacco Control Program; the Cancer Institute of New Jersey and the Robert Wood Johnson Foundation]

Caraballo, RS & Asman, K (2011). Epidemiology of menthol cigarette use in the United States. Tobacco Induced Diseases, 9 (Suppl 1): S1. [No funding source(s) provided. Authors affiliated with the Centers for Disease Control and Prevention]

Collins CC, Moolchan ET (2006) Shorter time to first cigarette of the day in menthol adolescent cigarette smokers. Addictive Behaviors 31:1460-4. [Funded by the National Institute on Drug Abuse, Intramural Research Program]

Everhart J, Ferketich AK, Browning K et al. (2009) Acculturation and misclassification of tobacco use status amont Hispanic men and women in the United States. Nicotine and Tobacco Research 11(3): 240-247. [Funding provided by the Summer Research Opportunities Program at the Ohio State University].

Fagan P, Moolchan ET, et al. (2010) Nicotine dependence and quitting behaviors among menthol and nonmenthol smokers with similar consumptive patterns. Addiction 105(suppl. 1):55-74. [Funded by the National Cancer Institute, Virginia Commonwealth University and the Massey Cancer Center]

Foulds JF, Gandhi KK, Steinberg MB, et al. (2006) Factors associated with quitting smoking at a tobacco treatment dependence treatment clinic. American Journal of Health Behavior 30(4):400–12. [Funding provided by The New Jersey Department of Health and Senior Services, as part of New Jersey's Comprehensive Tobacco Control Program; the Cancer Institute of New Jersey, The Robert Wood Johnson Foundation, the National Institute on Drug Abuse, and the American Legacy Foundation]

Dependence: Table of Referenced Sources

Author Name(s)	Article Title	Year Pub.	Funded By	Type of Study	Subject Description (Including Special population(s))	Sample Size (N)	Authors' Results/Conclusion(s) related to Menthol* (excerpted directly from article)
Ahijevych K, Parsley LA.	Smoke constituent exposure and stage of change in black and white women cigarette smokers.	1999	American Lung Association Research Grant; General Clinical Research Center M01 RR00034	Two-factor design	Black and White Women	N=95 total women (48 black with 27 smoking menthol cigarettes, and 47 white with 22 smoking menthol cigarettes)	Black women had significantly higher beliefs about the negative aspects of smoking than did White women; menthol smokers had a shorter time to first cigarette, indicating greater nicotine dependence.
Baker TB, Piper ME, McCarthy DE, et al.	Time to first cigarette in the morning as an index of ability to quit smoking: implications for nicotine dependence.	2007	National Institutes of Health	Data derived from four clinical trials and an epidemiology study	Data derived from smokers of three large clinical trials (including two with focused, real-time process measures) conducted in Madison and Milwaukee, WI, one clinical trial conducted in New Haven, CT, and one large international epidemiologic study.	N=463 (electronic diary study) N=608 (pharmacotherapy) N=410 (quitline) N=385 (naltrexone) N=9,058 (epi)	Results showed that much of the predictive validity of the FTND could be attributed to its first item, time to first cigarette in the morning, and this item had greater validity than any other single measure. [not menthol specific]
Bover MT, Foulds J, Steinberg MB, Richardson D,	Waking at night to smoke as a marker for tobacco	2008	The New Jersey Department of Health and Senior Services as part of New Jersey's	Not Specified	This study took place at the Tobacco Dependence Program (TDP) at University of	N=2312 consecutive eligible cigarette	Night-smoking was associated with a number of other patient characteristics, including African- American race or Hispanic ethnicity, having smoking-related

Author Name(s)	Article Title	Year Pub.	Funded By	Type of Study	Subject Description (Including Special population(s))	Sample Size (N)	Authors' Results/Conclusion(s) related to Menthol* (excerpted directly from article)
Marcella SW.	dependence: patient characteristics and relationship to treatment outcome.		Comprehensive Tobacco Control Program; the Cancer Institute of New Jersey and the Robert Wood Johnson Foundation		Medicine and Dentistry of New Jersey (UMDNJ)-School of Public Health. The TDP operates a tobacco dependence clinic in New Brunswick, New Jersey, USA and provides tobacco-dependence treatment, including a combination of therapeutic support (individual and group counseling) and withdrawal symptom management (including use of Food and Drug Administration-approved smoking cessation medications).	smokers who sought treatment at a specialist tobacco-dependence clinic declared a Target Quit Date, provided baseline information at assessment, and were then followed-up 4 and 26 weeks after their target quit date.	medical symptoms, having been treated for a behavioural health problem, smoking mentholated cigarettes, smoking within 30 min of waking in the morning, increased cigarettes smoked per day, and not having private health insurance.
Caraballo, RS & Asman, K	Epidemiology of menthol cigarette use in the United States.	2011	No funding source(s) provided. Authors affiliated with the Centers for Disease Control and Prevention.	Review and secondary analyses of national surveys	NSDUH: adolescents aged 12-17 years old who smoked in the past month and adult smokers (aged 18 years or older) who smoked in the past	NSDUH: 9,595 adolescents; 62,010 adults NYTS: 1,978 MS students and 6,163 HS	Menthol cigarettes are disproportionately smoked by adolescents, blacks/African Americans, adult females, those living in the Northeast of the United States and those with family incomes lower than $50,000. Based on self-reports of menthol cigarette use, menthol cigarette use among smokers

Dependence: Table of Referenced Sources (Continued)

Author Name(s)	Article Title	Year Pub.	Funded By	Type of Study	Subject Description (Including Special population(s))	Sample Size (N)	Authors' Results/Conclusion(s) related to Menthol* (excerpted directly from article)
					month NYTS: middle school (MS) and high school (HS) students with school year, past 30 day smoking, brand use, and menthol information. MTF: current smokers in 8th, 10th and 12th grade NHANES: 20 years and older who had Smoked and were non- Hispanic white, non- Hispanic black/African American, or Mexican American	students MTF: 20,863 8th graders; 30,722 10th graders; 40,914 12th Graders NHANES: 1571 individuals with UPC information	have increased from 2004 to 2008.
Collins CC, Moolchan ET.	Shorter time to first cigarette of the day in menthol adolescent cigarette smokers.	2006	National Institute on Drug Abuse, Intramural Research Program	Survey	Adolescent smokers recruited for a cessation treatment study, telephone survey	N=572	Adolescent menthol cigarette smokers had shorter TTF cigarette of the day when compared to non-menthol adolescent cigarette smokers, despite a lack of group differences in FTND scores or smoking rates (CPD).
Everhart J, Ferketich AK, Browning K et al.	Acculturation and misclassification of tobacco use status amont Hispanic men and	2009	Summer Research Opportunities Program at the Ohio State University	Cross-sectional survey (1999 – 2002 National Health and Nutrition	Self-identified "Mexican American" or "other Hispanic" and were at least 20 years old.	N=9965 (wave 1999-2000) N=11,039 (wave 2001-	A gender-specific association between misclassification and acculturation was found. Among males (n=1,175), the prevalence estimates of misclassification were 4.8%, 1.8%, and 2.2% for low,

Author Name(s)	Article Title	Year Pub.	Funded By	Type of Study	Subject Description (Including Special population(s))	Sample Size (N)	Authors' Results/Conclusion(s) related to Menthol* (excerpted directly from article)
	women in the United States.			Examination Surveys)		2002)	medium, and highly acculturated males, respectively (p< .02). Among females (n=1,345), the prevalence estimates of misclassification were 0.8%, 2.0%, and 4.9% for low, medium, and highly acculturated females, respectively (p< .03). [not menthol specific]
Fagan P, Moolchan ET et al.	Nicotine dependence and quitting behaviors among menthol and non-menthol smokers with similar consumptive patterns.	2010	The National Cancer Institute, Virginia Commonwealth University and the Massey Cancer Center	Cross-sectional survey (2003 and 2006/07 Tobacco Use Supplements to the Current Population Surveys)	Civilian non-institutionalized daily smokers aged 18 years and above.	N=11,671 (menthol smokers) N=33,644 (nonmenthol smokers) N=958 (no usual type)	...among adults, daily menthol smokers consuming six to 10 cigarettes per day were more likely than non-menthol smokers consuming six to 10 cigarettes per day to smoke their cigarette within the first 5 minutes after waking.
Foulds J, Gandhi KK, Steinberg MB, Richardson DL, Williams JM, Burke MV, Rhoads GG.	Factors associated with quitting smoking at a tobacco treatment dependence treatment clinic.	2006	The New Jersey Department of Health and Senior Services, as part of New Jersey's Comprehensive Tobacco Control Program; the Cancer Institute of New Jersey, The Robert Wood Johnson Foundation, the	Cohort	first 1021 patients who attempted to quit tobacco at a specialist tobacco dependence treatment outpatient clinic based at the Tobacco Dependence Program at the University of	N=1021	Forty-one percent of the patienta smoked menthol cigarettes. They were less likely to achieve abstinence in univariate analyses, and this item remained in the model predicting 4- week outcome.
			National Institute on Drug Abuse, and the American Legacy Foundation		Medicine and Dentistry of New Jersey-School of Public Health		

Dependence: Table of Referenced Sources (Continued)

Author Name(s)	Article Title	Year Pub.	Funded By	Type of Study	Subject Description (Including Special population(s))	Sample Size (N)	Authors' Results/Conclusion(s) related to Menthol* (excerpted directly from article)
Gandhi KK, Foulds J, Steinberg MB, Lu SE, Williams JM.	Lower quit rates among African American and Latino menthol cigarette smokers at a tobacco treatment clinic.	2009	New Jersey Department of Health and Senior Services, the Cancer Institute of New Jersey, the Robert Wood Johnson Foundation, National Institute on Drug Abuse, the American Legacy Foundation and the National Institute on Mental Health	Retrospective Cohort/ Population Studies	Specialized smoking cessation outpatient clinic in New Jersey: patients who set a quit date and attempted to quit smoking, between 1 January 2001 and 30 June 2005; African American, Latinos, Whites	N=1688 (787 Menthol, 910 Nonmenthol)	This study found lower short-term (4-week followup) quit rates among AA and Latino menthol smokers as compared with non-menthol smokers within the same racial/ ethnic subgroups.
Heatherton TF, Kozlowski LT, Frecker RC, Fagerström KO.	The Fagerström Test for Nicotine Dependence: a revision of the Fagerström Tolerance Questionnaire.	1991	No funding source(s) provided. Authors affiliated with Harvard University, Pennsylvania State University, Addiction Research Foundation, Ontario, and Pharmacia Leo Therapeutics AB, Sweden	Study	Smokers visiting the Ontario Science Centre	N=254	We found that the nicotine rating item and the inhalation item were unrelated to any of our biochemical measures and these two items were primary contributors to psychometric deficiencies in the PTQ. We also found that a revised scoring of time to the first cigarette of the day (TTP) and number of cigarettes smoked per day (CPD) improved the scale. [not menthol specific]
Hersey JC, Nonnemaker JM, Homsi G.	Menthol cigarettes contribute to the appeal and addiction potential of smoking for	2010	American Legacy Foundation and RTI International	Survey (2006 National Youth Tobacco Survey)	Middle and high school students who smoked in the past 30 days who reported that they had a usual brand of cigarette and who could identify	N=1458 (menthol smokers) N=1710 (nonmenthol smokers)	A logistic regression model of dependence, controlling for background (i.e., school level, gender, and race/ethnicity) and smoking level (i.e., years, frequency, and level of smoking) found that smoking menthol cigarettes was significantly associated with reduced time to needing a

Author Name(s)	Article Title	Year Pub.	Funded By	Type of Study	Subject Description (Including Special population(s))	Sample Size (N)	Authors' Results/Conclusion(s) related to Menthol* (excerpted directly from article)
	youth.				whether the usual brand was menthol or nonmenthol.		cigarette among smokers with a regular brand (odds ratio [OR]: 1.86, p = .003) and among established smokers (OR: 2.06, p = .001).
Hyland A,	Mentholated	2002	The National Cancer	Telephone	COMMIT study:	N=13,268	No clear associations were observed between
Garten S, Giovino GA, Cummings KM.	cigarettes and smoking cessation: findings from COMMIT.		Institute grant CA016056- 26	survey	Baseline smokers who reported whether their current cigarette brand or not in 1988, and had a known smoking status in 1993.	(3,184 menthol, 10084 non-menthol)	menthol cigarette use and indicators of nicotine dependence, even after controlling for race/ethnicity and other demographics..
Kozlowski LT, Porter CQ, Orleans CT, Pope MA, Heatherton T.	Predicting smoking cessation with self-reported measures of nicotine dependence: FTQ, FTND, and HSI.	1994	No funding source(s) provided. Authors affiliated with Pennsylvania State University	Experiment (two independent studies)	Smokers seeking treatment at the Ontario Lung Association	N=932 (study 1) N=1877 (study 2)	All tests made statistically reliable predictions of smoking cessation. ...samples of high scoring smokers will not be well differentiated from the mid-range to the high-end of the scores. [not menthol specific]
Lawrence DL, Rose A et al.	National patterns and correlates of menthol cigarette use in the United States.	2010	National Cancer Institute	Cross-sectional survey (2003 and 2006/07 Tobacco Use Supplements to the Current Population Survey)	Smokers at least 18 years old.	N=63,193	Use of mentholated cigarettes was higher among women than among men. Additional significant factors associated with mentholated cigarette smoking included being unmarried (never married: OR: 1.21, 99% CI: 1.09–1.34; divorced/separated: OR: 1.13, 99% CI: 1.03–1.23), being born in a US territory (OR: 2.01, 99% CI: 1.35–3.01), living in a non- metropolitan area (OR: 0.87, 99% CI:

Dependence: Table of Referenced Sources (Continued)

Author Name(s)	Article Title	Year Pub.	Funded By	Type of Study	Subject Description (Including Special population(s))	Sample Size (N)	Authors' Results/Conclusion(s) related to Menthol* (excerpted directly from article)
							0.80– 0.96), being unemployed (OR: 1.24, 99% CI: 1.06–1.44) and lower levels of education.
Muscat JE, Chen G, Knipe A, Stellman SD, Lazarus P, Richie JP Jr.	Effects of menthol on tobacco smoke exposure, nicotine dependence, and NNAL glucuronidation.	2009	No funding source(s) provided. Authors associated with Pennsylvania State College of Medicine	Community-based cross-sectional	Black and White adult smokers	N=525	Data indicate that menthol is not associated with a higher exposure to tobacco smoke carcinogens, but the findings on nicotine dependence are inconclusive. Menthol may not be more hazardous than other cigarette formulations for most smokers, although it cannot be ruled out at this time that some menthol smokers are possibly at increased risk for lung cancer because of selective inhibition of UDP-glucuronosyl transferase enzymes.
Okuyemi KS, Ahluwalia JS, Ebersole-Robinson M, Catley D, Mayo MS, Resnicow K.	Does menthol attenuate the effect of bupropion among African American smokers?	2003	National Cancer Institute grants (R01 CA77856, K07 CA90334, R24 CA95835-01)	Randomized Controlled Trial	African American smokers enrolled in a clinical trial that assessed the efficacy of sustained-release bupropion for smoking cessation. Menthol (n = 471) and non-menthol (n = 129) smokers were compared on smoking- related characteristics and abstinence rates at 6 weeks and 6 months.	N=600	African American menthol smokers had lower smoking cessation rates after 6 weeks of treatment with bupropion-SR than African- American non menthol smokers, thereby putting menthol smokers at greater risk from the health effects of smoking. Lower overall cessation rates among African Americans menthol smokers may partially explain ethnic differences in smoking-related disease risks.

Author Name(s)	Article Title	Year Pub.	Funded By	Type of Study	Subject Description (Including Special population(s))	Sample Size (N)	Authors' Results/Conclusion(s) related to Menthol* (excerpted directly from article)
Okuyemi KS, Ebersole-Robinson M, Nazir N, Ahluwalia JS.	African-American menthol and nonmenthol smokers: differences in smoking and cessation experiences.	2004	The National Institutes of Health (K07 CA90334) and the Cancer Research Foundation of America	Cross sectional survey	African-American smokers at an inner-city health center. Menthol smokers (n = 407) were compared to nonmenthol smokers (n = 73) in these characteristics.	N=480	Based on the consistency of the direction of the three measures of cessation success, the authors suggested that Black/African American individuals who smoke menthol cigarettes may be less likely to be successful in their quit attempts.
Piper ME, Piasecki TM, Federman EB, Bolt DM, Smith SS, Fiore MC, Baker TB.	A multiple motives approach to tobacco dependence: the Wisconsin Inventory of Smoking Dependence Motives (WISDM- 68).	2004	National Institutes of Health and a grant from the University of Missouri Research Board	Survey	Adults (18+) from Madison and Milwaukee, WI	N=775	Data collected from a large sample of smokers (N ™775) indicated that all 13 subscales of the Wisconsin Inventory of Smoking Dependence Motives (WISDM-68) have acceptable internal consistency, are differentially present across levels of smoking heaviness, and have a multidimensional structure. [not menthol specific]
Pletcher MJ, Hulley BJ, Houston T,	Menthol cigarettes, smoking	2006	Contracts N01-HC-48047, N01-HC-48048, N01-HC- 48049, N01-HC-48050,	Multi-center U.S. cohort study	African American and European American smokers aged 18 to 30	1544 (non-menthol smokers (n =	Menthol and nonmenthol cigarettes seem to be equally harmful per cigarette smoked in terms of atherosclerosis and pulmonary function decline,
Kiefe CI, Benowitz N, Sidney S.	cessation, atherosclerosis, and pulmonary function: the Coronary Artery Risk Development in Young Adults		and N01-HC-95095 from the National Heart, Lung, and Blood Institute	(CARDIA)	years and healthy at the time of enrollment in 1985	563) and menthol smokers (n = 972))	but menthol cigarettes may be harder to quit smoking.

Dependence: Table of Referenced Sources (Continued)

Author Name(s)	Article Title	Year Pub.	Funded By	Type of Study	Subject Description (Including Special population(s))	Sample Size (N)	Authors' Results/Conclusion(s) related to Menthol* (excerpted directly from article)
	(CARDIA) Study.						
Scharf DM, Dunbar MS, Shiffman S.	Smoking during the night: prevalence and smoker characteristics.	2008	Social Sciences and Humanities Research Council of Canada and National Institute on Drug Abuse	Treatment study	Heavy smokers enrolled in one of three smoking cessation studies	N=691	Night smoking is common, is associated with nicotine dependence, and it represents additional risk for cessation failure. [not menthol specific]
Shiffman S, Waters A, Hickcox M.	The nicotine dependence syndrome scale: a multidimensional measure of nicotine dependence.	2004	National Institutes on Health, GlaxoSmithKline and GlaxoSmithKline Consumer Healthcare	Factor analysis of three independent studies	Smokers participating in a smoking cessation study	N=317 (study 1) N=802 (study 2) N=93 (study 3)	...the NDSS presents a valid multidimensional assessment of nicotine dependence that may expand on current measure. [not menthol specific]
Stahre M, Okuyemi KS et al.	Racial/ethnic differences in menthol cigarette smoking, population quit ratios and utilization of evidence-based tobacco cessation treatments.	2010	Department of Veterans Affairs, Veterans Health Administration, Office of Research and Development and Health Services Research and Development	Cross-sectional survey (2005 National Health Interview Survey (NHIS) Cancer Control Supplement)	Current or former smokers, age 18 and over	N= 6511 (smoker) N= 6774 (former smoker)	Overall menthol smoking prevalence was significantly different by sex, region of the United States, race, marital status and average number of cigarettes smoked per day for both current and former smokers and age for former smokers only. For current and former smokers, non-menthol smokers reported a higher number of cigarettes smoked per day on average than menthol smokers. Menthol smoking status was not associated with differences in utilization of quit aids.

Author Name(s)	Article Title	Year Pub.	Funded By	Type of Study	Subject Description (Including Special population(s))	Sample Size (N)	Authors' Results/Conclusion(s) related to Menthol* (excerpted directly from article)
Yeager DS & Krosnick JA	The validity of self-reported nicotine product use in the 2001-2008 National Health and Nutrition Examination Survey.	2010	No funding source(s) provided. Authors affiliated with Stanford University	Study based on National Health and Nutrition Examination Survey (multiple waves)	Adult smokers age 20 and over	N=21,414	These analyses of NHANES data collected between 2001 and 2008 suggest that if any nicotine product users under-reported this behavior, the proportion of people who did so was exceedingly small. [not menthol specific]

* Note: these statements are taken directly from articles and may not include all relevant results/conclusions. [Bracketed notes added by FDA]

Gandhi KK, Foulds J, Steinberg MB, et al. (2009) Lower quit rates among African American and Latino menthol smokers at a tobacco treatment clinic. International Journal of Clinical Practice 63:360–7. [Funded by New Jersey Department of Health and Senior Services, the Cancer Institute of New Jersey, the Robert Wood Johnson Foundation, National Institute on Drug Abuse, the American Legacy Foundation and the National Institute on Mental Health]

Heatherton TF, Kozlowski LT, Frecker RC, Fagerström KO. (1991) The Fagerström Test for Nicotine Dependence: a revision of the Fagerström Tolerance Questionnaire. British Journal of Addiction 86(9):1119-27. [No funding source(s) provided. Authors affiliated with Harvard University, Pennsylvania State University, Addiction Research Foundation, Ontario, and Pharmacia Leo Therapeutics AB, Sweden]

Hersey JC, Nonnemaker JM, Homsi G (2010) Menthol cigarettes contribute to the appeal and addiction potential of smoking for youth. Nicotine and Tobacco Research 12(suppl 2):S136-46. [Funded by the American Legacy Foundation and RTI International]

Hyland A, Garten S, Cummings KM (2002) Mentholated cigarettes and smoking cessation: findings from COMMIT (Community Intervention Trial for Smoking Cessation). Tobacco Control 11(2):135–9. [Funded by the National Cancer Institute]

Kozlowski LT, Porter CQ, Orleans CT, Pope MA, Heatherton T. (1994) Predicting smoking cessation with self-reported measures of nicotine dependence: FTQ, FTND, and HSI. Drug Alcohol Dependence 34(3):211-6. [No funding source(s) provided. Authors affiliated with Penn State University]

Lawrence DL, Rose A et al. (2010) National patterns and correlates of mentholated cigarette use in the United States. Addiction 105(suppl 1):13–31. [Funded by the National Cancer Institute]

Muscat JE, Chen G, Knipe A, et al. (2009) Effects of menthol on tobacco smoke exposure, nicotine dependence, and NNAL glucuronidation. Cancer Epidemiology, Biomarkers, and Prevention 18:35–41. [No funding source(s) provided. Authors associated with Pennsylvania State College of Medicine]

Okuyemi KS, Ahluwalia JS, Ebersole-Robinson M, et al. (2003) Does menthol attenuate the effect of bupropion among African American smokers? Addiction 98(10):1387–1393. [Funded by the National Cancer Institute grants (R01 CA77856, K07 CA90334, R24 CA95835-01)]

Okuyemi KS, Ebersole-Robinson M, Nazir N, et al. (2004) African-American menthol and nonmenthol smokers: differences in smoking and cessation experiences. Journal of the National Medical Association 96(9):1208–11. [Funded by the National Institutes of Health (K07 CA90334) and the Cancer Research Foundation of America]

Piper ME, Piasecki TM, Federman EB, Bolt DM, Smith SS, Fiore MC, Baker TB (2004). A multiple motives approach to tobacco dependence: the Wisconsin Inventory of Smoking Dependence Motives (WISDM-68). Journal of Consulting and Clinical Psychology 72(2):139-54. [Funded by National Institutes of Health and a grant from the University of Missouri Research Board]

Pletcher MJ, Hulley BJ, Houston T, et al. (2006) Menthol cigarettes, smoking cessation, atherosclerosis, and pulmonary function: the Coronary Artery Risk Development in Young Adults (CARDIA) study. Archives of Internal Medicine 166(17):1915–22. [Funded by contracts N01-HC-48047, N01-HC-48048, N01-HC-48049, N01-HC-48050, and N01-HC-95095 from the National Heart, Lung, and Blood Institute]

Scharf DM, Dunbar MS, Shiffman S (2008) Smoking during the night: prevalence and smoker characteristics. Nicotine & Tobacco Research 10(1):167-78. [Funded by Social Sciences and Humanities Research Council of Canada and National Institute on Drug Abuse]

Shiffman S, Waters A, Hickcox M (2004) The nicotine dependence syndrome scale: a multidimensional measure of nicotine dependence. Nicotine & Tobacco Research 6(2):327-48. [Funded by the National Institutes on Health, GlaxoSmithKline and GlaxoSmithKline Consumer Healthcare]

Stahre M, Okuyemi KS, et al. (2010) Racial or ethnic differences in menthol cigarette smoking, population quit ratios and utilization of evidence-based tobacco cessation treatments. Addiction 105(suppl 1):75–83. [Funded by Department of Veterans Affairs, Veterans Health Administration, Office of Research and Development and Health Services Research and Development]

Yeager DS & Krosnick JA (2010) The validity of self-reported nicotine product use in the 2001-2008 National Health and Nutrition Examination Survey. Medical Care 48(12): 1128-1132. [No funding source(s) provided. Authors affiliated with Stanford University]

H. Cessation

Quitting smoking, even at later ages, can result in a significant reduction in disease risk and years of life lost (Doll et al., 2004). Therefore, any impact of menthol in cigarettes on smoking cessation has the potential to have a substantial impact on public health. This section evaluated the science comparing cessation success in menthol smokers and nonmenthol smokers. Articles that assessed differences in intention to quit, feelings regarding the likelihood of being able to quit, or the number of quit attempts without reference to cessation success are not a direct assessment of cessation and are not included. Additionally, studies of only former smokers or only current smokers are not included, as there is no relative measure of cessation success.

Cohort Studies

Hyland et al. (2002) conducted a large community-based cohort study to evaluate the association between menthol use and smoking cessation using data collected in the COMMIT study. The COMMIT study was a randomized community-based intervention trial identified by telephone survey for smoking cessation in 11 matched pairs of communities. The study population included 13,268 current smokers (25-64 years old) at baseline (1988). Researchers collected self- reported menthol cigarette use by brand type at baseline. The cessation outcome was defined as no smoking in the last six months. The study indicated that 24 percent of the overall population smoked menthol cigarettes (23% Whites and 57% African Americans). Baseline menthol cigarette use was not associated with quitting in 1993 (RR (95% CI): 1 (0.90-1.11)) in overall and race or ethnicity subgroups. This longitudinal study had a large community-based cohort sample with a strong definition of smoking cessation (six months abstinence at five years). The analysis was adjusted for demographics, nicotine dependence (e.g., TTFC), and smoking/quitting history. Since dependence may be an intermediate variable affecting cessation success, it is possible that the analyses were over-adjusted, which may result in a dilution of an association. In addition, there was a high loss to follow-up rate over five years (34% from baseline 1988 to 1993).

Pletcher et al. (2006) evaluated the associations between menthol cigarette use and smoking cessation behavior, coronary calcification, and changes in pulmonary function test among 1,544 current smokers who were participants in CARDIA. CARDIA is a population-based cohort study of risk factors for coronary artery diseases among healthy 18-30 years old African Americans and Whites. Smoking cessation behavior (including current smoking status, recent quit attempts, and cessation if recent quit attempt), sustained smoking cessation, and documented relapse were collected. Sustained smoking cessation was defined as no current smoking in the past two times examined. After adjusting for demographic and social factors, menthol smokers had statistically significant increased risk of relapse (OR (95% CI): 1.89 (1.17-3.05), p=0.009) as compared to nonmenthol smokers. Researchers identified a trend toward lower cessation in menthol smokers, however this did not reach statistical significance (OR (95% CI): 0.71 (0.49-1.02), p=0.06). The statistical analyses were robust, with repeated measures for outcomes such as quit attempts and cessation after quit attempts and longitudinal assessment for sustained smoking cessation. This large study had long-term follow up, and menthol status was collected at multiple time points. The sample population was diverse, though not nationally representative. Generalizability may be limited since the study included only young African American and White adults 18-30 years old at entry (mean age: 25 years). Statistical power was limited in subgroup analysis (e.g., White menthol smokers, African American nonmenthol smokers).

Blot et al. (2011) conducted a nested case-control study among 440 incident lung cancer cases and 2,213 controls enrolled in the Southern Community Cohort Study between 2002 and 2009. Researchers prospectively determined quitting smoking through computation of quit rates from the follow-up interviews for patients who were current smokers at entry into the cohort. Thus, a quitter was defined as a former smoker, but there was no measure of duration of quitting. After adjusting for demographic variables, there was no difference in the prevalence of having quit smoking between menthol and nonmenthol smoking African Americans (OR (95% CI): 1.03 (0.96-1.11)). However, among Whites, menthol smokers were more likely to have quit as compared to their nonmenthol-smoking counterparts (OR(95% CI): 1.55 (1.41-1.70)). Although there was a reasonable follow up period of over four years, full follow up was lacking for about 40 percent of the subjects. Cessation was biochemically verified via assessment of serum cotinine levels. Although multiple sites were used, generalizability may be limited since the sample was not nationally representative.

Okuyemi et al. (2003) evaluated the association between menthol cigarette smoking and cessation using data collected for a randomized clinical trial that assessed the efficacy of the medication bupropion-SR (treated for seven weeks) for smoking cessation. The study consisted of 600 African American smokers enrolled in an inner-city health center (• 18 years, •10 cpd) (471 menthol and 129 nonmenthol smokers). Compared to nonmenthol smokers, menthol smokers were less likely to be abstinent at six weeks (41.5% and 28.3%, respectively, p=0.006). However, the seven-day point prevalence abstinence rates at six weeks was not different between menthol and nonmenthol smokers who received placebo (20.5% for menthol vs. 23.3% for nonmenthol, p=0.63). Among the treatment group, menthol smokers had significantly lower abstinence rates than nonmenthol smokers at six weeks (36.2% vs. 60.3%, p<0.01). Thus it appears that the menthol smokers did not get the same benefit from the medication as the nonmenthol smokers did. The association between smoking cessation and menthol also differed by age. Among smokers 49 years old or younger, 24.9 percent of the menthol smokers were abstinent compared to 44.4 percent for nonmenthol smokers ($p<0.01$) but no difference was seen in smokers 50 years old or over. Nonmenthol smokers were twice as likely to quit smoking as menthol smokers (OR (95% CI): 2 (1.03-3.95)) among smokers who were 49 years old or younger at six weeks, but not in smokers who were 50 years old or over after controlling for treatment. The age-specific logistic regression results did not explicitly mention which factors were controlled. In the methods section, the author mentioned treatment was controlled in logistic regressions but it is not clear whether other factors such as sex, cpd, and duration of smoking were retained and adjusted in the stepwise regression. Generalizability may be limited since the sample consisted of those seeking treatment and was not nationally representative. The self-reported seven-day point prevalence cessation rates were biochemically confirmed.

Using the same dataset as Okuyemi et al. (2003), Harris et al. (2004) analyzed the predictors of seven-day cessation in a clinical trial cohort among 600 African Americans who randomly received the cessation medication bupropion SR or placebo for seven weeks and were followed for 27 weeks. Self-reported menthol use was one of the 21 baseline variables examined for the prediction of smoking cessation. The study outcome was biochemically-confirmed self-reported seven-day point prevalence abstinence at week seven, the end of the treatment phase. The study indicated that menthol smokers were less likely to quit smoking after 7 weeks of treatment compared to nonmenthol smokers (28.3% vs. 41.5%, $p=0.0062$) using a Chi square test (unadjusted); the effect was not present when researchers adjusted the analysis for demographic factors and factors related to dependence. Since dependence may be an intermediate variable affecting cessation success, it is possible that the analyses were over-adjusted, which resulted in a dilution of the association.Researchers used biochemical verification of self-reported cessation outcomes. Generalizability may be limited since the sample consisted of those seeking treatment and was not nationally representative.

Gandhi et al. (2009) evaluated the relationship between menthol cigarette smoking and short- term (4 weeks) and long-term (6 months) smoking cessation among 1,688 patients attending a tobacco treatment clinic in New Jersey. The outcome was a biochemically-verified seven-day point prevalence abstinence rate. The study demonstrated that African American and Latino menthol smokers had significantly lower odds of quitting (OR (95% CI): 0.32 (0.16-0.62) for African Americans; 0.43 (0.1-0.9) for Latinos) as compared to their nonmenthol counterparts at four weeks of follow-up. Researchers observed a similar trend at the six-month follow-up. No significant differences existed in the cessation rates of White menthol and nonmenthol smokers. Researchers adjusted analyses for demographic and dependence variables (e.g., TTFC, waking at night to smoke). Since dependence may be an intermediate variable affecting cessation success, it is possible that the analyses were over-adjusted, which may result in a dilution of association(s). Although this was a large study, there was a high loss to follow up at six months (approximately 42%). Since all those who were lost were included as cessation failures (i.e., still smoking), overall quit rates may be underestimated. Although seven-day point prevalence was biochemically verified, these data were incomplete or not clearly described for all subjects; half of the sample was followed up in person (carbon monoxide verification) but half were followed up via phone contact (no carbon monoxide verification). Generalizability may be limited since the sample consisted of those seeking treatment and was not nationally representative.

Foulds et al. (2006) evaluated factors associated with successful quitting using a sample of 1,021 patients at a free tobacco treatment clinic. Researchers evaluated abstinence at four-week and six-month follow-ups, and biochemically verified self-reported cessation. At the four-week follow up, data showed a trend toward menthol smokers having worse cessation outcomes, however this failed to reach significance (p=0.053). No differences existed at the six-month follow up. Analyses were adjusted for treatment, but other adjustments were unclear, and they may have been overadjusted (e.g., adjusted for dependence variables). This large, longitudinal study had a sample that mimics the U.S. population, however generalizability may be limited since the sample consisted of people seeking smoking cessation treatment.

Murray et al. (2007) investigated the health effect of menthol cigarette smoking among 5887 smokers 35-60 years old with mild to moderate airway obstruction who were selected to participate in a smoking cessation program and were followed for 11 years using the data from the Lung Health Study. In addition to disease-specific mortality, the outcomes included smoking cessation assessments that included the percentages of sustained quitters, of intermittent smokers and of continued smokers. Researchers assessed self-reported menthol cigarette use at baseline and annual follow-up visits for five years. The study indicated no significant difference existed between menthol use and the percentage of quitters during five years of follow-up, after controlling for age, sex, baseline cpd, FEV1% predicted, randomization group assignment, race, and years of education. Although this large clinical trial cohort study had a long follow up period (14 years), the researchers maintained an excellent follow-up rate (94% at five years and 83% 11 years after enrollment). Menthol preference was assessed annually for five years. The smoking cessation definition was fairly strict: sustained quitters were defined as those who were biochemically-confirmed quitters at five annual visits and who recalled no month in which they smoked more than one cpd at any annual visit. Although this was a national survey, the generalizability may be limited due to an under representation of African Americans and due to the inclusion solely of smokers with mild or moderate airway obstruction who received smoking cessation treatment.

Cropsey et al. (2009) analyzed the relationship between race, menthol cigarette use, and smoking cessation rates using data from a smoking cessation intervention trial among 233 female prisoner smokers (• 18 years old) . This 12-month clinical trial cohort assessed cigarette type (menthol or nonmenthol) after the subjects entered the intervention. Researchers verified outcomes using seven-day point prevalence abstinence at multiple time points. Menthol cigarette use was not associated with differences in smoking cessation rates. This is a small study of women only, with a very small number of White menthol smokers (approximately 6%). Cessation was biochemically verified. Menthol use was only assessed while in prison, however use patterns may have changed (e.g., differences in brand availability). Despite being a controlled sample, there was a high loss to follow-up. Any generalizability potential is limited.

Cross-Sectional Studies

Fu et al. (2008) conducted a cross-sectional survey to evaluate the association between menthol cigarette use and smoking cessation among 1,343 older smokers involved in an aided quit attempt. They used data from a multi-center randomized clinical smoking cessation trial that evaluated the effectiveness of phone call intervention versus usual care. Self-reported menthol use was assessed at the six-month survey post randomization to treatment group. The outcome was self-reported seven-day point prevalence smoking abstinence. The study indicated that smoking menthol cigarettes was not associated with smoking cessation among these older smokers (OR (95% CI): 1.31 (0.95-1.82)). Analyses were adjusted for demographic variables, test site, and TTFC. Since dependence may be an intermediate variable affecting cessation, it is possible that the analyses were over-adjusted. Cessation was also self-reported with no biochemical verification. There was a low response rate at the six-month follow up survey, with a loss of 25 percent. Generalizability may be limited since the sample was composed of those seeking treatment, mostly older males (77% > 50 years old), and not nationally representative.

Muscat et al. (2002) conducted a cross-sectional study to analyze the associations between smoking status and menthol cigarette use among 19,545 current and former African American and White smokers (3,005 menthol and 16,540 nonmenthol) using data collected in a case-control study designed for characterizing tobacco-related cancers. The study was conducted in several hospitals in New York, Pennsylvania, and the District of Columbia between 1981 and 1999. Menthol status was self-reported based on last brand cigarette smoked. The primary outcome was self-reported smoking status (current vs. quit), which may be subject to misclassification. Menthol smoking was not associated with current versus quitting status (prevalence odds ratio (95% CI): 1.1 (0.8-1.4) in African Americans and 1.1 (1.0-1.3) in Whites).The odds ratios appear to have been rounded to the nearest tenth, which makes some of the findings difficult to interpret. Interpretation of some study results was questionable. For example, the authors stated that smokers of menthol cigarettes were significantly more likely to have been former smokers (African Americans), while the data shown in Table 1 indicated that menthol smokers were more likely to be current smokers (70.4% menthol smokers were current smokers vs. 64.3% nonmenthol smokers were current smokers ($p < 0.01$)). Although the sample size was reasonable, the study period spanned 18 years. The definition of an ex-smoker (someone who did not smoke at least one cigarette every day for the past 12 months) was weak and may lead to misclassification. Generalizability may be limited since the sample consisted of older, hospitalized patients, and was not nationally representative. More importantly, the utility of the findings of this study are limited due to significant methodological flaws.

Gundersen et al. (2009) analyzed the association between menthol smoking and cessation among a nationally representative sample of adult current and former smokers (n=7,815) using the 2005 National Health Interview Survey (NHIS). Self-reported menthol use was based on the usual brand of cigarettes smoked in the past 12 months for current smokers or 12 months prior to quitting for former smokers. A former smoker was defined as having smoked 100 or more cigarettes in a lifetime but now "not smoking at all." African Americans and Hispanics were combined under a category labeled "non-White.". The study indicated that non-White menthol smokers were significantly less likely to have quit smoking compared to nonmenthol smoking counterparts (odds ratio (95% CI): 0.55 (0.43-0.71)). The odds ratios (95% CI) were 0.78 (0.56- 1.09) for African Americans and 0.61 (0.39-0.97) for Hispanics. White menthol smokers, in contrast, were more likely to have quit ($p<0.05$), with an odds ratio of 1.17 (1-1.36).

Stahre et al. (2010) examined the relationship between menthol smoking, the population quit ratio, and utilization of smoking cession aid among 6,511 current and 6,774 former smokers who participated in the 2005 NHIS-CCS. Researchers collected data on the menthol status of the participants' usual brand. The quit ratio was defined as the total number of former smokers divided by the total number of ever smokers, whereas quitters were defined as people who reported quitting within the previous 12 months. The quit ratio for African American menthol smokers was significantly lower than their nonmenthol counterparts (34% vs. 49%, $p < 0.001$). No significant difference was found in other racial groups including Whites, Asian Americans, American Indian/Alaska Natives and Hispanics. The NHIS sample was large and nationally representative. It is unknown whether smoking cessation lasted for a short time (e.g., one day) or continued long-term (e.g., months).

Levy et al. (2011) evaluated data from the 2003 and 2006-2007 CPS-TUS. This large, nationally representative survey included data from 34,260 individuals in the 2003 survey and 31,250 individuals in the 2006-2007 survey. The likelihood of quitting was 3.5% lower for quitting in the past year and 6% lower for quitting in the past 5 years in menthol compared with nonmenthol smokers. Although the CPS-TUS is a nationally representative dataset, there are limitations with this study, including data transformation, and calculation of prevalence differences. Thus, it may be difficult to interpret the data as presented or draw conclusions from this study.

Given the limitations of Levy et al. (2011), FDA performed independent analyses of the 2006/2007 CPS-TUS dataset. FDA assessed data related to cessation among smokers and former smokers who had last smoked less than five years ago. Menthol smokers had a lower prevalence of cessation as compared to nonmenthol smokers for smokers overall (OR = 0.87, 95% CI = 0.820.93), and among whites (OR = 0.87, 95% CI = 0.80-0.94), but not among African Americans (OR = 0.84, 95% CI = 0.65-1.08) or Hispanics (OR = 0.98, 95% CI = 0.74-1.29). The association with lower cessation for menthol smokers was more pronounced among males (OR = 0.83, 95% CI = 0.75-0.93) than among females (OR = 0.93, 95% CI = 0.85-1.02).

Conclusion

In all studies available for evaluation, the use of or preference for a menthol brand was based solely on self-report. Although this could be associated with misclassification, self-report is the standard of this research field and not considered detrimental to the study results. Furthermore, Caraballo et al. (2011) noted that while evidence exists of some self-report bias in reporting menthol or nonmenthol cigarette use, especially among adolescents, this is not necessarily problematic since it is likely that this type of bias is fairly constant over time.

Of the nine cohort studies reviewed, three studies (Hyland et al., 2002; Cropsey et al. 2009; Murray et al., 2007) failed to find any differences in the cessation or relapse rates of menthol versus non-menthol smokers. However, one of those studies may have over-adjusted their analyses (Hyland et al., 2002) and the generalizability of another was extremely limited due to the use of prisoners (Cropsey et al., 2009). A fourth study (Blot et al., 2011) found no difference between African American smokers but that White menthol smokers were more likely to have quit. Of the remaining five cohort studies, four found worse cessation outcomes for menthol smokers as compared to their nonmenthol counterparts (Pletcher et al., 2006; Okuyemi et al., 2003; Harris et al., 2004), and one had a trend towards menthol smokers having worse outcomes (Foulds et al., 2006). Of the six reviewed cross sectional studies, two (Fu et al., 2008; Muscat et al., 2002) failed to find significant differences between menthol and non-menthol smokers. Of these, the utility of one (Muscat et al., 2002) was found to be extremely limited due to severe methodological flaws. Of the remaining four studies, three found that menthol smokers had worse cessation outcomes as compared to their nonmenthol smoking counterparts, while one (Gundersen et al., 2009), found that African-American and

Latino menthol smokers had worse cessation outcomes as compared to their nonmenthol smoking counterparts while the reverse was true for White smokers.

Several of the studies that found no significant association between menthol and cessation success may have overadjusted their analyses by including adjustments for dependence factors such as TTFC. Since dependence may be an intermediate factor impacting cessation success, it may not be appropriate to control for the level of dependence. This is consistent with the observation that menthol smokers appear to be more nicotine dependent as compared to nonmenthol smokers. Furthermore, the data regarding African American menthol smokers are fairly consistent; they are less likely to be successful in quitting smoking as compared to their nonmenthol counterparts. Although there is a suggestion that White menthol smokers may have greater quitting success, this is not consistent, even using large nationally representative datasets. From the available studies, the weight of evidence supports the conclusion that menthol in cigarettes is likely associated with reduced success in smoking cessation, especially among African American menthol smokers.

References

Blot WJ, Cohen SS, Aldrich M, McLaughlin JK, Hargreaves MK, Signorello LB (2011) Lung cancer risk among smokers of menthol cigarettes. Journal of the National Cancer Institute 103:810-6. [Funded by National Cancer Institute]

Caraballo, RS & Asman, K (2011). Epidemiology of menthol cigarette use in the United States. Tobacco Induced Diseases, 9 (Suppl 1): S1. [No funding source(s) provided. Authors affiliated with the Centers for Disease Control and Prevention]

Cropsey KL, Weaver MF, Eldridge GD, et al. (2009) Differential success rates in racial groups: results of a clinical trial of smoking cessation among female prisoners. Nicotine and Tobacco Research 11(6):690–7. [Funded by National Institute on Drug Abuse grant K23 DA15774]

Doll R, Peto R, Boreham J et al. (2004) Mortality in relation to smoking: 50 years' observation on male British doctors. British Medical Journal 26;328(7455):1519. [Funded by the Medical Research Council, the British Heart Foundation, and Cancer Research UK]

Foulds JF, Gandhi KK, Steinberg MB, et al. (2006) Factors associated with quitting smoking at a tobacco treatment dependence treatment clinic. American Journal of Health Behavior 30(4):400–12. [Funding provided by grant from the New Jersey Department of Health and Senior Services, as part of New Jersey's Comprehensive Tobacco Control Program; the Cancer Institute of New Jersey, The Robert Wood Johnson Foundation, the National Institute on Drug Abuse, and the American Legacy Foundation]

Foulds J, Hooper MW, Pletcher MJ, Okuyemi KS (2010) Do smokers of menthol cigarettes find it harder to quit smoking? Nicotine and Tobacco Research 12(suppl 2): S102-9. [No funding source(s) provided. Authors affiliated with Pennsylania State College of Medicine, University of Miami, University of California, San Francisco, University of Minnesota]

Cessation: Table of Referenced Sources

Author Name(s)	Article Title	Year Pub.	Funded By	Type of Study	Subject Description (Including Special population(s))	Sample Size (N)	Authors' Results/Conclusion(s) related to Menthol* (excerpted directly from article)
Blot WJ, Cohen SS, Aldrich M, McLaughlin JK, Hargreaves MK, Signorello LB.	Lung cancer risk among smokers of menthol cigarettes.	2011	The National Cancer Institute	Prospective	12,373 smokers who participated in a follow up of the Southern Community Cohort Study	440 incident lung cancer case patients and 2213 matched control subjects	During an average of 4.3 years of follow-up, 21% of participants smoking at baseline had quit, with menthol and nonmenthol smokers having equal odds of quitting (OR = 1.02, 95% CI = 0.89 to 1.16).
Caraballo, RS & Asman, K.	Epidemiology of menthol cigarette use in the United States.	2011	No funding source(s) provided. Authors affiliated with the Centers for Disease Control and Prevention	Review and secondary analyses of national surveys	NSDUH: adolescents aged 12-17 years old who smoked in the past month and adult smokers (aged 18 years or older) who smoked in the past month NYTS: middle school (MS) and high school (HS) students with school year, past 30 day smoking, brand use, and menthol information. MTF: current smokers in 8th, 10th and 12th grade NHANES: 20 years and older who had Smoked and were non- Hispanic white,	NSDUH: 9,595 adolescents; 62,010 adults NYTS: 1,978 MS students and 6,163 HS students MTF: 20,863 8th graders; 30,722 10th graders; 40,914 12th Graders NHANES: 1571 individuals with UPC information	Menthol cigarettes are disproportionately smoked by adolescents, blacks/African Americans, adult females, those living in the Northeast of the United States and those with family incomes lower than $50,000. Based on self-reports of menthol cigarette use, menthol cigarette use among smokers have increased from 2004 to 2008.

Author Name(s)	Article Title	Year Pub.	Funded By	Type of Study	Subject Description (Including Special population(s))	Sample Size (N)	Authors' Results/Conclusion(s) related to Menthol* (excerpted directly from article)
					non- Hispanic black/African American, or Mexican American		
Cropsey KL, Weaver MF, Eldridge GD, Villalobos GC,	Differential success rates in racial groups: results of a clinical	2009	National Institute on Drug Abuse (grant K23DA15774)	Original study = randomizied control trial. Extracted data	White and Black female prisoners, aged •18, smoking at least 5 cpd.	N=233 cases N= 289 controls	Smoking mentholated cigarettes was not associated with these differences in quit rates.
Best AM, Stitzer ML.	trial of smoking cessation among female prisoners.			using case control design			
Doll R, Peto R, Boreham J et al.	Mortality in relation to smoking: 50 years' observation on male British doctors.	2004	Medical Research Council, the British Heart Foundation, and Cancer Research UK	Prospective study starting in 1951	British doctors	N=34,439	The excess mortality associated with smoking chiefly involved vascular, neoplastic, and respiratory diseases that can be caused by smoking. [Not menthol specific]
Foulds J, Gandhi KK, Steinberg MB, Richardson DL, Williams JM, Burke MV, Rhoads GG.	Factors associated with quitting smoking at a tobacco treatment dependence treatment clinic.	2006	The New Jersey Department of Health and Senior Services, as part of New Jersey's Comprehensive Tobacco Control Program; the Cancer Institute of New Jersey, The Robert Wood Johnson Foundation, the National Institute on Drug Abuse, and the American	Cohort	first 1021 patients who attempted to quit tobacco at a specialist tobacco dependence treatment outpatient clinic based at the Tobacco Dependence Program at the University of Medicine and Dentistry of New Jersey-School of	N=1021	Forty-one percent of the patients smoked menthol cigarettes. They were less likely to achieve abstinence in univariate analyses, and this item remained in the model predicting 4- week outcome.

Cessation: Table of Referenced Sources (Continued)

Author Name(s)	Article Title	Year Pub.	Funded By	Type of Study	Subject Description (Including Special population(s))	Sample Size (N)	Authors' Results/Conclusion(s) related to Menthol* (excerpted directly from article)
			Legacy Foundation		Public Health		
Foulds J, Hooper MW, Pletcher MJ, Okuyemi KS.	Do smokers of menthol cigarettes find it harder to quit smoking?	2010	No funding source(s) provided. Authors affiliated with Pennsylvania State College of Medicine, University of Miami, University of California, San Francisco, University of Minnesota	Review	Ten published, peer-reviewed studies	Not Applicable	Half of the studies found evidence that menthol smoking is associated with lower odds of cessation, while the other half found no such effects. The pattern of results in these studies suggest that the association between smoking menthol cigarettes and difficulty quitting is stronger in (a) racial/ethnic minority populations, (b) younger smokers, and (c) studies carried out after 1999.
Fu SS, Kodl MM, Joseph AM, Hatsukami DK, Johnson EO, Breslau N,	Racial/Ethnic disparities in the use of nicotine replacement therapy and quit	2008	Veterans Affairs Health Services Research and Development research career development award and Veterans Affairs	Large, randomized intervention study	Adults ages 25 -44 years from 3 metropolitan areas in the Midwest were randomly sampled	N=27,031 baseline total; Caucasian (n= 7,907),	No association between adult use of menthol cigarettes and cessation success
Wu B, Bierut L.	ratios in lifetime smokers ages 25 to 44 years.		Health Services Research and Development postdoctoral research fellowship; National Cancer Institute and University of Minnesota Transdisciplinary Tobacco Use Research Center		using Health Maintenance Organization membership lists in Detroit, MI and Minneapolis, MN and a driver's license registry in St. Louis, MO; sample was limited to lifetime smokers (individuals who had ever smoked	African American (n=955), Latino (n= 246), and Asian (n=108) race/ethnicity. Lifetime smokers who were	

Author Name(s)	Article Title	Year Pub.	Funded By	Type of Study	Subject Description (Including Special population(s))	Sample Size (N)	Authors' Results/Conclusion(s) related to Menthol* (excerpted directly from article)
					>100 cigarettes).	multiracial or of other race (n=387) were excluded	
Gandhi KK, Foulds J, Steinberg MB, Lu SE, Williams JM.	Lower quit rates among African American and Latino menthol cigarette smokers at a tobacco treatment clinic.	2009	New Jersey Department of Health and Senior Services, the Cancer Institute of New Jersey, the Robert Wood Johnson Foundation, National Institute on Drug Abuse, the American Legacy Foundation and the National Institute on Mental Health	Retrospective Cohort/ Population Studies	Specialized smoking cessation outpatient clinic in New Jersey: patients who set a quit date and attempted to quit smoking, between 1 January 2001 and 30 June 2005; African American,Latinos, Whites	N=1688 (787 Menthol, 910 Nonmenthol)	This study found lower short-term (4-week followup) quit rates among AA and Latino menthol smokers as compared with non-menthol smokers within the same racial/ ethnic subgroups.
Gundersen DA, Delnevo CD, Wackowski O.	Exploring the relationship between race/ethnicity, menthol smoking, and cessation, in a nationally representative sample of adults.	2009	No funding source(s) provided. Authors affiliated with University of Medicine and Dentistry of New Jersey	Retrospective analysis of cross-sectional study	Sample of those who indicated that they do not currently use other tobacco products and have made a quit attempt..	N=7815	Menthol smoking can lead to poorer cessation outcomes, but only for non-white smokers.
Harris KJ, Okuyemi KS, Catley D, Mayo MS, Ge B, Ahluwalia	Predictors of smoking cessation among African-Americans	2004	Grants RO1 CA77856, K07 CA87714, R24 CA95835 and K07 CA90334 from the National Cancer	Double-blind placebo-controlled, randomized trial	1,498 smokers in a mid- western city who identified themselves as black or African-American were	N=600	Other than bupropion treatment, the strongest predictors for success included not smoking menthol cigarettes

Cessation: Table of Referenced Sources (Continued)

Author Name(s)	Article Title	Year Pub.	Funded By	Type of Study	Subject Description (Including Special population(s))	Sample Size (N)	Authors' Results/Conclusion(s) related to Menthol* (excerpted directly from article)
JS.	enrolled in a randomized controlled trial of bupropion.		Institute		screened, and 981 were eligible and invited to participate.		
Hyland A, Garten S, Giovino GA, Cummings KM.	Mentholated cigarettes and smoking cessation: findings from COMMIT.	2002	The National Cancer Institute grant CA016056- 26	Telephone survey	COMMIT study: Baseline smokers who reported whether their current cigarette brand or not in 1988, and had a known smoking status in 1993.	N=13,268 (3,184 menthol, 10084 non-menthol)	No clear associations were observed between menthol cigarette use and indicators of nicotine dependence, even after controlling for race/ethnicity and other demographics..
Levy DT, Blackman K, Tauras J, Chaloupka F, Villanti A, Niaura R, Vallone DM, Abrams DB.	Quit attempts and quit rates among menthol and nonmenthol smokers in the United States	2011	Legacy	Tobacco Use Supplement to the Current Population Survey	Participants (18+ yo) who responded to 2003 and 2006–2007 waves	N=34260 for 2003 wave N=31250 for 2007 wave	Menthol smokers are more likely to make quit attempts, but are less successful at staying quit.
Murray RP, Connett JE, Skeans MA, Tashkin DP.	Menthol cigarettes and health risks in Lung Health Study data.	2007	Grant HR 46002 from the Division of Lung Disease; National Heart, Lung, and Blood Institute; National Institutes of Health	Randomized Controlled Trial	Adult smokers in a clinical trial of smoking cessation and ipratropium in the prevention of chronic obstructive pulmonary disease.	N=5,887	We conclude that our data contain no evidence that mentholation of cigarettes increases the hazards of smoking.
Muscat JE, Richie JP Jr,	Mentholated cigarettes and	2002	US Public Health Service grants CA-32617, CA-	Cohort/ Population	Hospital between 1981 and 1999: 19 545	N=19,545 subjects,	The risk of quitting was not associated with cigarette menthol flavour.

Author Name(s)	Article Title	Year Pub.	Funded By	Type of Study	Subject Description (Including Special population(s))	Sample Size (N)	Authors' Results/Conclusion(s) related to Menthol* (excerpted directly from article)
Stellman SD.	smoking habits in whites and blacks.		68384 and CA-17613		subjects. Eleven per cent of subjects were black, including 16 540 (84.6%) smokers of non-mentholated cigarettes and 3005 (15.4%) smokers of mentholated cigarettes; Current smokers vs Former smoker; Among blacks, no difference in heavy smoking of menthol vs non-menthol.	11% of subjects were black, including 16,540 (84.6%) smokers of non-mentholated cigarettes and 3005 (15.4%) smokers of mentholated.	
Okuyemi KS, Ahluwalia JS, Ebersole-Robinson M, Catley D, Mayo MS, Resnicow K.	Does menthol attenuate the effect of bupropion among African American smokers?	2003	National Cancer Institute grants R01 CA77856, K07 CA90334, R24 CA95835- 01	Randomized Controlled Trial	African American smokers enrolled in a clinical trial that assessed the efficacy of sustained-release bupropion for smoking cessation. Menthol (n = 471) and non-menthol (n = 129) smokers were compared on smoking- related characteristics and abstinence rates at 6 weeks and 6 months.	N=600	African American menthol smokers had lower smoking cessation rates after 6 weeks of treatment with bupropion-SR than African- American non menthol smokers, thereby putting menthol smokers at greater risk from the health effects of smoking. Lower overall cessation rates among African Americans menthol smokers may partially explain ethnic differences in smoking-related disease risks.

Cessation: Table of Referenced Sources (Continued)

Author Name(s)	Article Title	Year Pub.	Funded By	Type of Study	Subject Description (Including Special population(s))	Sample Size (N)	Authors' Results/Conclusion(s) related to Menthol* (excerpted directly from article)
Pletcher MJ, Hulley BJ, Houston T, Kiefe CI, Benowitz N, Sidney S.	Menthol cigarettes, smoking cessation, atherosclerosis, and pulmonary function: the Coronary Artery	2006	Contracts N01-HC-48047, N01-HC-48048, N01-HC- 48049, N01-HC-48050, and N01-HC-95095 from the National Heart, Lung, and Blood Institute	Multi-center U.S. cohort study (CARDIA)	African American and European American smokers aged 18 to 30 years and healthy at the time of enrollment in 1985	1544 (non-menthol smokers (n = 563) and menthol smokers (n = 972))	Menthol and nonmenthol cigarettes seem to be equally harmful per cigarette smoked in terms of atherosclerosis and pulmonary function decline, but menthol cigarettes may be harder to quit smoking.
	Risk Development in Young Adults (CARDIA) Study.						
Stahre M, Okuyemi KS et al.	Racial/ethnic differences in menthol cigarette smoking, population quit ratios and utilization of evidence-based tobacco cessation treatments.	2010	Department of Veterans Affairs, Veterans Health Administration, Office of Research and Development and Health Services Research and Development	2005 National Health Interview Survey (NHIS) Cancer Control Supplement	18+ yo for which menthol cigarette status was known.	N=12,004	Menthol cigarette smoking is associated negatively with successful smoking cessation among African Americans

* Note: these statements are taken directly from articles and may not include all relevant results/conclusions. [Bracketed notes added by FDA]

Fu SS, Kodl MM, Joseph AM, et al. (2008) Racial or ethnic disparities in the use of nicotine replacement therapy and quit ratios in lifetime smokers ages 25 to 44 years. Cancer Epidemiology, Biomarkers, and Prevention 17(7):1640–1647. [Funded by Veterans Affairs Health Services Research and Development research career development award and Veterans Affairs Health Services Research and Development postdoctoral research fellowship; National Cancer Institute and University of Minnesota Transdisciplinary Tobacco Use Research Center]

Gandhi KK, Foulds J, Steinberg MB, et al. (2009) Lower quit rates among African American and Latino menthol smokers at a tobacco treatment clinic. International Journal of Clinical Practice 63:360–367. [Funded by New Jersey Department of Health and Senior Services, the Cancer Institute of New Jersey, the Robert Wood Johnson Foundation, National Institute on Drug Abuse, the American Legacy Foundation and the National Institute on Mental Health]

Gundersen DA, Delnevo CD, Wackowski O (2009) Exploring the relationship between race or ethnicity, menthol smoking, and cessation, in a nationally representative sample of adults. Preventive Medicine 49(6):553-7. [No funding source(s) provided. Authors affiliated with University of Medicine and Dentistry of New Jersey]

Harris KJ, Okuyemi KS, Catley D, et al. (2004) Predictors of smoking cessation among African-Americans enrolled in a randomized controlled trial of bupropion. Preventive Medicine 38(4):498–502. [Funded by Grants RO1 CA77856, K07 CA87714, R24 CA95835 and K07 CA90334 from the National Cancer Institute]

Hyland A, Garten S, Giovino, GA, Cummings KM (2002) Mentholated cigarettes and smoking cessation: findings from COMMIT (Community Intervention Trial for Smoking Cessation). Tobacco Control 11(2):135–9. [Funded by The National Cancer Institute grant CA016056-26]

Levy DT, Blackman K, Tauras J, Chaloupka F, Villanti A, Niaura R, Vallone DM, Abrams DB (2011) Quit attempts and quit rates among menthol and nonmenthol smokers in the United States. American Journal of Public Health, 101: 1241-1247. [Funded by Legacy]

Murray RP, Connett JE, Skeans MA, Tashkin, DP (2007) Menthol cigarettes and health risks in Lung Health Study data. Nicotine and Tobacco Research, 9(1):101–7. [Funded by Grant HR 46002 from the Division of Lung Disease; National Heart, Lung, and Blood Institute; National Institutes of Health]

Muscat JE, Richie JP Jr, et al. (2002) Mentholated cigarettes and smoking habits in Whites and Blacks. Tobacco Control 11(4):368–71. [Funded by US Public Health Service grants CA-32617, CA-68384 and CA-17613]

Okuyemi KS, Ahluwalia JS, Ebersole-Robinson M, et al. (2003) Does menthol attenuate the effect of bupropion among African American smokers? Addiction 98(10):1387–1393. [Funded by National Cancer Institute grants R01 CA77856, K07 CA90334, R24 CA95835- 01]

Pletcher MJ, Hulley BJ, Houston T, et al. (2006) Menthol cigarettes, smoking cessation, atherosclerosis, and pulmonary function: the Coronary Artery Risk Development in Young Adults (CARDIA) study. Archives of Internal Medicine 166(17):1915–22. [Funded by Contracts N01-HC-48047, N01-HC-48048, N01-HC-48049, N01-HC-48050, and N01-HC-95095 from the National Heart, Lung, and Blood Institute]

Stahre M, Okuyemi KS et al. (2010) Racial or ethnic differences in menthol cigarette smoking, population quit ratios and utilization of evidence-based tobacco cessation treatments. Addiction 105(suppl. 1):75–83. [Funded by Department of Veterans Affairs, Veterans Health Administration, Office of Research and Development and Health Services Research and Development]

Disease Risk

Data are clear that smoking tobacco results in an increased risk of disease for smokers, and research has identified causal links between smoking tobacco and risk for lung cancer, esophageal and oropharyngeal cancers, cardiovascular disease and respiratory outcomes, and many others. As part of FDA's analyses, scientists investigated case studies related to menthol and nonmenthol cigarette smoking and the above specific disease risks to determine if menthol affects disease risk for users.

Lung Cancer

Kabat and Hebert (1991) conducted a hospital-based, case-control study among current smokers in eight hospitals located in four U.S. cities. They found no difference in lung cancer risk between menthol smokers (short-term 1-14 years or long-term ?15 years) and nonmenthol smokers (males: OR (95% CI) 0.98 (0.70-1.38) and 1.14 (0.82-1.59); females, 0.76 (0.53-1.16) and 0.82 (0.52-1.28) for menthol ? 15 years and menthol 1-14 years respectively). Researchers detected no association in stratified analysis by histological types of lung cancer after controlling for cpd, duration of smoking, inhalation, race, education, age, and BMI. This appears to be the first epidemiologic study that evaluated the associations between menthol cigarette use and lung cancer risk. The racial or ethnic composition of this study was comparable to White and African Americans in the general population. Generalizability may be limited due to the relatively low prevalence of menthol use by African American participants as compared to the general African American smoking population. Most of the participants were at least 50 years old, however since lung cancer typically does not occur at younger ages, this is not considered a weakness. There is limited power for stratified analysis by histological type (e.g., large cell carcinoma), and the hospital-based controls may have had conditions potentially related to smoking (including colon and breast cancer), which may reduce an association. Menthol cigarette use status was determined by specifically asking about specific brands of cigarettes, which may reduce the potential for misclassification.

Sidney et al. (1995) conducted a cohort study among 11,761 Northern California Kaiser Permanente Insurers current smokers 30-89 years old who had smoked for at least 20 years. The study found that the prevalence of menthol cigarette use was highest among African American smokers, followed by Asian American and White smokers. Menthol smokers were younger and more likely to be females than nonmenthol smokers. Menthol smokers had a statistically significantly higher lung cancer risk than nonmenthol smokers among men (RR (95% CI): 1.45 (1.03-2.02)), but not among women (0.75 (0.51-1.11)). Relative risks were calculated adjusting for age, sex, race, education, cpd, and duration of smoking; the multivariate model did not adjust for other potential factors, such as family history of lung cancer. After more than eight years of follow up, researchers noted a loss of about 25 percent due to members terminating the insurance program which may lead to selection bias. Generalizability may be limited since the difference was only seen in men, and the participant pool was limited to Northern California Kaiser Permanente Insurerers customers only, a pool that was not nationally representative.

Carpenter et al. (1999) examined the association between menthol cigarette use and lung cancer using data from a population based case-control study that evaluated genetic markers for lung cancer risk in Los Angeles County, California. The subjects were current and former smokers 40-84 years old. The study found no difference in lung cancer risk between menthol and nonmenthol smokers (OR(95% CI): 1.04 (0.62, 1.75)). The study also found no difference in lung cancer risk between menthol smokers and nonmenthol smokers by race. The analysis adjusted for matching factors, total pack-years, and years since quitting. Due to the low response rate of controls (731:3193) the remaining controls may not be representative of the general population from which the cases were drawn. Generalizability is limited, as the African American sample reported smoking menthol cigarettes at rates lower than the national estimate.

Brooks et al. (2003) conducted a hospital-based case-control study using data collected in the Slone Epidemiology Center Case-Control Surveillance Study in the eastern United States. The analysis was restricted to subjects 40-74 years old who had smoked for at least 20 years, had no history of cancer, and were interviewed between 1981 and 2000. Analyses were adjusted for demographic factors and smoke-related factors (e.g., duration of smoking, cpd, years since quitting, proportion of years smoking filtered cigarettes, etc.). The study found no difference in lung cancer risk between long-term menthol smokers and nonmenthol smokers (OR (95% CI): 0.97 (0.70-1.34)). Risks also did not differ by race or sex. Menthol status was characterized by brand and dose of exposure (i.e., duration of menthol cigarette use). Due to differences in how cases and controls were identified, researchers adjusted the data for the time of interview to account for bias. The study was restricted to long-term smokers to minimize the potential for selection bias for controls, however this may limit generalizability. A significant amount of missing data makes establishing exposures difficult; brand information could be identified in 60 percent of total duration of smoking. Most lung cancer patients were discovered at a time when menthol cigarettes were not popular so menthol status was not known for many patients. The authors assumed these cases smoked nonmenthol cigarettes. However, this may result in misclassification of the exposure and bias the estimates. A possible selection bias may exist in cases since the study included lung cancer cases in patients who were diagnosed with lung cancer 12 months before their current admission instead of only newly diagnosed patients. Thus, the cases may include long-time survivors who may not have general characteristics for all lung cancer patients. The controls were hospitalized for diseases determined to be unrelated to cigarette smoking, however diagnoses could include breast and colon cancers, which may be related to smoking. Data collection was limited to the brand most recently smoked (or currently smoking) and also the brand reportedly smoked the longest. Data from both questions were only obtained from 17 percent of the subjects, so researchers included subjects who could provide brand information for at least 60 percent of the total duration of smoking.

Stellman et al. (2003) reported results from a hospital-based, case-control study that was conducted between 1984 and 1998. The study found no associations between menthol cigarette use status and lung cancer risk among current smokers for white males (OR (95% CI): 0.83 (0.63-1.09)), African American males (1.34 (0.79-2.29)), white females (0.61 (0.44-1.06)), and African American females (0.79 (0.41-1.54)). Odds ratios were adjusted for age at diagnosis, pack-years of smoking, education years, and BMI. The study did not report odds ratios for current smokers overall, by sex, or by race. The hospital-based controls may have had conditions related to smoking that would reduce the association. Generalizability is limited, as subjects were hospitalized and not nationally representative.

Murray et al. (2007) investigated the health effects of menthol cigarette smoking among 5,887 adult smokers 35-60 years old with mild to moderate airway obstruction who participated in a smoking cessation program as part of the Lung Health Study. This long-term cohort study had annual assessments for five years. Menthol cigarette use was not significantly associated with mortality caused by coronary heart disease, cardiovascular disease, lung cancer (hazard ratio (95% CI):0.96 (0.70-1.32)), and any causes during 14 years of follow-up. Researchers adjusted estimates for age, sex, race, years of education, cpd, and predicted respiratory volume (FEV1% predicted), and randomization group assignment. Menthol status was checked annually. Generalizability may be limited as the sample was not nationally representative.

Etzel et al. (2008) analyzed results from a case-control study of African American smokers in the Houston area to identify lung cancer risk factors to be included in a lung cancer risk prediction model. The study did not find statistically significant differences in lung cancer risk between menthol and nonmenthol smokers in the case-control data, although the risk estimates trended toward being lower for current smokers (OR 0.69 (0.46-1.03)) and ever smokers (0.81 (0.60- 1.09)), but not for former smokers 0.99 (0.621.56)). Menthol cigarette use was not retained in the final multivariable epidemiologic risk model for African Americans. The sample is not nationally representative. This novel model of lung cancer risk prevention has not yet been validated by others in the field.

Blot et al. (2011) conducted a nested case-control study among 440 incident lung cancer cases and 2,213 controls enrolled in the Southern Community Cohort Study between 2002 and 2009. Researchers matched cases and controls on age, sex, and race, and they adjusted estimates for pack-years of smoking, educational attainment, household income, use of other tobacco products, health insurance coverage, close family history of lung cancer, and BMI. The risk of lung cancer incidence for both current smokers and former smokers was substantially higher than for nonsmokers. In a multivariate analysis adjusted for pack-years of smoking, there was a statistically significant association between menthol smoking and lower lung cancer risks for incidence (OR 0.65 (0.47-0.90)) and mortality (HR 0.69 (0.49-0.95)) among current menthol smokers compared to current nonmenthol smokers. The study also found statistically significant lower incidence risks for menthol smoking among current female smokers (OR 0.43 (0.24-0.75)) and current African American smokers (OR 0.52 (0.34-0.78), but not among current male smokers (OR 0.77 (0.49-1.23)) and current White smokers (OR 0.84 (0.43-1.64).

Among a set of secondary data analyses conducted in 2010 that have not been peer-reviewed, Muscat analyzed data from a community cross-sectional study of 525 African American and White smokers. The analysis found a statistically significant lower risk of lung cancer among current menthol smokers 50 years old and over (OR 0.76, p-value=0.049). There was a trend toward an association between menthol smoking status and lower risk of lung cancer among all current smokers (OR 0.82, p-value=0.110).

In addition to peer-reviewed articles and secondary data analyses, FDA also evaluated the association between menthol smoking and disease risk using data from the 1987 National Health Interview Survey that was linked to the National Death Index for mortality follow-up. Mortality data were available for approximately 5,000 participants who were current menthol and nonmenthol smokers at the time of interview. FDA estimated mortality hazard ratios for menthol smokers compared to nonmenthol smokers, adjusting for demographic and smoking characteristics. The hazard ratio for lung cancer mortality for menthol smokers overall was 0.69 (95% CI: 0.45-1.06). The hazard ratio for lung cancer mortality for menthol smokers 50 years old and over was 0.59 (95% CI = 0.36-0.96). No differences existed in overall mortality from all causes of death, other than lung cancer, for menthol and nonmenthol smokers.

In an industry supported study, Lee (2011) conducted a systematic review and meta-analysis of eight epidemiological studies examining the relationship between lung cancer risk and menthol smoking. The meta-analysis included the seven articles previously discussed in this section as well as a conference abstract (Jockel, Pohlabeln, and Jahn, 2004) that was conducted in Germany and for which the results have only been reported in English in a journal abstract. The overall adjusted relative risk estimate for menthol smoking compared to nonmenthol smoking from the meta-analysis was 0.93 (95% CI 0.84-1.02, n=8). A statistically significant lower risk was observed in females (RR 0.80, 0.67-0.95, n=5 studies) and in studies published since 2001 (0.88, 0.77-0.99, n=5 studies). No difference in risk was observed in males (1.01, 0.84-1.22, n=5 studies) or in studies published between 1991 and 2000 (1.00, 0.86-1.15, n=3). Estimates of relative risk for menthol smokers compared to nonmenthol smokers trended toward being lower for whites (0.87, 0.75-1.03, n=4) and African Americans (0.90, 0.73-1.10, n=4 studies), but the differences failed to reach significance.

Oropharyngeal Cancer

Kabat and Hebert (1994) conducted a hospital-based, case-control study of tobacco-related cancers among current smokers in eight hospitals in four U.S. cities. This was a moderately sized study, with 194 male and 82 female newly diagnosed oropharyngeal cancer cases, and 845 male and 411 female controls. After adjusting for demographic factors, as well as cpd, BMI, alcohol intake, filtered or unfiltered cigarette use, and duration of smoking, they found no association between menthol cigarette use and oropharyngeal cancer risk (OR (95% CI): 0.9 (0.5-1.6)) for male menthol smokers and 0.7 (0.5-1.7) for females menthol smokers compared to nonmenthol smokers. Although the authors stated that menthol cigarette use was positively associated with pharynx cancer in males 1.7 (0.8-3.4), the difference was not statistically significant. Menthol use was self-reported. The control cases were hospitalized with conditions thought not to be related to smoking, however it included cancers that could be smoking-related (e.g., breast cancer, colon cancer). The sample size in subgroups was small, with limited power. Generalizability may be limited since the sample was not nationally representative and limited to hospitalized patients.

Esophageal Cancer

In a letter to the editor, Hebert and Kabat (1988) reported results of an analysis of case-control study data of esophageal cancer and found no effect of menthol smoking on esophageal cancer risk. The risks for esophageal cancer for men and women who smoked menthol cigarettes for 10 years or more versus nonmenthol smokers were not significantly different (men = OR (95% CI): 0.70 (0.29-1.73); women = OR (95% CI): 1.53 (0.61-3.86)). This is a relatively small study, with 96 female and 216 male cases and 157 female and 305 male controls. It is not clear from the letter if the authors controlled for factors such as alcohol consumption and socioeconomic status in the analysis.

In a follow-up to the 1988 letter to the editor, Hebert and Kabat (1989) again sought to investigate the relationship between menthol cigarette smoking and esophageal cancer. They analyzed a larger dataset from 20 hospitals in nine U.S. cities in the American Health Foundation Comprehensive Tobacco Questionnaire, a large, matched, case-control study. This time, investigators found a trend toward reduced risk (p=0.08) among male menthol smokers (<10 yrs) versus male never smokers (OR (95% CI): 0.50 (0.23-1.07)), but this trend failed to reach significance. There was no increased risk for those who had been menthol smokers for more than 10 years. Logistic analysis for females showed a non-statistically significant trend toward increased risk for those who had been menthol smokers for more than 10 years (OR (95% CI: 2.3 (0.93-5.720) (p=0.07)). In this investigation, researchers included major risk factors for esophageal cancer for analysis, such as lifetime exposure to tobacco (cpd, menthol vs. nonmenthol) and alcohol (duration, amount). Statistical analysis included adjustment for demographic factors.

Multiple Cancers

Freidman et al. (1998) conducted a cohort study among 5,770 men and 5,990 women 30-89 years old who were enrolled in Kaiser Permanente health insurance from 1979-1985 in Northern California, with follow-up through 1994. The subjects had each smoked for at least 20 years. The study examined relative risks for upper aerodigestive cancer, pancreatic cancer, renal adenocarcinoma, other urinary tract cancer, uterine cervical cancer, and all of these cancers combined among menthol smokers compared to nonmenthol smokers. Analyses were controlled for race and age. There were no significant differences, although the relative risks for menthol smoking for seven of the nine estimates (five cancer sites by sex) trended toward being reduced. The overall relative risk for all smoking-related cancers was not significantly different between male menthol and nonmenthol smokers (0.76 with 95% CI 0.52-1.11) or female menthol and nonmenthol smokers (0.79 with 95% CI 0.53-1.18). The overall relative risk for both sexes combined was not presented; it is not clear if this result would have shown a statistically significant lower risk of these cancers for menthol smokers compared to nonmenthol smokers.

Among a set of secondary data analyses conducted in 2010 that have not been peer-reviewed, Stellman and Neugut produced a follow-up to their 2003 study by analyzing data on cancer risk from the American Health Foundation hospital-based, multi-center, case-control study (3,728 cases and 4,888 controls). The researchers estimated the odds ratios for the association between menthol smoking and cancer risk of the oral cavity, larynx, lung, esophagus, and bladder and among the overall population and in subgroups stratified by sex, controlling for age, race, educational attainment, BMI, and pack-years of smoking. Nine of the 10 odds ratios for the cancers by sex were less than 1.0 and the tenth, lung cancer among males, was 1.0, although the differences were not statistically significant. The odds ratio for lung cancer for female menthol smokers versus female nonmenthol smokers was 0.8 (95% CI 0.6-1.0). Since the authors did not report odds ratios to the nearest hundredth, it is not possible to determine how close this result was to statistical significance. That is, if the 1.0 was a result of rounding up, the odds ratio would reach significance, indicating reduced lung cancer risk for female menthol smokers, but if it was a result of rounding down, it would indicate overlapping data and therefore no significant differences.

Multiple Non-Cancer Diseases

Pletcher et al. (2006) evaluated the associations between menthol cigarette use, coronary calcification and changes in pulmonary function test among 1,544 current smokers who were participants in CARDIA. CARDIA is a population-based longitudinal cohort study of risk factors for coronary artery diseases among healthy African Americans and Whites 18-30 years old. The subjects were followed for 15 years. The study found no difference in the association between menthol or nonmenthol exposure (in pack-years) and the prevalence of coronary calcification and 10-year decline in lung function. This is one of only two studies in this section that assessed menthol use on multiple occasions, finding that menthol status was relatively stable, suggesting little misclassification. Although the sample was diverse, it was not nationally representative, which may limit generalizability. While this is a large study, sample sizes in certain groups were small (e.g., African American nonmenthol smokers).

Murray et al. (2007) examined the associations between menthol cigarette use and health risks among 5,887 Lung Health Study participants with early signs of obstructive lung impairment. They conducted analyses of mortality from selected causes and concluded menthol cigarette use was not significantly associated with mortality caused by coronary heart disease, cardiovascular disease, and any causes during 14 years of follow-up. Estimates were adjusted for age, sex, race, educational attainment, cpd, predicted respiratory volume, and randomization group assignment.

This is a fairly large study with long-term follow up, and researchers assessed menthol use at multiple time points. Generalizability may be limited, as the sample is not nationally representative and limited to people with mild or moderate airway obstruction who participated in a smoking cessation program. Among a set of secondary data analyses conducted in 2010 that have not been peer-reviewed, Hyland and Kasza analyzed data from the International Tobacco Control Four Country Survey, with data from the United States, United Kingdom, Canada and Australia. Data were collected from 7,532 individuals between 2002 and 2008. This study had a large and nationally representative sample population. Hyland and Kasza used case-control data collected between 2005 and 2010 by Roswell Park Cancer Institute and interview data collected between 1957 and 1965 by Roswell Park Memorial Institute to analyze the association between menthol smoking and risks of lung cancer and COPD.

Adjusted relative risks for lung cancer or COPD trended toward being lower for female menthol smokers (OR 0.48, 0.23-1.02) and smokers overall (0.68, 0.38-1.22) compared to nonmenthol smokers, however the differences were not statistically significant. No difference was observed between male menthol and male nonmenthol smokers (1.16, 0.43-3.10). Analysis of data collected during the 1957-1965 time period indicated no menthol:nonmenthol differences for smokers overall (1.15, 0.73-1.81) or by sex. Relative risks were adjusted for age, race, and pack-years of smoking.

Other Health Characteristics

Mendiondo et al. (2010) examined the health characteristics between menthol and nonmenthol smokers using data from the 2005 NHIS-CCS, a large, nationally representative, cross-sectional survey. The study demonstrated that former menthol smokers had slightly higher BMI (OR (95% CI): 1.01(1.00-1.02)) and were more likely to have visited the emergency room due to asthma (OR 2.30: 1.04, 5.09).

Conclusion

Although menthol or nonmenthol classification and cigarette use data were self-reported and could be associated with misclassification, self-report of this kind of data are the standard of this research field and not considered detrimental to the study results. Furthermore, the data do not support the claim that a substantial number of adult respondents intentionally under-report tobacco use (Everhart et al., 2009; Yeager & Krosnick, 2010). Furthermore, as noted by Caraballo et al. (2011), although there is evidence that there is some self-report bias in reporting menthol:nonmenthol cigarette use, especially among adolescents, this is not necessarily problematic since it is likely that this type of bias is fairly constant over time.

Eleven studies (Brooks et al., 2003; Carpenter et al., 1999; Etzel et al., 2008; Freidman et al., 1998; Hebert and Kabat, 1988; Hebert and Kabat, 1989; Kabat and Hebert, 1991; Kabat and Hebert, 1994; Murray et al., 2007; Pletcher et al., 2006; Stellman et al., 2003) failed to find any significant differences in disease risk between menthol and nonmenthol smokers. One study found a greater disease risk in some groups (Sidney et al., 1995). Two studies (Blot et al., 2011; Lee, 2011) suggest that, in some groups, menthol smoking may be associated with lower cancer risk as compared to nonmenthol smoking. It is possible, but not clear at this time, that this association might be related to historical differences in cigarette design features (such as tip ventilation between menthol and nonmenthol cigarettes) or other demographic factors. No physiological cause for an association between cancer risk and menthol in cigarettes has been established. From the available studies, the weight of evidence supports the conclusion that menthol in cigarettes is not associated with an increase in disease risk to the user.

References

Blot WJ, Cohen SS, Aldrich M, McLaughlin JK, Hargreaves MK, Signorello LB (2011) Lung cancer risk among smokers of menthol cigarettes. Journal of the National Cancer Institute 103:810-6. [Funded by National Cancer Institute]

Brooks DR, Palmer JR, Strom BL, Rosenberg L (2003) Menthol cigarettes and risk of lung cancer. American Journal of Epidemiology 158:609-16. [Funded by by National Institutes of Health and by the US Food and Drug Administration]

Carpenter CL, Jarvik ME, Morgenstern H, McCarthy WJ, London SJ (1999) Menthol cigarette smoking and lung-cancer risk. Annals of Epidemiology 9:114-20. [Funded by the State of California Tobacco-Related Disease Research Program and the National Institutes of Health; the California Public Health Foundation which is supported by the California Department of Health Services]

Etzel CJ, Kachroo S, Liu M, D'Amelio A, Dong Q, Cote ML, Wenzlaff AS, Hong WK, Greisinger AJ, Schwartz AG, Spitz MR (2008) Development and validation of a lung cancer risk prediction model for African-Americans. Cancer Prevention Research (Philadelphia) 1:255-65. [Funded by National Cancer Institute grant K07CA093592; National Cancer Institute grants CA55769, CA123208, CA60691, and CA87895; National Cancer Institute contract N01-PC35745; Flight Attendant Medical Research Institute]

Disease Risk: Table of Referenced Sources

Author Name(s)	Article Title	Year Pub.	Funded By	Type of Study	Subject Description (Including Special population(s))	Sample Size (N)	Authors' Results/Conclusion(s) related to Menthol* (excerpted directly from article)
Blot WJ, Cohen SS, Aldrich M, McLaughlin JK, Hargreaves MK, Signorello LB.	Lung cancer risk among smokers of menthol cigarettes.	2011	The National Cancer Institute	Prospective	12,373 smokers who participated in a follow up of the Southern Community Cohort Study	440 incident lung cancer case patients and 2213 matched control subjects	A lower lung cancer incidence was noted in menthol vs nonmenthol smokers (for smokers of <10, 10–19, and •20 cigarettes per day, compared with never smokers, OR = 5.0 vs 10.3, 8.7 vs 12.9, and 12.2 vs 21.1, respectively). These trends were mirrored for lung cancer mortality.
Brooks DR, Palmer JR, Strom BL, Rosenberg L.	Menthol cigarettes and risk of lung cancer.	2003	The National Institutes of Health and the US Food and Drug Administration	Case-control	40-74 years of age who had no history of cancer, had smoked cigarettes for at least 20 years, and had been interviewed during the period 1981-2000 fpr the Slone Epidemiology Center Case Control Surveillance Study	N=643ses N=4110 controls	The lung cancer risk for long-term smokers of menthol cigarettes was similar to that for smokers of nonmenthol cigarettes(odds ratio= 0.97,95% confidence interval: 0.70, 1.34). Odds ratios were also close to 1. 0 in separate analyses of male, female, Black, and White subjects. The results of this study do not support the hypothesis that smoking menthol cigarettes increases the risk of lung cancer relative to smoking nonmenthol cigarettes.
Carpenter CL, Jarvik ME, Morgenstern H, McCarthy WJ, London SJ.	Mentholated cigarette smoking and lung-cancer risk.	1999	The State of California Tobacco-Related Disease Research Program and the National Institutes of Health; the California Public Health Foundation which is supported by the California Department of Health Services	Case-control	Incident cases of lung cancer were identified between 1991 and 1994 from 35 hospitals in Los Angeles County, CA; African Americans and Caucasians ages 40-84 yrs, with no prior cancer other than melanoma of skin	Number of incident cases= 337 and Population control=478	Our results suggest that lung cancer risk for smoking mentholated cigarettes resembles risk of smoking non-mentholated cigarettes.

Author Name(s)	Article Title	Year Pub.	Funded By	Type of Study	Subject Description (Including Special population(s))	Sample Size (N)	Authors' Results/Conclusion(s) related to Menthol* (excerpted directly from article)
Etzel CJ, Kachroo S, Liu M, D'Amelio A, Dong Q, Cote ML, Wenzlaff AS, Hong WK,	Development and validation of a lung cancer risk prediction model for African-Americans.	2008	National Cancer Institute grant K07CA093592; National Cancer Institute grants CA55769, CA123208, CA60691, and CA87895; National Cancer	Case-control	African-American, Men and Women, from The University of Texas M. Anderson Cancer Center and the Midrael DeBakey VA Medical	Cases N=491 Controls N=497	In our analysis, we observed no significant risks of lung cancer among former or current smokers who reported smoking mentholated cigarettes (OR range 0.69 -.0.99)
Greisinger AJ, Schwartz AG, Spitz MR.			Institute contract N01-PC35745; Flight Attendant Medical Research Institute		Center, both in Houston, from 1995 to 2005. All cases with newly diagnosed, histopathologically confirmed, and untreated lung cancer were eligible for the study. Case exclusion criteria for the study included prior hemotherapy or radiotherapy or recent blood transfusion. We recruited our control population from Houston area community centers and the Kelsey-Seybold Clinic, Houston's largest multispecialty physicians group practice.		

Author Name(s)	Article Title	Year Pub.	Funded By	Type of Study	Subject Description (Including Special population(s))	Sample	Authors' Results/Conclusion(s) related to Menthol* (excerpted directly from article)
Everhart J, Ferketich AK, Browning K et al.	Acculturation and misclassification of tobacco use status among Hispanic men and women in the United States.	2009	Summer Research Opportunities Program at the Ohio State University	Cross-sectional survey	Data from self-reported "Mexican American" or "other Hispanic" participants of the 1999-2002 National Health and Nutrition Examination Surveys who were at least 20 years old.	N=3982 for the 1999-2000 wave N=3293 for the 2001-2001 wave	Among males ($n = 1,175$), the prevalence estimates of misclassification were 4.8%, 1.8%, and 2.2% for low, medium, and highly acculturated males, respectively ($p < .02$). Among females ($n = 1,345$), the prevalence estimates of misclassification were 0.8%, 2.0%, and 4.9% for low, medium, and highly acculturated females, respectively ($p < .03$). [not menthol specific]
Friedman GD, Sadler M, Tekawa IS,	Mentholated cigarettes and non-lung smoking	1998	National Cancer Institute grant R35 CA 49761	Retrospective Survey	In 1979-1985, 79,946 subscribers of the Kaiser Permanente	N=5770 men And N=5990 women,	Risk was not increased among persons who currently smoked mentholated compared with plain cigarettes for all of the non-lung smoking
Sidney S.	related cancers in California, USA.				Medical Care Program in northern CA, age 30- 89 years, completed a detailed questionnaire about smoking habits and were followed up through 1994.	currently smoking cigarettes and for at least 20 years, no smoking related cancer at entry, recorded whether their current cigarette was mentholated. .	related cancers combined or for most sites studied

Disease Risk: Table of Referenced Sources (Continued)

Author Name(s)	Article Title	Year Pub.	Funded By	Type of Study	Subject Description (Including Special population(s))	Sample Size (N)	Authors' Results/Conclusion(s) related to Menthol* (excerpted directly from article)
Hebert JR, Kabat GC.	Menthol cigarettes and esophageal cancer.	1988	No funding source(s) provided. Authors affiliated with the American Health Foundation	Case-control	Male and female menthol smokers	Cases: N=96 female, N=216 male; Control: N=157 female, N=305 male	We analyzed existing data from a case-control study ofesophageal cancer and found no menthol effect.
Hebert JR, Kabat GC.	Menthol cigarette smoking and oesophageal cancer.	1989	National Cancer Institute and American Cancer Society	Hospital-based, case-control	Patients were interviewed in 20 hospitals in 9 US cities from 1969 to 1984; Smokers were included in cases and control	N=172 cases N=184 controls	Our results do not support the hypothesized relationship between menthol cigarette smoking and oesophageal cancer.
Jöckel K-H, Pohlabeln H, Jahn I.	Use of menthol cigarettes and risk of lung cancer.	2004	No funding source(s) provided. Author affiliated with the Institut fur Medizinishche Informatik	Hospital-based study	Not specified	1004 incident lung cancer cases (839 males and 165 females) and the same number of population controls	The present study gives no indication for an additional risk of ever smoking menthol cigarettes if total amount of smoking is taken into account.
Kabat GC, Hebert JR.	Use of mentholated cigarettes and lung cancer risk.	1991	National Cancer Institute Program Project Grant CA32617 and Center Grant CAI7613	Case-control	Current cigarette Smokers interviewed between 1985 and 1990.	N=588 male lung cancer cases and 914 male control patients;	No significant association was observed between either short-term (1-14 years) or long- term (15+ years) menthol use and lung cancer in logistic regression analyses adjusting for covariates. For specific histological types of lung cancer there was

Author Name(s)	Article Title	Year Pub.	Funded By	Type of Study	Subject Description (Including Special population(s))	Sample Size (N)	Authors' Results/Conclusion(s) related to Menthol* (excerpted directly from article)
						N=456 female lung cancer cases and 410 female controls	no indication of an association with menthol usage.
Kabat GC, Hebert JR.	Use of mentholated cigarettes and oropharyngeal cancer.	1994	National Cancer Institute Program Project Grant CA32617 and Center Grant CAI7613	Case-control	Current smokers	N=194 male and 82 female newly diagnosed, histologically confirmed cases of oropharyngeal cancer; 845 male and 411 female controls	Use of mentholated cigarettes is unlikely to be an important independent factor in oropharyngeal cancer.
Lee PN	Systematic review of the epidemiological evidence comparing lung cancer risk in	2011	Lorillard Tobacco Company	Meta-analysis	Eight epidemiological studies	Not Applicable	The data do not suggest any effect of mentholation on lung cancer risk.
	smokers of menthol and unmenthol cigarettes						
Mendiondo MS, Alexander LA, Crawford	Health profile differences for menthol and	2010			Current and former smokers 18+ years old	N=12,004	Overall, current menthol and non-menthol smokers have similar health profiles.

Disease Risk: Table of Referenced Sources (Continued)

Author Name(s)	Article Title	Year Pub.	Funded By	Type of Study	Subject Description (Including Special population(s))	Sample Size (N)	Authors' Results/Conclusion(s) related to Menthol* (excerpted directly from article)
T.	nonmenthol smokers: findings from the National Health Interview Survey.		No funding source(s) provided. Authors affiliated with University of Kentucky	Cross-sectional study (2005 National Health Interview Survey and its cancer control supplement)			
Murray RP, Connett JE, Skeans MA, Tashkin DP.	Menthol cigarettes and health risks in Lung Health Study data.	2007	Grant HR 46002 from the Division of Lung Disease; National Heart, Lung, and Blood Institute; National Institutes of Health	Randomized Controlled Trial	Adult smokers in a clinical trial of smoking cessation and ipratropium in the prevention of chronic obstructive pulmonary disease.	N=5,887	We conclude that our data contain no evidence that mentholation of cigarettes increases the hazards of smoking.
Pletcher MJ, Hulley BJ, Houston T, Kiefe CI, Benowitz N, Sidney S.	Menthol cigarettes, smoking cessation, atherosclerosis, and pulmonary function: the Coronary Artery Risk Development in Young Adults (CARDIA) Study.	2006	Contracts N01-HC-48047, N01-HC-48048, N01-HC-48049, N01-HC-48050, and N01-HC-95095 from the National Heart, Lung, and Blood Institute	Multi-center U.S. cohort study (CARDIA)	African American and European American smokers aged 18 to 30 years and healthy at the time of enrollment in 1985	1544 (non-menthol smokers (n = 563) and menthol smokers (n = 972))	Menthol and nonmenthol cigarettes seem to be equally harmful per cigarette smoked in terms of atherosclerosis and pulmonary function decline, but menthol cigarettes may be harder to quit smoking.

Author Name(s)	Article Title	Year Pub.	Funded By	Type of Study	Subject Description (Including Special population(s))	Sample Size (N)	Authors' Results/Conclusion(s) related to Menthol* (excerpted directly from article)
Sidney S, Tekawa IS, Friedman GD, Sadler MC, Tashkin DP.	Mentholated cigarette use and lung cancer.	1995	Grants R01 CA 36704 and R35 CA 49761 from the US National Cancer Institute	Cohort	Members of the Northern California Kaiser Permanente Medical Care Program, Oakland (5771 men and 3990 women), aged 30 to 89 years, who underwent a multiphasic health checkup in 1979 through 1985 and reported that they were current cigarette smokers who had smoked for at least 20 years.	N=11,761	This study suggests that there is an increased risk of lung cancer associated with mentholated cigarette use in male smokers but not in female smokers.
Stellman SD, Chen Y, Muscat JE, Djordjevic MV, Richie JP Jr, Lazarus P, Thompson S, Altorki N, Berwick M, Citron ML, Harlap S, Kaur TB, Neugut AI, Olson S, Travaline JM,	Lung cancer risk in white and black Americans.	2003	US Public Health Service grants CA-68384, CA-91401, and CA-17613	Comparative , case- control	White males, white females, black males, black females	N=1,710 white male and 1,321 white female cases of histologically confirmed lung cancer, 254 black male and 163 black female cases, and 8,151 controls.	Lung cancer risks were similar for whites and blacks with similar smoking habits, except possibly for blacks who were very heavy smokers; this sub-group is unusual in the general population of African American smokers. Explanations of racial disparities in lung cancer risk may need to account for modifying factors including type of cigarette (yield, mentholation), diet, occupation, and host factors such as ability to metabolize mainstream smoke carcinogens.

Disease Risk: Table of Referenced Sources (Continued)

Author Name(s)	Article Title	Year Pub.	Funded By	Type of Study	Subject Description (Including Special population(s))	Sample Size (N)	Authors' Results/Conclusion(s) related to Menthol* (excerpted directly from article)
Witorsch P, Zhang ZF.							
Yeager DS & Krosnick JA.	The validity of self-reported nicotine product use in the 2001-2008 National Health and Nutrition Examination Survey.	2010	No funding source(s) provided. Authors affiliated with Stanford University	Area-probability sample survey	NHANES respondents 20+ years old who participated in 2001–2002, 2003–2004, 2005– 2006, and 2007–2008 surveys	N=4000+ respondents for each wave	These data do not support the claim that a substantial number of adult respondents intentionally under- report nicotine consumption in face-to-face interviews. [not menthol specific]

*Note: these statements are taken directly from articles and may not include all relevant results/conclusions.

Everhart J, Ferketich AK, Browning K et al. (2009) Acculturation and misclassification of tobacco use status among Hispanic men and women in the United States. Nicotine and Tobacco Research 11(3): 240-247. [Funding provided by the Sumemr Research Opportunities Program at the Ohio State University].

Friedman GD, Sadler M, Tekawa IS, Sidney S (1998) Menthol cigarettes and non-lung smoking related cancers in California, USA. Journal of Epidemiology and Community Health 52:202. [Funded by National Cancer Institute grant R35 CA 49761]

Hebert JR, Kabat GC (1988) Menthol cigarettes and esophageal cancer. American Journal of Public Health 78:986-7. [No funding source(s) provided. Authors affiliated with the American Health Foundation]

Hebert JR, Kabat GC (1989) Menthol cigarette smoking and oesophageal cancer. International Journal of Epidemiology 18:37-44. [Funded by National Cancer Institute and American Cancer Society]

Jöckel K-H, Pohlabeln H, Jahn I (2004) Use of menthol cigarettes and risk of lung cancer. Biometrical Journal 46:33. [No funding source(s) provided. Author affiliated with the Institut fur Medizinishche Informatik]

Kabat GC, Hebert JR (1991) Use of menthol cigarettes and lung cancer risk. Cancer Research 51:6510-3. [Funded by National Cancer Institute Program Project Grant CA32617 and Center Grant CAI7613]

Kabat GC, Hebert JR (1994) Use of menthol cigarettes and oropharyngeal cancer. Epidemiology 5:183-8. [Funded by National Cancer Institute Program Project Grant CA32617 and Center Grant CAI7613]

Lee PN (2011) Systematic review of the epidemiological evidence comparing lung cancer risk in smokers of menthol and unmenthol cigarettes. BMC Pulmonary Medicine 11:18. [Funded by the Lorillard Tobacco Company]

Mendiondo MS, Alexander LA, Crawford T (2010) Health profile differences for menthol and nonmenthol smokers: findings from the National Health Interview Survey. Addiction 105(suppl 1):124-40. [No funding source(s) provided. Authors affiliated with University of Kentucky]

Murray RP, Connett JE, Skeans MA, Tashkin DP (2007) Menthol cigarettes and health risks in Lung Health Study data. Nicotine & Tobacco Research 9:101-7. [Funding provide by Grant HR 46002 from the Division of Lung Disease; National Heart, Lung, and Blood Institute; National Institutes of Health]

Pletcher MJ, Hulley BJ, Houston T, Kiefe CI, Benowitz N, Sidney S (2006) Menthol cigarettes, smoking cessation, atherosclerosis, and pulmonary function: the Coronary Artery Risk Development in Young Adults (CARDIA) Study. Archives of Internal Medicine 166:1915-22. [Funded by Contracts N01-HC-48047, N01-HC-48048, N01-HC-48049, N01-HC-48050, and N01-HC-95095 from the National Heart, Lung, and Blood Institute]

Sidney S, Tekawa IS, Friedman GD, Sadler MC, Tashkin DP (1995) Menthol cigarette use and lung cancer. Archives of Internal Medicine 155:727-32. [Funded by Grants R01 CA 36704 and R35 CA 49761 from the US National Cancer Institute]

Stellman SD, Chen Y, Muscat JE, Djordjevic MV, Richie JP, Lazarus P, Thompson S, Altorki N, Berwick M, Citron ML, Harlap S, Kaur TB, Neugut AI, Olson S, Travaline JM, Witorsch P, Zhang ZF (2003) Lung cancer risk in white and black Americans.

Annals of Epidemiology 13:294-302. [Funded by US Public Health Service grants CA-68384, CA-91401, and CA-17613]

Yeager DS & Krosnick JA (2010) The validity of self-reported nicotine product use in the 2001-2008 National Health and Nutrition Examination Survey. Medical Care 48(12): 1128-1132. [No funding source(s) provided. Authors affiliated with Stanford University]

In: Health Effects of Menthol Cigarettes
Editors: Mark C. Eldridge and Edward Forester
ISBN: 978-1-62948-291-0

Chapter 2

Reference Addendum: Preliminary Scientific Evaluation of the Possible Public Health Effects of Menthol versus Nonmenthol Cigarettes*

Food and Drug Administration

Introduction

The "Preliminary Scientific Evaluation of the Possible Public Health Effects of Menthol versus Nonmenthol Cigarettes" was submitted for Peer Review in August 2011. Since that time, several peer-reviewed articles have been published that relate to this topic. This reference addendum provides a summary of updated research relevant to the full scientific review.

On March 27, 2013, a systematic literature search was conducted in the PubMed database using the search term "menthol" and including articles published between July 1, 2011 and March 27, 2013.

As with the full scientific review, only original peer-reviewed publications were used. Basic information on menthol has been included here only as background; as with the full scientific review, this addendum is not intended to be a comprehensive review of menthol itself but rather menthol as related to its use in menthol cigarettes. General methodology caveats (e.g., self-report) and descriptions (e.g., TRPM8 channels, large national surveys) were discussed in the full scientific review, and will not be duplicated here.

NOTE: The 2012 SGR, "Preventing Tobacco Use Among Youth and Young Adults", did not contain any information on the public health effects of menthol versus nonmenthol cigarettes that was not included in the original report.

---

* This is an edited, reformatted and augmented version of a Food and Drug Administration publication, dated 2013.

Smoke Chemistry and Nonclinical Toxicology

Seven additional articles regarding the association between menthol in cigarettes and smoke chemistry and nonclinical toxicity were reviewed.

Smoke Chemistry

One study compared the Federal Trade Commission (FTC)-measured nicotine levels of menthol and nonmenthol cigarette brands smoked by smokers who participated in the 2001-2006 National Health and Nutrition Examination Survey (NHANES), a nationally representative household survey. Participants either provided a cigarette pack or information on their usual brand, and Universal Product Code information was used to verify menthol versus nonmenthol classification.

The researchers found that the brands of menthol cigarettes smoked by African Americans had a higher average FTC nicotine level than the menthol cigarettes smoked by White smokers (Caraballo et al., 2011).

In another study, cigarettes with four different menthol levels were created and smoked through a linear-port smoking machine. The collected total particulate matter (TPM) was analyzed for menthol, nicotine, tobacco-specific nitrosamines (TSNAs), polynuclear aromatic hydrocarbons, cotinine, and quinolone, and whole smoke was collected for measurement of volatile organic compounds.

Although differences in the amount of menthol present in the TPM existed, there were no differences in any of the other target constituents. Thus, while menthol in TPM increased in a linear fashion, the other measured constituents remained unchanged (Gordon et al., 2011).

Using the Health Canada method of machine smoking, Bodnar and colleagues (2012) compared levels of 19 constituents in 61 brand styles of fire-standard compliant cigarettes. The researchers found few differences in the measured levels of constituents between menthol and nonmenthol cigarettes.

In some cases, for some styles, there were greater levels of a constituent (e.g., 2-aminonaphathalene, catechol) in menthol cigarettes, while levels of other constituents (e.g., benzo[a]pyrene, catechol, crotonaldehyde) were greater for nonmenthol cigarettes. There was no consistent direction of difference and, in the case of catechol, the difference occurred in the opposite direction when "full flavor" and "lights" were compared (Bodnar, Morgan, Murphy, & Ogden, 2012).

Brinkman and colleagues (2012) examined participant-specific mainstream smoke for 4-(methylnitrosamino)-1-(3-pyridyl)-1-butanone (NNK), nicotine, ultrafine and fine particulate matter by simulated use (used topography measurements) using a programmable linear smoking machine.

Overall, the researchers found no differences in fine particulate matter between menthol and nonmenthol test cigarettes. However, a significantly larger mass of ultrafine particulate was collected from the menthol cigarettes ($p<0.05$) (Brinkman et al., 2012).

Menthol as a Singular Compound – Toxicology, Pharmacology and Therapeutic Applications

Another study found that, when added to mucoadhesive patches, menthol increased permeability of the oral mucosa, as measured with a porcine buccal tissue preparation. This allowed greater absorption of fenretinide, a chemopreventive compound (Wu et al., 2012).

Antiproliferative Effects of Menthol as a Singular Compound

Valero and colleagues (2012) examined the effects of menthol on cell survival and cell proliferation of normal and cancerous human prostate cell lines. The prostate-derived cell lines were cultured, expression of TRMP8 receptors was confirmed, and proliferation was estimated using the methyl tetralam (MTT) assay (which assesses metabolic activity). Menthol increased metabolic activity but there was no consistent change in growth after stimulation of TRPM8 channels with menthol (Valero, Mello de, Stuhmer, Viana, & Pardo, 2012).

In Vitro Toxicity of Menthol Tobacco Exposure

Fowler and colleagues (2012) treated six cell types (rodent cell lines V79, CHL and CHO, p-53 competent human peripheral blood lymphocytes, TK6 human lymphoblastoid cells, and the human liver cell line HepG2) with racemic menthol. Treatment with menthol was cytotoxic.

However, the authors suggest that this is a "false positive" since there was no genotoxic effect as measured by micronucleus induction. The authors note that testing was limited by cytotoxicity, and even though required levels of cytotoxicity were induced, micronucleus induction was not (Fowler et al., 2012). Thus, the dose-response curve may have been too narrow to detect micronucleus induction.

Conclusion

The addition of these articles did not change the finding of the full scientific review, namely that the weight of evidence supports the conclusion that, from a nonclinical toxicity standpoint, menthol in cigarettes is not associated with either increased or decreased smoke toxicity.

Physiology

Seventeen additional articles regarding the association between menthol in cigarettes and physiological response to tobacco smoke were reviewed.

Sensory Effects

The effect of menthol on cough threshold was evaluated in 13 subjects (12 nonsmokers) during single-inhalation capsaicin challenges. Inhalation of menthol vapor prior to measuring cough thresholds resulted in reduced sensitivity to cough in some subjects. That is, for some, but not all, of the subjects, the amount of capsaicin needed to trigger a cough response was increased following menthol vapor exposure.

The authors concluded that adding menthol to cigarettes may increase the tolerability of tobacco smoke by reducing the sensitivity of an airway defense mechanism (coughing) (Wise, Breslin, & Dalton, 2012).

A study of 14 patients with chronic cough and airway sensitivity to environmental irritants and 15 control subjects evaluated the effect of inhaling nebulized menthol on cough threshold provoked with capsaicin inhalation. Inhaled menthol reduced cough sensitivity to the inhaled capsaicin and influenced inspiratory flows in the patients, an effect that did not occur in the control group ($p<0-05$).

Furthermore, in people with chronic cough (without asthma, chronic obstructive pulmonary disease or infection), pre-inhalation of menthol reduced the threshold to capsaicin-stimulated cough ($p<0.05$).

The authors state that "the use of menthol in different cigarette brands could be questioned since it could conceal the natural irritation following smoking" (Millqvist, Ternesten-Hasseus, & Bende, 2013).

The somatosensory effects of topically-applied capsaicin and menthol were assessed in a cross-over study with 15 subjects. When menthol was topically applied to the gingiva, nine subjects reported mild levels of pain.

Pain ratings were lower than those reported following application of capsaicin, and were also more short-lived. Menthol elicited hypersensitivity to both cold and warm stimuli (Lu, BaadHansen, List, Zhang, & Svensson, 2013).

A laboratory study involving 22 adults (age 21-46 years) investigated the effect of menthol on stimulated nasal irritation. In this study, participants simultaneously sniffed clean air into one nostril while sniffing a chemical vapor into the other. Acetic acid and allyl isothiocyanate produced nasal irritation, and menthol pretreatment had different effects. Menthol exposure prior to stimulation with acetic acid resulted in decreased sensitivity to irritation but prompted increased sensitivity to allyl isothiocyanate ($p<0.005$). Thus, menthol can modify irritating stimuli differently (Wise, Preti, Eades, & Wysocki, 2011).

In another study, researchers applied the irritant capsaicin to the nasal mucosa in order to assess threshold to cough and urge to cough. When menthol alone was applied, subjects reported a refreshing feeling and cooling sensation. Menthol administration decreased cough sensitivity produced by capsaicin ($p<0.05$), such that higher levels of capsaicin were needed to produce coughing, and fewer coughs were produced ($p<0.01$). Urge to cough also increased with higher capsaicin concentrations ($p<0.01$), indicating that subjects were less sensitive to capsaicin.

Subjects reported that menthol reduced the intensity of capsaicin irritation of the nasal mucosa, thus increasing capsaicin tolerability (Buday et al., 2012).

A randomized cross-over study by Pereira and colleagues (2013) investigated the effect of inhaled menthol on upper airway resistance during quiet breathing. The upper airway resistance of ten participants was examined following exposure to menthol and was compared to regular room air. Nine out of 10 participants reported that that they could breathe more easily on the menthol test day; however, upper airway resistance was not significantly affected (Pereira, Sim, Driver, Parker, & Fitzpatrick, 2013). The discordance between sensation and physiological response has been noted in the full scientific review.

Twenty subjects participated in a lateralization test of menthol, eucalyptol, mustard oil, a mixture of menthol and eucalyptol, and a mixture of menthol and mustard oil. After exposure, participants identified which nostril was presented with the target odorant. They also rated the intensity and pleasantness of each odorant, and attached three descriptors. All odorants activated the trigeminal system and were easily accurately lateralized ($p<0.001$). Menthol was described as cool, fresh and tickling. Agonists of different trigeminal receptors had clearly dissociated lateralization scores.

Thus, activation of the trigeminal nerve by TRPM8 agonists (menthol, eucaluptol) elicited a different response than the TRPM1 agonist mustard oil (Frasnelli, Albrecht, Bryant, & Lundstrom, 2011).

Ashley et al. (2012) conducted a study in Japan and Poland to investigate mouth level exposure (MLE) to nicotine using filter analysis. In this cross-over study, 800 subjects (regular nonmenthol smokers, occasional and regular menthol smokers) smoked each of five types of test cigarettes (nonmenthol and four levels of natural or synthetic menthol, matched for their usual tar level) and completed questionnaires assessing the sensory characteristics of the test cigarettes.

Both Japanese and Polish smokers who occasionally smoked menthol cigarettes reported increased perceived irritation as compared to those who regularly smoked menthol cigarettes ($p<0.05$). In all Japanese smokers, the level of menthol loading affected the perceived strength of menthol taste and intensity of cooling ($p<0.05$); this effect was less notable among the Polish smokers.

Both Japanese and Polish smokers reported differences in how synthetic and natural menthol cigarettes were perceived (Ashley, Dixon, Sisodiya, & Prasad, 2012). Taken together, these data suggest that use of synthetic or natural menthol may impact the sensory characteristics of the cigarette. Since the cigarette styles were matched for the country, product differences may have contributed to country-related differences.

Mechanisms of Menthol Action

Using isolated dorsal root ganglion neurons from rats, the effects of heat, anthralic acid (ACA) and 2- aminoethyl diphenylborinate (2-APB), both putative TRPM8 channel blockers, on stimulation of TRPM8 currents by noxious cold or menthol. Menthol consistently produced TRPM8 currents, confirming its activity at that receptor. Heat inhibited TRPM8 channel currents.

Unlike the currents produced by noxious cold, currents produced by menthol were blocked by neither ACA nor 2-APB (Naziroglu & Ozgul, 2012). According to the authors, this study confirms that menthol activates TRPM8 channels; however, it is unclear whether one or both of the putative TRPM8 blockers are acting at the TRPM8 site, given conflicting reports of their blocking actions.

TRPM8 channel sensitivity to menthol was investigated using tetrameric TRPM8 constructs. Using electrophysiological and intracellular Ca2+ as measurements for current activity in HEK293 cells transfected with TRPM8 channels, researchers assessed the stoichiometry of menthol ligand attachment. Up to four menthol molecules can independently bind to a single TRPM8 channel, with each bound molecule producing a similar energetic stabilization of the open channel, resulting in a step- wise stabilization of the open state (Janssens & Voets, 2011). This provides more specific information about how menthol interacts with the TRPM8 channel.

An *in vitro* model of CYP2A6 and CYP2A13 activity (part of the metabolism pathway of nicotine and NNK) was used to assess relative inhibition produced by several compounds, including menthol. When activity was stimulated with coumarin, menthol was less potent as an inhibitor than the other tested compounds. There was no evidence that menthol inactivated CYP2A6 or CYP2A13. The authors concluded that menthol may not influence nicotine and NNK metabolism in smokers (Kramlinger, von Weymarn, & Murphy, 2012).

Cheang and colleagues (2013) investigated the effect of treatment with menthol on rat aortae and mesenteric and coronary arteries. Menthol induced relation (e.g., dilation) in the three types of arteries in a concentration-dependent manner. Using a smooth muscle cell line, the researchers determined that this effect was mediated by inhibition of calcium influx (Cheang et al., 2013). This demonstrates menthol activity at a receptor other than the TRPM8 receptor.

A study by Willis and colleagues (2011) used a mouse model to study the sensory irritation response elicited by acrolein, acetic acid and cyclohexane vapors (smoke irritants). The irritation produced by these chemicals was reversed by menthol, even at concentrations lower than in menthol cigarette smoke ($p<0.005$). The TRPM8 receptor mediated this effect; other TRPM8 agonists also abolished the irritant effect, and menthol's effects were reversed by a TRPM8 antagonist. Menthol also acted via the capsaicin receptor. The authors concluded that menthol may facilitate smoke inhalation (Willis, Liu, Ha, Jordt, & Morris, 2011).

Hans and colleagues (2012) investigated how nicotinic receptors are modulated by menthol. Menthol reversibly bound to both native and recombinant nicotinic receptors in a concentration-dependent manner ($p<0.005$). Single channel and whole-cell recordings from nicotinic receptors expressed in HEK tsA201 cells established that menthol acts as a negative allosteric modulator (Hans, Wilhelm, & Swandulla, 2012). This finding suggests that menthol directly interacts with nicotinic receptors.

Using PET scans, Brody and colleagues (2012) compared the relative densities of a2134 nicotinic acetylcholine receptors (AChRs) of menthol ($n=22$) and nonmenthol ($n=41$) smokers. Menthol smokers exhibited greater densities in the brainstem, cerebellum and corpus callosum ($p<0.05$), but not the thalamus or prefrontal cortex. According to the author, this may be a result of greater exposure, and may help explain why menthol smokers have a more difficult time quitting compared to nonmenthol smokers (Brody et al., 2012).

Effect of Menthol on Smoking Topography

In a cross-over study by Brinkman and colleagues (2012), nine participants smoked either menthol or nonmenthol cigarettes for one week. During a single laboratory session, smoking topography measurements were taken. When smoking the menthol test cigarettes, participants had greater volume of inhaled smoke, took longer puffs and took more time while smoking ($p<0.05$). This suggests that, when smoking menthol cigarettes, there was greater exposure to smoke. There were no inter-puff interval differences or differences in inspiration time (Brinkman et al., 2012).

In a laboratory study, Strasser and colleagues (2013) randomized 32 adult smokers to an experimental group (menthol Camel Crush for 15 days followed by nonmenthol Camel Crush for 15 days) or a control group (usual brand for 30 days).

Every five days, laboratory assessments of smoking topography (total puff volume of each of two cigarettes) were taken. Compared to baseline, the experimental group evidenced a slight increase in total puff volume when smoking menthol Camel Crush cigarettes, compared to a larger increase under the nonmenthol Camel Crush condition ($p=0.02$) (Strasser et al., 2013). That is, although both conditions produced increased puff volumes, there was a smaller increase under the menthol Camel Crush condition.

It is unclear whether these differences are the result of the brand or the presence/absence of menthol versus nonmenthol. It is unknown if there was an influence of time since usual brand on smoking behavior since there was no randomization to avoid order effects; menthol Camel Crush always preceded nonmenthol Camel Crush, and increased exposure to Camel Crush generally and/or greater time away from usual brand may impact behavior.

Conclusion

The addition of these articles did not change the conclusion presented in the full scientific review: the weight of evidence supports the conclusion that menthol in cigarettes is likely associated with altered physiological responses to tobacco smoke.

Biomarkers

Eleven additional articles evaluating the association between menthol in cigarettes and biomarkers of exposure were reviewed.

Biomarkers of Exposure to Carbon Monoxide (CO)

In the Strasser et al. study described above, laboratory assessments of biomarkers of exposure (including breath carbon monoxide [CO] before and after smoking each of two cigarettes) were taken every five days. CO measurements decreased from baseline in Camel Crush smokers ($p=0.033$), with no differences between the Camel Crush conditions (Strasser et al., 2013).

It is unknown if there was an influence of time since usual brand on smoking behavior since there was no randomization to avoid order effects; menthol Camel Crush always preceded nonmenthol Camel Crush, and increased exposure to Camel Crush generally and/or greater time away from usual brand may impact behavior.

Using data and biospecimens from the Total Exposure Study, a large cross-sectional study of smokers at least 21 years, levels of carboxyhemoglobin of 1044 menthol and 2297 nonmenthol smokers were compared. There was no difference (Sarkar, Wang, & Liang, 2012). It is unclear what, if any, adjustments were made for this analysis.

Biomarkers of Exposure to Nicotine

A nonclinical study by Abobo and colleagues (2012) examined the effect of menthol on the pharmacokinetics of nicotine. Rats were exposed to mainstream smoke under either a single-cigarette smoke inhalation procedure (1 puff/minute for 10 minutes) or a multiple-cigarette smoke inhalation procedure (equivalent to 17 cigarettes via 10 puffs every 12 hours). Following both the single- and multiple-cigarette smoke inhalation procedures, menthol cigarette smoke resulted in lower maximum plasma levels of nicotine and cotinine ($p<0.05$). Following the multiple-cigarette smoke inhalation procedure, menthol appeared to influence nicotine metabolism as indicated by a shorter relative half-life. The authors suggest that the reduced maximum levels of nicotine associated with menthol smoke may be impacted by differences in aversiveness (i.e., the rats inhale less menthol smoke as compared to nonmenthol smoke), and/or an altered nicotine half-life (Abobo, Ma, & Liang, 2012).

In a cross-over study, Brinkman and colleagues (2012) found no differences in urine levels of cotinine in subjects who smoked either menthol or nonmenthol test cigarettes for a week each ; When MLE to nicotine was estimated by quantifying solanesol levels in cigarette butts, menthol cigarettes had higher levels than nonmenthol cigarettes ($p<0.05$) (Brinkman et al., 2012).

In the study by Ashley et al. (2012) described above, Japanese smokers in the higher tar group (4 mg tar yield) exhibited no effects of menthol loading or type of menthol on nicotine MLE. In the lower tar group (1 mg tar yield), the occasional menthol smokers had higher nicotine MLE when smoking the high loading natural menthol cigarette as compared to the nonmenthol cigarette.

Among Polish smokers, smokers in the lower tar group with the low synthetic menthol cigarettes had higher MLE to nicotine as compared to the high synthetic nicotine product (Ashley et al., 2012). Taken together, these data suggest that use of synthetic or natural menthol may impact MLE to nicotine. As noted earlier, since the cigarette styles were matched for the country, product differences may have contributed to country-related differences.

MLE was also assessed by Nelson and colleagues (2011). In this study, 1330 subjects who smoked their usual brand-style of cigarettes collected their butts for two days. A subset of this group repeated the test cycle as a check of replicability. Saliva samples were collected after two days when the subjects returned their butts. Six of the 26 brands included in this study were menthol brands.

There were no differences in MLE per cigarette for menthol brands as compared to nonmenthol brands (Nelson, Chen, Dixon, & Steichen, 2011). There were three times as many test-cycles with nonmenthol cigarettes as menthol cigarettes; such a skewed sample may have implications regarding confidence in the statistical analyses. There was no information on the possible inclusion of menthol as an additive to the nonmenthol brands; even low levels of menthol may impact smoking behavior and, therefore, MLE of nicotine.

In the study described above, Strasser and colleagues (2013) conducted laboratory assessments of biomarkers of exposure (including nicotine and cotinine on days five, 20 and 35) every five days.

The researchers found no effect of menthol/nonmenthol on nicotine or cotinine levels (Strasser et al., 2013). It is unknown if there was an influence of time since usual brand on smoking behavior since there was no randomization to avoid order effects; menthol Camel Crush always preceded nonmenthol Camel Crush, and increased exposure to Camel Crush generally and/or greater time away from usual brand may impact behavior.

In a study of adult smokers, Benowitz and colleagues (2011) compared the plasma nicotine levels of 60 menthol smokers to those of 67 nonmenthol smokers. Plasma nicotine levels and urine nicotine equivalents were significantly higher in regular compared to menthol cigarette smokers ($p<0.05$) (Benowitz, Dains, Dempsey, Wilson, & Jacob, 2011). Over 70% of African American smokers smoked menthol cigarettes, compared to 25% of White smokers; thus, race/ethnicity may be a factor mediating these results.

Using 1999-2004 NHANES data, Jones and colleagues (2012) investigated possible associations between current menthol versus nonmenthol cigarette smokers and peripheral artery disease. As part of this study, serum cotinine levels were compared. Menthol cigarette smokers (n=310) were observed to have higher serum cotinine compared to nonmenthol cigarette smokers (n=734).

As noted by the authors, a cautious interpretation is warranted since this was a descriptive finding and the data were not adjusted for smoking patterns, sociodemographic characteristics, smoking history (e.g., pack years), or other factors (Jones, Apelberg, Samet, & Navas-Acien, 2012).

A large cross-sectional study of 221 menthol and 274 nonmenthol smokers examined the association between menthol and nicotine update as measured by plasma cotinine levels. Although several covariates were associated with cotinine levels (e.g., time to first cigarette, race, age, BMI, cigarettes per day [cpd]), smoking menthol cigarettes was not ($p=0.66$) (Muscat, Liu, Stellman, & Richie, Jr., 2012).

Using data and biospecimens from the previously described Total Exposure Study, total urinary cotinine, glucuronide metabolite ratios for nicotine (nicotine-N-glucuronide/free nicotine) and cotinine (cotinineN-glucuronide/free cotinine, *trans* 3'-hydroxy cotinine-O-glucuronide/*free* trans 3'-hydroxy cotinine) were calculated for 1044 menthol and 2297 nonmenthol smokers.

There was no difference in total levels of serum cotinine. Although there was no overall difference reported, menthol was a significant factor ($p=0.0145$) for the cotinine metabolite ratios; they were higher among menthol smokers as compared to nonmenthol smokers. There was also a menthol x age effect on *trans* 3'-hydroxy cotinineO-glucuronide ratios, however this effect was not described (Sarkar et al., 2012). Although other factors were found to be significant (e.g., race, age, cpd), it is unclear what, if any, adjustments were made for these analyses.

Menthol and Nonmenthol Smokers

An analysis of data from 1918 menthol and nonmenthol smokers who participated in the 2001-2006 NHANES compared serum cotinine levels of non-Hispanic adult smokers (age 20 years) who reported smoking a menthol brand of cigarettes (n=677) with those who reported smoking a nonmenthol brand (n=1241). After adjusting for cpd, there were no differences between the serum cotinine levels of menthol smokers as compared to nonmenthol smokers (Caraballo et al., 2011). Sample sizes were sufficiently large that the uneven subpopulations are not a concern (Caraballo et al., 2011).

Rostron (2012) used data from the 2007-2010 NHANES to analyze data on total urinary cotinine concentrations of 1452 everyday smokers and compare levels found between everyday menthol and nonmenthol smokers. There were no differences in cotinine levels of menthol and nonmenthol smokers, despite menthol smokers generally smoking fewer cpd. The author noted that nicotine exposure as measured by cotinine generally increased with cpd across race/ethnicity groups for U.S. smokers, but he did not compare menthol subpopulations (e.g., African American menthol smokers compared to White menthol smokers) and nonmenthol subpopulations (African American nonmenthol smokers compared to White nonmenthol smokers). Less than 30% of those surveyed smoked menthol cigarettes, suggesting that sample size may be a limitation (Rostron,B, 2012b).

Biomarkers of Exposure to TSNAs

Jones et al. (2013) used data from 1999-2010 NHANES to compare urine 4-(methylnitrosamino) -1-(3- pyridyl)-1-butanol (NNAL) levels in menthol smokers versus nonmenthol smokers. After adjusting for demographic factors, serum cotinine levels were similar for menthol and nonmenthol smokers (Jones, Apelberg, Tellez-Plaza, Samet, & Navas-Acien, 2013).

In a study of adult smokers, Benowitz and colleagues (2011) compared the urine NNAL levels of 60 menthol smokers to those of 67 nonmenthol smokers and found no differences in urine NNAL levels (Benowitz et al., 2011).

A cross-over study involving participants who smoked menthol and nonmenthol test cigarettes for a week each found no significant differences in urinary levels of NNAL or the carcinogen metabolite 1- hydroxypyrene. When MLE to NNK was estimated by quantifying solanesol levels in cigarette butts, menthol cigarettes were associated with higher estimated MLE NNK levels than nonmenthol cigarettes (Brinkman et al., 2012).

An analysis of 2007-2010 NHANES data on 1447 everyday smokers compared the total urinary NNAL concentrations (adjusted for urinary creatinine levels) of menthol and nonmenthol smokers. Overall, menthol use was associated with lower NNAL concentrations ($p<0.05$), an effect that was primarily driven by White smokers. However, menthol smokers overall, and White menthol smokers specifically, also smoked fewer cpd and cpd was not included as a control variable. The author notes that NNAL generally increased with cpd across race/ethnicity groups for U.S. smokers. Less than 30% of those surveyed smoked menthol cigarettes, suggesting that sample size may be a limitation. Since the same analysis found that lower cpd did not result in differences in cotinine levels, the pharmacokinetic profiles of these constituents may differ (Rostron,B, 2012b).

Using data and biospecimens from the previously described Total Exposure Study, total serum NNAL, and glucuronide metabolite ratios for NNAL (NNAL-O- and N-glucuronide/free NNAL) were calculated for 1044 menthol and 2297 nonmenthol smokers. There was no difference in total levels of NNAL or the glucuronide metabolite ratio (Sarkar et al., 2012).

Conclusion

The addition of these articles did not change the finding of the full scientific review that the weight of evidence supports the conclusion that menthol in cigarettes is likely not associated with increased or decreased levels of biomarkers of exposure.

Patterns of Use

Five additional articles related to the association between menthol in cigarettes and smoking patterns were reviewed.

Tobacco Use Supplement to the Current Population Survey (CPS-TUS)

In a cross-sectional study, Delnevo and colleagues (2011) analyzed data from 2003 and 2006/7 Tobacco Use Supplement to the Current Population Survey (TUS-CPS) and compared the smoking cessation prevalence of menthol and nonmenthol smokers. Five different sample restrictions (using other tobacco products, ever making a quit attempt, etc.) were used, so the sample size ranged from 71,193 to 24,465 participants. Overall, menthol smokers were more likely to be female and aged 18-24 years (Delnevo, Gundersen, Hrywna, Echeverria, & Steinberg, 2011).

National Survey on Drug Use and Health (NSDUH)

Hickman and colleagues (2012) analyzed data from 24,157 people who participated in the 2008 and 2009 National Survey on Drug Use and Health (NSDUH). Data were categorized for menthol or nonmenthol use, and for level of psychological distress (none/mild, moderate, severe). The overall prevalence of menthol cigarette use was 33.3%. Menthol use was more prevalent among young adults, African Americans, Native Hawaiians/Pacific Islanders, those with severe psychological distress, lower education level, lower income level, and those who were unmarried and uninsured. The authors suggest that menthol's anesthetic and bronchodialation effects may influence metabolism of psychotropic medications. This study agrees with previously discussed prevalence data (Hickman, III, Delucchi, & Prochaska, 2012).

National Health and Nutrition Examination Survey (NHANES)

Data from 1943 smokers who participated in the 2001-2006 National Health and Nutrition Examination Survey (NHANES) were analyzed. Serum cotinine levels of non-Hispanic adult smokers (III20 years) who reported smoking a menthol brand of cigarettes (n=677) were compared with those who reported smoking a nonmenthol brand (n=1218). Less than 20% of White smokers smoked menthol cigarettes, compared to more than 70% of African American smokers (Caraballo et al., 2011).

Another analysis using 1999-2010 NHANES data estimated that 74.3% of smokers smoked nonmenthol cigarettes compared with 25.7% who smoked menthol cigarettes. This finding is similar to that of Caraballo et al. (2011), but may be more representative of current use patterns since this analysis is based upon more recent datasets (Jones et al., 2013).

National Youth Cessation Survey

The National Youth Smoking Cessation Survey (NYSCS) data were collected in 2003 from 2582 16-24 year olds who had ever smoked 20 lifetime cigarettes and had smoked within the past 30 days. From baseline to the two-year follow-up, more baseline menthol smokers switched to nonmenthol cigarettes than vice versa (Villanti et al., 2012).

Conclusion

The addition of these articles did not change finding in the full scientific review, namely that the weight of evidence supports the conclusion that menthol in cigarettes is associated with particular patterns of smoking.

Marketing and Consumer Perception of Risk

Five additional articles related to menthol cigarette marketing and consumer perception of risk were reviewed.

Marketing

Marketing Strategies

Researchers performed a cross-sectional analysis of tobacco retail advertising in a California community with a greater proportion of African Americans than in California as a whole, and a "menthol share of voice" (the proportion of all cigarette advertisements in a store that featured menthol brands) was calculated. On average, the menthol share of voice was higher in this community (36.9%) than the state average (25.7%) (Dauphinee, Doxey, Schleicher, Fortmann, & Henriksen, 2013).

Henriksen and colleagues (2012) examined 407 stores within walking distance of 91 California high schools and counted advertisements for menthol and nonmenthol cigarettes, and for promotions and prices for Newport (leading menthol brand) and Marlboro (leading nonmenthol brand).

The proportion of advertisements for menthol cigarettes increased with the proportion of African-American students. For each 10 percentage-point increase in the proportion of African American students, there was an increase of 5.9 percent in menthol share of voice, and stores were 1.5 times more likely to advertise a Newport promotion. The menthol share of voice increased by 11.6 percentage points with each 10 percentage-point increase in the proportion of neighborhood residents aged 10–17 years. Although this is not a national study, it supports the notion that at least some menthol brands target some African American neighborhoods, as well as those with younger demographics (Henriksen, Schleicher, Dauphinee, & Fortmann, 2012).

Tobacco advertising prevalence and placement at the point of sale by neighborhood and store characteristics in the ethnically and economically diverse St. Paul, MN area was assessed using data from a cross-sectional assessment of the advertising environment in 654 licensed tobacco vendors (conducted in 2007) and demographic data taken from the Year 2000 US census. Sixty percent of the establishments had an average of six menthol cigarette advertisements.

About 10% of those had health words such as "low tar", "light", "natural or "additive free" in their advertisements, and 47.5% had advertisements of price deals. For total number of menthol ads, the proportion African American,

Asian, below 150% of the poverty line, on public assistance, and under the age of 18 years were associated with more advertisements, the proportion White was associated with fewer advertisements ($p<0.05$). Gas/convenience stores had more menthol advertisements than all other types of stores except for tobacco shops and liquor stores (Widome, Brock, Noble, & Forster, 2012).

Consumer Perceptions

A study of brand recognition among 2589 6th through 9th graders (ages 11-15) in California found that the top three recognized brands were Camel (52%), Marlboro (36%) and Newport (32%).

However, there was disproportionate recognition of Newport by African American students, with over double the brand recognition levels for those students. This held true after adjustment for smoking by parents and peers. This analysis was based on a cross-sectional sample from the longitudinal Survey of Teen Opinions about Retail Environments (STORE) (Dauphinee et al., 2013).

In another study, adult smokers (n=923) who participated in the New Zealand International Tobacco Control (ITC) project survey were classified as either menthol or nonmenthol users and queried on their beliefs about the harmfulness of menthol cigarettes. Current menthol users and smokers from the Pacific region of New Zealand believed that menthols were less harmful than nonmenthol cigarettes.

Although these results reflect New Zealand's cultural and advertising histories, these results are applicable to the U.S. in that both countries have a documented history of advertising that links healthfulness and menthol cigarettes (Wilson, Weerasekera, Peace, & Edwards, 2011).

Conclusion

The addition of these articles did not change the finding of the full scientific review that 1) the weight of evidence supports the conclusion that the marketing of menthol cigarettes is likely associated with brand preference and use among adolescents and the African American community and 2) the weight of evidence is not sufficient to support a conclusion that consumer perceptions are associated with the use of menthol cigarettes

Initiation and Progression to Regular Use

Four additional articles regarding the association between menthol and smoking initiation and progression to regular use were reviewed.

First Smoking Experience

The study by Dauphinee et al. (2013) described above evaluated the relationship between brand recognition and smoking initiation. A greater proportion of students who recognized Newport (a menthol brand) brand at baseline initiated smoking; they were 49% more likely to initiate. Brand recognition of Camel (menthol) or Marlboro (nonmenthol) did not predict initiation. Recognition of Newport explained some of the variance attributed to the finding that African American students were more likely to initiate smoking (22%) compared to other students (15%), as recognition of Newport predicted smoking initiation regardless of race. Although the original survey (STORE) was longitudinal, it has only been administered three times, and some students only participated in two of the three waves. There was disproportionate loss-to-follow-up among boys, Hispanic students, younger students, and students in lower grade levels. It is also unknown how smoking behavior was evaluated (e.g., experience versus regular smoking).

Despite these limitations, this study provides support that there may be additional factors in the relationship of exposure to advertising on smoking initiation. Although Newport was third in brand recognition, it was the only brand recognition that was associated with future smoking behavior (Dauphinee et al., 2013).

A cross-sectional study of 928 treatment-seeking women in the Boston area was performed by Rosenbloom and colleagues (2012). Menthol (n=123) and nonmenthol (n=121) smoking women recalled the age at which they started smoking. There was no difference; both groups started smoking at around 16 years of age. Since the participants were asked generally about the age they started smoking, it is unclear whether they were reporting the age when they had their first cigarette or when they became regular smokers (Rosenbloom, Rees, Reid, Wong, & Kinnunen, 2012).

Faseru and colleagues (2013) compared the baseline characteristics of 540 African American light (10 cpd) smokers participating in a clinical smoking cessation study. There was no difference between menthol and nonmenthol smokers in the age of first cigarette smoked. Given the specific population included as participants (African American light smokers), generalizability is limited. In addition, drastically uneven numbers of menthol (452) and nonmenthol (88) smokers might have skewed the results (Faseru et al., 2013).

Progression to Regular Smoking

The Faseru study cited above also found no difference in the age at which menthol and nonmenthol smokers started smoking regularly (Faseru et al., 2013).

Using data from the longitudinal American Legacy Longitudinal Tobacco Use Reduction Study (ALLTURS), a three-wave longitudinal school-based survey of middle- and high school students, Nonnemaker and colleagues (2012) calculated the odds of escalating from non-established to established smoking. Menthol was associated with a higher likelihood of progressing to established smoking (odds ratio [OR] = 1.8, confidence interval [CI]: 1.02-3.16). Of the 638 participants, it is unclear how many were menthol versus nonmenthol smokers (Nonnemaker et al., 2013).

Conclusion

The addition of these articles does not alter the finding of the full scientific review, namely that the weight of evidence supports the conclusion that menthol in cigarettes is likely associated with increased initiation and progression to regular smoking of cigarettes.

Dependence

Nine additional articles related to the association between menthol cigarette use and tobacco dependence were reviewed.

Time to First Cigarette (Ttfc)

The study by Rosenbloom and colleagues (2012) described above found a significant effect of menthol on ttfc. Menthol smokers were more likely to smoke within the first five minutes of waking (49%) as compared to nonmenthol smokers (36%) ($p<0.01$). The authors concluded that menthol smokers showed evidence of greater tobacco dependence compared to nonmenthol smokers (Rosenbloom et al., 2012).

A survey of Minnesota Quitline users who registered for services and had a phone or mail survey follow-up 7 months post-registration was analyzed for self-reported cessation success of menthol (n=1172) versus nonmenthol (n=5085) participants. Baseline demographic data found a difference in ttfc, with a greater percentage of menthol smokers reporting smoking within the first 5 minutes of waking, and lower percentage reporting smoking their first cigarette more than 5 minutes after waking ($p<0.05$) (D'Silva, Boyle, Lien, Rode, & Okuyemi, 2012).

A large cross-sectional study of 221 menthol and 274 nonmenthol smokers examined the association between menthol and ttfc. There was a relationship between menthol and shorter ttfc ($p<0.02$), which was driven by African American smokers. This suggests that while menthol smokers may be more dependent, this effect is driven by African American menthol smokers. That is, the differences between a single subpopulation's menthol and nonmenthol smokers was strong enough to drive overall population differences, however it is unclear what is driving this difference between African American menthol and nonmenthol smokers (Muscat et al., 2012).

Cigarettes per Day (cpd)

During a cross-over study by Brinkman and colleagues (2012), nine subjects were given either menthol or nonmenthol cigarettes to smoke for a week each. On average, participants smoked fewer menthol cpd. However, of the nine participants, only one reported a study method brand as their usual brand. Therefore, it is difficult to generalize this finding to national menthol versus nonmenthol smoking populations (Brinkman et al., 2012).

The cross-sectional study by Rosenbloom and colleagues (2012) evaluated menthol preference on cpd. Although race effects were found, there was no effect of menthol preference on cpd (menthol = 16.8 cpd; nonmenthol =18.8 cpd) (Rosenbloom et al., 2012).

The demographics of menthol and nonmenthol smokers participating in a PET scan study allowed comparison of self-reported cpd by group. There were no differences between the menthol (n=22) and nonmenthol (n=41) groups, with menthol smokers smoking 19.9 ±5.8 cpd and nonmenthol smokers smoking 18.4 ±3.7 cpd (Brody et al., 2012).

Scales of Nicotine Dependence

The study by Brody et al. (2012) cited above allowed comparison of Fagerstrom Test of Nicotine Dependence (FTND) score by group. The researchers found no differences between the menthol (n=22) and nonmenthol (n=41) groups (Brody et al., 2012).

Faseru and colleagues (2013), in the study described earlier, found no difference in the FTND scores between menthol and nonmenthol smokers (Faseru et al., 2013).

Using data from ALLTURS study described earlier, Nonnemaker and colleagues (2012) calculated a scale of nicotine dependence based on five questions that focus on ttfc on weekdays, ttfc on weekends, and craving. Participants who initiated with menthol cigarettes had higher nicotine dependence scores ((3 1.25, CI: 0.1-2.4) (Nonnemaker et al., 2013).

The association between menthol use status and Heaviness of Smoking Index (HSI) was examined as part of the baseline characteristics of 183 (83 menthol, 100 nonmenthol) smokers from a longitudinal study examining risk perceptions over time among community smokers attempting to quit. The HSI of menthol smokers was no different from that of nonmenthol smokers (p=0.579) (Reitzel et al., 2013).

Industry Documents Research

Verger (2011) reviewed publicly available tobacco industry documents on the topic of menthol and nicotine dependence. The documents mainly focused on menthol's sensory and physiological effects and how these effects may interact with nicotine. According to these documents, the cooling and anesthetic effects of menthol may alleviate nicotine's irritating effects. Menthol may also act synergistically with nicotine, may stimulate the trigeminal nerve, and may make low tar, low nicotine tobacco products more acceptable. According to the documents, menthol level (but not nicotine level) affects level of "impact" felt by the user (Verger, 2011).

Conclusion

The addition of these articles does not change the conclusion of the full scientific review, namely that the weight of evidence supports the conclusion that menthol in cigarettes is likely associated with increased dependence.

Cessation

Seven additional studies addressing the link between menthol and smoking cessation were reviewed.

Cohort Studies

The association between menthol use status and biochemically-verified short term abstinence was examined by Reitzel and colleagues (2013) in the study described above. Smoking status was assessed via self-report and exhaled CO at weeks 1, 2 and 3 post-quit. There was no effect of menthol status on continuous short-term abstinence (p=0.44); however, this was moderated by race. After adjusting for demographic factors, menthol use was significantly associated with short-term continuous abstinence among White smokers (p=0.05), but not African American smokers. White menthol smokers were five times less likely to maintain abstinent as compared to White nonmenthol smokers (OR = 0.21m CI 0.05 0.98) (Reitzel et al., 2013).

Cross-Sectional Studies

Data collected as part of a randomized clinical trial were analyzed for race/ethnicity effects on postpartum maintenance of smoking abstinence. Participants smoked prior to pregnancy (n=123 menthol; n=121 nonmenthol) and stopped either during their pregnancy or within two months of becoming pregnant. The outcome measure was continuous abstinence since delivery date, and was assessed at eight and 26 weeks postpartum. Although responses were self-reported, there was cotinine verification of smoking abstinence. White menthol users, but not menthol smokers of other race/ethnic subgroups, were less likely to maintain continuous abstinence rates.

Analyses were adjusted for a variety of factors, including cpd and ttfc. As discussed in the full scientific review, since level of dependence may be an intermediate factor impacting cessation success, thus, these analyses may have been overadjusted (Reitzel et al., 2011).

The smoking cessation prevalence of menthol and nonmenthol smokers was compared by Delnevo and colleagues (2011). This cross-sectional study analyzed data from 2003 and 2006/7 TUS-CPS. Adjusted odds of cessation were calculated using multiple logistic regressions. Overall, menthol smokers were less likely to be former smokers than were nonmenthol smokers (AOR 0.91, 95% CI 0.87, 0.96), an effect that was relatively small but consistent (Delnevo et al., 2011).

An analysis of data from a survey of Minnesota Quitline users, described above, found no significant difference in quit status reported during the follow-up; menthol was not a significant predictor of 30-day abstinence (D'Silva et al., 2012).

Data from the 2003 and 2006/7 TUS-CPS were used to examine quit rates among menthol and nonmenthol smokers. Although menthol smokers were more likely to have made a quit attempt, they were either 4% (2003) or 12% (2006/7) less likely to have quit successfully in the past year. The final sample sizes are unclear, since the study authors did not indicate the number of subjects who met the inclusion requirements (Levy et al., 2011).

A randomized double-blind, placebo-controlled smoking cessation study investigated the efficacy of bupropion in promoting cessation in adult African American light (<_10 cpd) treatment-seeking smokers (n=540). Cotinine-verified seven-day point prevalence abstinence at week 7 (end of drug treatment) and week 26 were compared. Compared to continuing smokers, those who were abstinent were more likely to smoke nonmenthol cigarettes at week 7 (p=0.001) and week 26 (p=0.005).

However, being a menthol or nonmenthol smoker did not alter the efficacy of bupropion, which was higher than placebo at week 7 (24% versus 13%), but not at week 26 (13% versus 10%). Thus, although smoking menthol cigarettes was negatively associated with successful abstinence, it did not affect response to pharmacotherapy (Faseru et al., 2013).

Industry Documents Research

In a study of publicly available tobacco industry documents, Anderson (2011) reviewed documents on the topic of menthol and smoking cessation behavior. The documents mainly focused on the cooling and anesthetic effects of menthol. According to the documents, these effects may mask the short-term negative physiological effects of smoking such as throat pain, burning, cough. Documents also suggest that these sensory effects may also allow some smokers who were dissatisfied with the smoking experience to continue to smoke, and discourage them from quitting (Anderson, 2011).

Conclusion

The addition of these articles did not change the conclusion of the full scientific review, namely that the weight of evidence supports the conclusion that menthol in cigarettes is likely associated with reduced success in smoking cessation, especially among African American menthol smokers.

Disease Risk

Four additional articles related to menthol and disease risk were reviewed.

Lung Cancer

Using data from the 1987 National Health Interview Survey Cancer Control Supplement (with links to the National Death Index), Rostron (2012) estimated lung cancer mortality hazards for menthol and nonmenthol smokers. Menthol cigarette use had a lower hazard ratio (HR) for lung cancer mortality (HR = 0.59, CI 0.37-0.95) among 50+ year olds as compared use of nonmenthol cigarettes, but there was no similar association with other causes of mortality.

The author concluded that it is unknown how differences in smoking behavior and/or cigarette design may have impacted these findings. (Rostron,B, 2012a). These findings were commented on by Villanti et al. (Villanti, Giovino, Burns, & Abrams, 2013) with a rebuttal by Rostron (Rostron, 2013).

Multiple Cancers

Kabat and colleagues (2012) used data on age-adjusted incidence rates of lung, esophageal, oropharyngeal, and laryngeal cancers from the Surveillance, Epidemiology, and End Results (SEER) program.

Although not directly comparing menthol and nonmenthol smokers, Kabat and colleagues inferred that menthol did not alter multiple types of cancer risk since the market share of menthol cigarettes has remained stable over the past two decades, whereas cancer incidences have changed over the past 35 years, and these changes differ greatly depending on race and sex. The authors conclude that if menthol cigarettes had a "discernible effect" on the risk of smoking-related cancers, the incidence of these cancers in African Americans, especially African American females, would be higher, since this group smokes menthol cigarettes at a higher prevalence than White smokers (Kabat, Shivappa, & Hebert, 2012).

Multiple Non-Cancer Diseases

Using data from the 1999-2004 NHANES, Jones and colleagues (2012) investigated possible associations between current menthol versus nonmenthol cigarette smokers and peripheral artery disease. An ankle-brachial blood pressure index (ABI) calculation was made for 734 nonmenthol smoking adults and 310 menthol smoking adults who were at least 40 years old.

This calculation is a highly specific marker for subclinical peripheral artery disease. After adjusting for risk factors, demographics, pack-years of smoking and serum cotinine, there was no significant difference in the association between smoking and peripheral artery disease for current smokers of menthol and nonmenthol cigarettes.

Although there were half as many menthol smokers as nonmenthol smokers, it is unlikely that small sample size contributed to the negative results since even a directional trend did not exist ($p=0.59$) (Jones et al., 2012).

Data from the 2001-2008 NHANES was used to examine possible relationships between menthol smoking and the odds of stroke, hypertension, myocardial infarction, congestive heart failure, and COPD. The data were adjusted for demographic factors, and smoking quantity and duration. There were increased odds of stroke in menthol smokers (OR= 2.25, CI: 1.33-3.78), particularly women and non-African Americans, as compared to the nonmenthol smoking counterparts.

This increase was slightly reduced, but still significant, when data were adjusted for being diagnosed by a health professional, self-reported hypertension, diabetes mellitus and dyslipidemia (OR=2.19, CI: 1.05-4.58). There were no significant differences in the odds of any of the other diseases and smoking either menthol or nonmenthol cigarettes. The author suggests that the menthol cigarette-stroke association may be underestimated since former smokers were not included in the analysis (Vozoris, 2012).

Conclusion

The addition of these articles did not change the conclusion of the full scientific review: the weight of evidence supports the conclusion that menthol in cigarettes is not associated with an increase in disease risk to the user.

Overall Conclusion

None of the additionally reviewed peer-reviewed articles altered the findings of the full science report.

Reference Addendum

Author Name(s)	Article Title	Year Pub.	Funded By	Type of Study	Subject Description (Including Special Population(s))	Sample Size (N)	Authors' Results/Conclusion(s) Related to Menthol* (excerpted directly from article)
Abobo CV, Ma J, Liang D.	Effect of menthol on nicotine pharmacokinetics in rats after cigarette smoke inhalation.	2012	NIH Grants and the state tobacco settlement funds (Texas)	Nonclinical	Rats	N=8/group	Consistent with the findings after single-cigarette exposure, multiple-mentholated cigarette exposures caused significant reductions in the mean maximum nicotine plasma concentration... Similar to that observed after single cigarette smoke inhalation, menthol appreciably reduced the mean maximum plasma concentration of cotinine The mean elimination half-lives after multiple -nonmentholated and –mentholated cigarette smoke exposures were significantly different (49.4 vs. 37.3 min; Table 2). We found that single inhalation of mentholated cigarette significantly decreased the maximum plasma level and the area under the curve of nicotine but not the terminal half-life of nicotine.
Anderson SJ.	Menthol cigarettes and smoking cessation behaviour: a review of tobacco industry documents.	2011	Contract from DHHS HHSN261201000035I	Documents	N/A	509 documents qualitatively analyzed, 46 documents included	Menthol's cooling and anaesthetic effects mask the short-term negative physiological effects of smoking such as throat pain, burning and cough. This provides superficial physical relief as well as psychological assurance against concerns about the health dangers of smoking that would otherwise motivate smokers to quit.

Reference Addendum (Continued)

Author Name(s)	Article Title	Year Pub.	Funded By	Type of Study	Subject Description (Including Special Population(s))	Sample Size (N)	Authors' Results/Conclusion(s) Related to Menthol* (excerpted directly from article)
Ashley M, Dixon M, Sisodiya A, Prasad K.	Lack of effect of menthol level and type on smokers' estimated mouth level exposures to tar and nicotine and perceived sensory characteristics of cigarette smoke.	2012	British American Tobacco (BAT)	Human subjects	Smokers (age 21-65) who smoked at least 10 cpd	N=800 menthol and nonmenthol smokers (this was a "target"; number of actual completers wasn't given)	There were no effects of menthol loading or type on mean nicotine MLE in the 4 mg tar yield smoker groups, but within the 1 mg tar yield smoker groups the occasional menthol smokers obtained higher mean nicotine MLE when smoking the high loading natural menthol product (J1N 11.6) compared with smoking the non-menthol cigarette (J1 0). The only significant effect of menthol loading on mean nicotine MLE was in the regular 1 mg tar yield group where the low synthetic menthol loading product (P1S 3.9) produced higher mean nicotine MLE than the high synthetic menthol product (P1S 6.1 and the high natural menthol product (P1N 6.3). . . . for the two occasional menthol smoker groups, the addition of menthol to the products was associated with a marked and significant increase in perceived irritation. The effects of menthol loading on the intensities of the strength of menthol taste and the cooling effect were less clear-cut than those observed in the Japanese smoker groups. However, in

Author Name(s)	Article Title	Year Pub.	Funded By	Type of Study	Subject Description (Including Special Population(s))	Sample Size (N)	Authors' Results/Conclusion(s) Related to Menthol* (excerpted directly from article)
							most groups there were trends towards higher intensities of menthol taste and cooling effect with increasing menthol loading, but unlike the results from the Japanese study these differences were not significant in all cases.
Benowitz NL, Dains KM, Dempsey D, Wilson M, Jacob P.	Racial differences in the relationship between number of cigarettes smoked and nicotine and carcinogen exposure.	2011	NIH Grants	Human laboratory study	Healthy adult (age 18-65) smokers who smoked an average of •10 cpd for the past year or longer	N=127	Plasma nicotine levels were significantly higher in regular compared to menthol cigarette smokers.
Bodnar JA, Morgan WT, Murphy PA, Ogden MW.	Mainstream smoke chemistry analysis of samples from the 2009 US cigarette	2012	R.J. Reynolds Tobacco Co.	Nonclinical	N/A	N/A	Menthol cigarette mean constituent yields were observed to be within the range of the non-menthol cigarettes of similar "tar" categories.
Abobo CV, Ma J, Liang D.	Effect of menthol on nicotine pharmacokinetics in rats after cigarette smoke inhalation.	2012	NIH Grants and the state tobacco settlement funds (Texas)	Nonclinical	Rats	N=8/group	Consistent with the findings after single-cigarette exposure, multiple-mentholated cigarette exposures caused significant reductions in the mean maximum nicotine plasma concentration... Similar to that observed after single cigarette smoke inhalation, menthol appreciably reduced the mean maximum plasma concentration of cotinine The mean elimination half-lives after multiple -nonmentholated and –

Reference Addendum (Continued)

Author Name(s)	Article Title	Year Pub.	Funded By	Type of Study	Subject Description (Including Special Population(s))	Sample Size (N)	Authors' Results/Conclusion(s) Related to Menthol* (excerpted directly from article)
							mentholated cigarette smoke exposures were significantly different (49.4 vs. 37.3 min; Table 2). We found that single inhalation of mentholated cigarette significantly decreased the maximum plasma level and the area under the curve of nicotine but not the terminal half-life of nicotine.
Anderson SJ.	Menthol cigarettes and smoking cessation behaviour: a review of tobacco industry documents.	2011	Contract from DHHS HHSN261201000035I	Documents	N/A	509 documents qualitatively analyzed, 46 documents included	Menthol's cooling and anaesthetic effects mask the short-term negative physiological effects of smoking such as throat pain, burning and cough. This provides superficial physical relief as well as psychological assurance against concerns about the health dangers of smoking that would otherwise motivate smokers to quit.
Ashley M, Dixon M, Sisodiya A, Prasad K.	Lack of effect of menthol level and type on smokers' estimated mouth level exposures to tar and nicotine and perceived sensory characteristics of market.	2012	British American Tobacco (BAT)	Human subjects	Smokers (age 21-65) who smoked at least 10 cpd	N=800 menthol and nonmenthol smokers (this was a "target"; number of actual completers	There were no effects of menthol loading or type on mean nicotine MLE in the 4 mg tar yield smoker groups, but within the 1 mg tar yield smoker groups the occasional menthol smokers obtained higher mean nicotine MLE when smoking the high loading natural menthol product (J1N 11.6) compared with smoking the non-menthol cigarette (J1 0).
Brinkman MC, Chuang JC,	Exposure to and deposition of fine	2012	Contract from the Centers for Disease	Nonclinical and Laboratory	Smokers (age 18-30) who smoked at least 1	N=9	... there were no significant differences measured in daily MLE [mouth level

Author Name(s)	Article Title	Year Pub.	Funded By	Type of Study	Subject Description (Including Special Population(s))	Sample Size (N)	Authors' Results/Conclusion(s) Related to Menthol* (excerpted directly from article)
Gordon SM, Kim H, Kroeger RR, Polzin GM, Richter PA.	and ultrafine particles in smokers of menthol and nonmenthol cigarettes.		Control and Prevention (CDC)		pack/day for at least 6 months		exposure] and participant specific mainstream smoke when participants smoked the two test cigarettes. There were no significant differences in the level of urinary cotinine between the menthol and the nonmenthol cigarettes. Urinary 1-HOP levels were not significantly different between the two test cigarettes. The menthol test cigarette showed a significantly higher number (11%) and mass (33%) of ultrafine particles than the nonmenthol test cigarette. Participants smoked significantly fewer menthol cigarettes/day... as compared to nonmenthol test cigarettes. ...participants took longer puffs (0.24 s) and required a longer period of time (25 s) for each menthol cigarette, which resulted in a larger volume of smoke inhaled per menthol cigarette (73 ml/cigarette) as compared to nonmenthol.
Brody AL, Mukhin AG, La Charite J, Ta K, Farahi J, Sugar CA, Mamoun MS, Vellios E, Archie M, Kozman M,	Up-regulation of nicotinic acetylcholine receptors in menthol cigarette smokers.	2012	Tobacco-Related Disease Research Program, NIH grant, Veterans Affairs Type I Merit Review Award, endowment from the Richard Metzner Chair in Clinical	Clinical study	Healthy adult smokers (10-40 cpd)	N=22 menthol smokers, N=41 nonmenthol smokers	Menthol and non-menthol cigarette smokers did not differ on any demographic or rating scale measure, other than race/ethnicity... Follow-up tests revealed between-group differences for the brainstem, cerebellum and corpus callosum...

Reference Addendum (Continued)

Author Name(s)	Article Title	Year Pub.	Funded By	Type of Study	Subject Description (Including Special Population(s))	Sample Size (N)	Authors' Results/Conclusion(s) Related to Menthol* (excerpted directly from article)
Phuong J, Arlorio F, Mandelkern MA.			Neuropharmacology				
Buday T, Brozmanova M, Biringerova Z, Gavliakova S, Poliacek I, Calkovsky V, Shetthalli MV, Plevkova J.	Modulation of cough response by sensory inputs from the nose - role of trigeminal TRPA1 versus TRPM8 channels.	2012	VEGA no 1/0031/11 and Centre of Experimental and Clinical Respirology II (CEKR) co-financed from EU sources	Human laboratory study	Healthy non-smoking adults (average age 23)	N=18	Both menthol isomers after nasal administration significantly modulated urge to cough, cough threshold, and total cough response probably via the reduction of airway irritation induced during capsaicin challenge.
Caraballo RS, Holiday DB, Stellman SD, Mowery PD, Giovino GA, Muscat JE, Eriksen MP, Bernert JT, Richter PA, Kozlowski LT.	Comparison of serum cotinine concentration within and across smokers of menthol and nonmenthol cigarette brands among non-Hispanic black and non-Hispanic white U.S. adult smokers, 2001-2006.	2011	No funding source(s). Authors affiliated with the Centers for Disease Control and Prevention, RTI International, Georgia State University, Columbia University, State University of New York at Buffalo, Penn State College of Medicine	Cohort survey (NHANES 2001-2006)	Smokers (age •20) who had smoked on the day of or the day prior to the NHANES visit	N=1943	Smoking a menthol cigarette brand versus smoking a nonmenthol cigarette brand was not associated ($P< 0.05$) with mean serum cotinine concentration in either black or white smokers. ...only a minority (19.4%) of the sample of white smokers smoked menthol cigarettes, whereas the majority (73.9%) of black smokers smoked a menthol brand. Menthol cigarettes smoked by black smokers (1.24 mg) were on an average higher in FTC nicotine levels to the menthol cigarettes (0.94 mg) smoked by white smokers ($P < 0.01$).
Cheang WS, Lam MY,	Menthol relaxes rat aortae,	2013	National Basic Research Program of China, a	Nonclinical	Rat tissue, cell culture	N/A	The present study demonstrates that menthol relaxes rat arteries through

Author Name(s)	Article Title	Year Pub.	Funded By	Type of Study	Subject Description (Including Special Population(s))	Sample Size (N)	Authors' Results/Conclusion(s) Related to Menthol* (excerpted directly from article)
Wong WT, Tian XY, Lau CW, Zhu Z, Yao X, Huang Y.	mesenteric and coronary arteries by inhibiting calcium influx		research grant from Research Grants Council of Hong Kong, and CUHK Focused Investment Scheme B.				loweringCa2þ influx probably vianifedipine-sensitiveCa2þ channels in vascular smooth muscle. This effect appears independent of the reported TRPM8 activation.
Dauphinee AL, Doxey JR, Schleicher NC, Fortmann SP, Henriksen L.	Racial differences in cigarette brand recognition and impact on youth smoking.	2013	NIH grant	Longitudinal study with some cross-sectional analyses	6th-9th grade students(age 11-15) in Vallejo, California	N=2589	On average, the proportion of cigarette ads that featured a menthol brand (menthol share of voice) was 36.9% (SD = 18.3), which was higher than the average for the state (25.7% (SD = 26.1)... ...provide the brand name: 52% for Camel, 36% for Marlboro, and 32% for Newport. The odds of smoking initiation increased by 49% for students who recognized the Newport brand at baseline.
Delnevo CD, Gundersen DA, Hrywna M, Echeverria SE, Steinberg MB.	Smoking-cessation prevalence among U.S. smokers of menthol versus non-menthol cigarettes.			Cross-sectional TUS-CPS	Black, White and Hispanic current smokers and those who have quit in the past 5 years	N=71,193 to 24,465 (depending on sample restrictions)	...there was a small but consistent relationship between menthol cigarettes and cessation, whereby smokers of menthol cigarettes were signif3/4cantly less likely to have quit smoking than smokers of non-menthol cigarettes.
D'Silva J, Boyle RG, Lien R, Rode P, Okuyemi KS.	Cessation outcomes among treatment-seeking menthol and nonmenthol smokers.	2012	No funding source(s). Authors were affiliated with ClearWay Minnesota; University of Minnesota; Professional Data Analysts; Minnesota	Cross-sectional survey with single follow-up	Cigarette smokers who called the Minnesota Quitline and registered for services	N=1172 menthol smokers, N=5085 nonmenthol smokers	...the odds of quitting for menthol smokers was not signif3/4cantly different from nonmenthol smokers (OR 1.29, 95% CI 0.77, 2.15) after controlling for the other covariates.

Reference Addendum (Continued)

Author Name(s)	Article Title	Year Pub.	Funded By	Type of Study	Subject Description (Including Special Population(s))	Sample Size (N)	Authors' Results/Conclusion(s) Related to Menthol* (excerpted directly from article)
			Department of Health				
Faseru B, Choi WS, Krebill R, Mayo MS, Nollen NL, Okuyemi KS, Ahluwalia JS, Cox LS.	Factors associated with smoking menthol cigarettes among treatment-seeking African American light smokers.	2011	NIH Grant	Clinical trial	Treatment-seeking African-American light (”10 cpd) smokers	N=452 menthol, N=88 nonmenthol	Table 1 Baseline characteristics of AA menthol and non-menthol smokers in KIS III.
Faseru B, Nollen NL, Mayo MS, Krebill R, Choi WS, Benowitz NL, Tyndale RF, Okuyemi KS, Ahluwalia JS, Sanderson Cox L.	Predictors of cessation in African American light smokers enrolled in a bupropion clinical trial.	2013	NIH Grants; NRSA grant, American Cancer Society Institutional Research Grant	Clinical trial	Treatment-seeking African-American light (”10 cpd) smokers	N=540	Our current study has demonstrated a robust effect of menthol on smoking cessation. African American light smokers of menthol cigarettes were less likely to quit smoking compared to non-menthol cigarette smokers.
Fowler P, Smith K, Young J, Jeffrey L, Kirkland D, Pfuhler S, Carmichael P.	Reduction of misleading ("false") positive results in mammalian cell genotoxicity assays. I. Choice of cell type.	2012	European Cosmetic Industry Association, UK National Centre for the 3Rs (NC3Rs)	Nonclinical	6 *in vitro* cell lines	N/A	It was cytotoxic, inducing at least 50% reduction in RI at the top concentrations scored, but there were no increases in MN frequency. In other cases (e.g., d,l-menthol), testing was limited by cytotoxicity, and even though required levels of cytotoxicity were induced, MN were not.
Frasnelli J, Albrecht J, Bryant B,	Perception of specific trigeminal	2011	Postdoctoral fellowship from the Canadian Institutes of Health	Human laboratory study	Healthy adults with no reductions in sense of smell	N=20	All stimuli clearly activated the trigeminal system as demonstrated by the ease subjects had in lateralizing them.

Author Name(s)	Article Title	Year Pub.	Funded By	Type of Study	Subject Description (Including Special Population(s))	Sample Size (N)	Authors' Results/Conclusion(s) Related to Menthol* (excerpted directly from article)
Lundström JN.Frasnelli J, Albrecht J, Bryant B, Lundström JN.	chemosensory agonists.		Research				The scores for menthol and eucalyptol showed the highest correlation (r20 0.79; P< 0.001), Eucalyptol and menthol were described as predominantly cool (2.4 p and 2.3 p, respectively), fresh (both 1.4 p) and tickling (0.5 p and 0.7 p, respectively).
Gordon SM, Brinkman MC, Meng RQ, Anderson GM, Chuang JC, Kroeger RR, Reyes IL, Clark PI.	Effect of cigarette menthol content on mainstream smoke emissions.	2011	Battelle internal research and development funds	Nonclinical	N/A	N/A	Menthol in the TPM samples obtained from the cigarettes at each of the menthol levels investigated showed a linear increase with applied menthol concentration, but the amounts of nicotine, target TSNAs, PAHs, cotinine, and quinolone in the cigarettes remained essentially unchanged. Similarly, yields of the targeted VOCs in mainstream smoke from the MEN cigarettes that were measured in real-time on a puff-by-puff basis in whole smoke were largely unaffected by the levels of menthol present in the cigarettes.
Hans M, Wilhelm M, Swandulla D.	Menthol suppresses nicotinic acetylcholine receptor functioning in sensory neurons via allosteric modulation.	2012	Altria Client Services, Inc.	Nonclinical	Nicotinic acetylcholine receptors (native and recombinant)	N/A	...we show that nAChRs expressed in sensory neurons are reversibly inhibited by menthol with an IC50 of 111 lM. Single channel recordings from human a4b2 nAChR in HEK tsA201 cells revealed that menthol causes an increase in single channel amplitude, a shorting of channel open time and a prolongation of its close time. We conclude that the mechanism underlying the menthol-

Reference Addendum (Continued)

Author Name(s)	Article Title	Year Pub.	Funded By	Type of Study	Subject Description (Including Special Population(s))	Sample Size (N)	Authors' Results/Conclusion(s) Related to Menthol* (excerpted directly from article)
							mediated inhibition of nAChR is due to an allosteric modulation of the nAChR by menthol.
Henriksen L, Schleicher NC, Dauphinee AL, Fortmann SP.	Targeted advertising, promotion, and price for menthol cigarettes in California high school neighborhoods.	2012	California's Tobacco-Related Disease Research Program grant	Cross-sectional study	Stores within walking distance of California high schools	N=407	For each 10 percentage point increase in the proportion of Black students, the proportion of menthol advertising increased by 5.9 percentage points... The menthol share of voice increased by 11.6 percentage points with each 10 percentage-point increase in the proportion of neighborhood residents ages 10–17 years. For each 10 percentage-point increase in the proportion of Black students, the odds of a store advertising a Newport promotion were 1.5 times greater
Hickman NJ 3rd, Delucchi KL, Prochaska JJ.	Menthol use among smokers with psychological distress: findings from the 2008 and 2009 National Survey on Drug Use and Health.	2012	NIH grants	Nationally representative cohort study (NSDUH)	Current smokers (age 18) who answered the item on menthol use	N=24157	The prevalence of menthol smoking among this national sample of current smokers was 33.3%. The prevalence of menthol use was higher among individuals with severe psychological distress, women, young adults, African Americans, Native Hawaiians/Pacific Islanders, persons with fewer years of education and lower income, the unmarried and uninsured.
Janssens A, Voets T.	Ligand stoichiometry of the cold- and	2011	Grants from the Belgian Federal Government, the Research Foundation-	Nonclinical	TRPM8 ion channels expressed in HEK293 cells	N/A	This indicates that TRPM8 can simultaneously bind up to four menthol molecules, resulting in a stepwise

Author Name(s)	Article Title	Year Pub.	Funded By	Type of Study	Subject Description (Including Special Population(s))	Sample Size (N)	Authors' Results/Conclusion(s) Related to Menthol* (excerpted directly from article)
	menthol-activated channel TRPM8.		Flanders, and the Research Council of the KU Leuven				stabilization of the open state.
Jones MR, Apelberg BJ, Samet JM, Navas-Acien A.	Smoking, menthol cigarettes, and peripheral artery disease in U.S. adults.	2012	NIH Grants	Nationally representative survey from 1999-2004 (NHANES)	Adults (age • 40)	N=5973	Serum cotinine and blood cadmium concentrations were also higher in smokers of menthol cigarettes compared to smokers of nonmenthol cigarettes... We observed no significant difference in the association between smoking and peripheral artery disease for current smokers of nonmenthol and menthol cigarettes (p value for heterogeneity = 0.59).
Jones MR, Apelberg BJ, Tellez-Plaza M, Samet JM, Navas-Acien A.	Menthol cigarettes, race/ethnicity, and biomarkers of tobacco use in U.S. adults: the 1999-2010 National Health and Nutrition Examination Survey (NHANES).	2012	NIH grants	Cohort nationally representative survey from 1999-2010 (NHANES)	Adult current smokers (including White, African American and Mexican American smokers)	N=4603	In a representative sample of U.S. adult smokers, current menthol cigarette use was associated with increased concentration of blood cadmium, an established carcinogen and highly toxic metal, but not with other biomarkers. A total of 3,210 (74.3%) participants smoked nonmenthol cigarettes compared with 1,393 (25.7%) participants who smoked menthol cigarettes... After further adjustment for race/ethnicity, the corresponding ratios were markedly decreased and no longer statistically significant for serum cotinine (1.03; 95% CI, 0.9)
Kabat GC, Shivappa N, HÃ©bert JR.	Mentholated cigarettes and smoking-related	2012	NIH Grants	Multiple years of SEER data	Case and controls: lung. esophageal, oropharyngeal,	Not given/Not appropriate	Given the large differences in exposure to mentholated cigarettes by race and sex, if menthol had a discernible effect

Reference Addendum (Continued)

Author Name(s)	Article Title	Year Pub.	Funded By	Type of Study	Subject Description (Including Special Population(s))	Sample Size (N)	Authors' Results/Conclusion(s) Related to Menthol* (excerpted directly from article)
	cancers revisited: an ecologic examination.				laryngeal cancer		on the risk of smoking-related cancers, one might expect to see one or both of the following patterns: (1) higher incidence rates among Blacks of both sexes compared to their White counterparts; (2) differences in the temporal trends between Blacks and Whites of both sexes.
Kramlinger VM, von Weymarn LB, Murphy SE.	Inhibition and inactivation of cytochrome P450 2A6 and cytochrome P450 2A13 by menthofuran, Î2-nicotyrine and menthol.	2012	NIH Grants	Nonclinical	*In vitro*	N/A	Inhibition of CYP2A6 by menthol was 100 times less potent (Ki of 100mM). There was no indication that menthol inactivated CYP2A6 or CYP2A13.
Levy DT, Blackman K, Tauras J, Chaloupka FJ, Villanti AC, Niaura RS, Vallone DM, Abrams DB.	Quit attempts and quit rates among menthol and nonmenthol smokers in the United States.	2011	Legacy	Nationally representative cross-sectional TUC-CPS from 2003 and 2006/7	Adult smokers who had smoked at least 100 cigarettes and are either current or former smokers	Unknown	Table 1 presents the proportions of smokers and former smokers who quit within the past 5 years by cigarette type. In both 2003 and 2007, about 70% smoked nonmenthol, 26% smoked menthol, and 4% had no preference. Although they had a higher likelihood of a quit attempt, menthol smokers compared with nonmenthol smokers were 4% less likely to have quit successfully in the past year in 2003 and 12%less likely in 2007.

Author Name(s)	Article Title	Year Pub.	Funded By	Type of Study	Subject Description (Including Special Population(s))	Sample Size (N)	Authors' Results/Conclusion(s) Related to Menthol* (excerpted directly from article)
Lu S, Baad-Hansen L, List T, Zhang Z, Svensson P.	Somatosensory profiling of intra-oral capsaicin and menthol in healthy subjects	2013	NIH research grant	Human laboratory study	Healthy adults (mean age 31.5±7.5)	N=15	More than half (9/15) of the subjects reported mild levels of pain during menthol application. Our study showed that topical application of menthol on the gingiva elicited cold and warmth hyperesthesia...
Millqvist E, Ternesten-Hasséus E, Bende M.	Inhalation of menthol reduces capsaicin cough sensitivity and influences inspiratory flows in chronic cough.	2013	Grants from the Regional Health Care Authority of West Sweden, the Swedish Asthma and Allergy Association and the Swedish Heart and Lung Foundation	Human laboratory study	Patients: non-smokers with histories of cough and other airway symptoms induced by environmental irritants (average age 51). Controls: healthy nonsmokers (average age 52).	N=14 (patients) N=15 (controls)	We conclude that in patients with chronic cough that is not caused by asthma, COPD or infections, pre-inhalation of menthol reduces cough sensitivity to inhaled capsaicin and influences inspiratory flows.
Muscat JE, Liu HP, Stellman SD, Richie JP Jr.	Menthol smoking in relation to time to first cigarette and cotinine: results from a community-based study.	2012	NIH Grants; contracts from DHHS; Pennsylvania Department of Health	Human laboratory study	Daily smokers (•5 cpd for one or more years)	N=495	. Overall there was a trend between menthol smoking and a shorter TTFC (P < 0.02). When analyzed by race, the trend was significant in black subjects (P < 0.04). The time to first cigarette (P < 0.01) but not menthol (P = 0.66) was significantly associated with cotinine levels.
Naziro÷lu M, Ozgül C.	Effects of antagonists and heat on TRPM8 channel currents in dorsal root ganglion neuron activated by	2012	No funding source(s). Authors affiliated with University of Suleyman Demirel, Turkey	Nonclinical	Rat dorsal root ganglia	N/A	In the current study, TRPM8 channels were activated by menthol.

Reference Addendum (Continued)

Author Name(s)	Article Title	Year Pub.	Funded By	Type of Study	Subject Description (Including Special Population(s))	Sample Size (N)	Authors' Results/Conclusion(s) Related to Menthol* (excerpted directly from article)
	nociceptive cold stress and menthol.						
Nelson PR, Chen P, Dixon M, Steichen T.	A survey of mouth level exposure to cigarette smoke in the United States.	2011	No funding source(s). Authors affiliated with R.J. Reynolds Tobacco Company	Human study	Healthy smokers (•7 cpd) who smoked one of the selected brand styles as their usual brand style	N= 1330	The regression lines for the menthol cigarettes fell slightly below those for the non-menthol cigarettes suggesting a trend towards slightly lower MLEs per cigarette for the menthol brand-styles. However, differences in the slopes and intercepts of the regression lines were not statistically significant.
Nonnemaker J, Hersey J, Homsi G, Busey A, Allen J, Vallone D.	Initiation with menthol cigarettes and youth smoking uptake.	2012	DHHS contract	Cross-sectional survey	Middle and high school students from 83 schools in seven communities and five states	N=638 (progression analysis) or N=399 (dependence analysis)	The models reveal a positive and statistically significant association between menthol at initiation [odds ratio (OR) = 1.8, confidence interval (CI): 1.02–3.16) and escalation to established smoking. As shown, initiation with menthol is associated positively and significantly with nicotine dependence (b = 1.25, CI: 0.1–2.4).
Pereira EJ, Sim L, Driver H, Parker C, Fitzpatrick M.	The effect of inhaled menthol on upper airway resistance in humans: A randomized controlled crossover study.	2013	Research grants from the Ontario Thoracic Society, William M. Spear Foundation, Queen's University and Clinical Teachers Association at Queen's University	Human laboratory study	Healthy adults (age 21±0.5 years)	N=10	...90% of participants reported that they could breathe easier on the menthol test day. The present study demonstrated that cold receptor stimulation of the upper airway with inhaled menthol does not alter UAR [upper airway respiration] in conscious resting human subjects.

Author Name(s)	Article Title	Year Pub.	Funded By	Type of Study	Subject Description (Including Special Population(s))	Sample Size (N)	Authors' Results/Conclusion(s) Related to Menthol* (excerpted directly from article)
Reitzel LR, Li Y, Stewart DW, Cao Y, Wetter DW, Waters AJ, Vidrine JI.	Race moderates the effect of menthol cigarette use on short-term smoking abstinence.	2013	NIH Grant; CDC grant, The University of Texas MD Anderson Cancer Center	Cohort study	Current smokers (age 18-65), smoking •5 cpd for at least a year, willingness to quit	N=183	The main effects of menthol use status on continuous short-term smoking abstinence were not significant... Menthol use was significantly associated with short-term continuous smoking abstinence among White participants... White menthol users were about 5 times less likely to maintain continuous smoking abstinence than White nonmenthol users (odds ratio = 0.21, 95% CI = 0.05–0.98).
Reitzel LR, Nguyen N, Cao Y, Vidrine JI, Daza P, Mullen PD, Velasquez MM, Li Y, Cinciripini PM, Cofta-Woerpel L, Wetter DW.	Race/ethnicity moderates the effect of prepartum menthol cigarette use on postpartum smoking abstinence.	2011	NIH Grants	Clinical trial	Women who smoked prior to pregnancy and quit either during pregnancy or within 2 months of becoming pregnant	N= 123 menthol smokers, 121 nonmenthol smokers	White menthol users were less likely to maintain continuous abstinence than White non-menthol users.
Rosenbloom J, Rees VW, Reid K, Wong J, Kinnunen T.	A cross-sectional study on tobacco use and dependence among women: Does menthol matter?	2012	NIH Grant, the Harvard School Office for Enrichment Programs and the Harvard School of Dental Medicine	Cross-sectional study	Women smokers	N=198 African American, N=730 White	A greater proportion of menthol smokers smoked their first cigarette within five minutes of waking ($p < 0.01$)... The ANOVAs conducted showed no significant menthol preference main effects on cigarettes per day, age of smoking initiation...
Rostron B.	NNAL exposure by race and menthol cigarette use among US	2012 (epub)	No funding source(s). Author affiliated with FDA	Nationally representative survey (NHANES)	NHANES smoker participants from 2007- 2010 (age •20)	N=1614	Menthol cigarette use was associated with lower NNAL concentrations among smokers overall. This difference was principally due to lower NNAL

Reference Addendum (Continued)

Author Name(s)	Article Title	Year Pub.	Funded By	Type of Study	Subject Description (Including Special Population(s))	Sample Size (N)	Authors' Results/Conclusion(s) Related to Menthol* (excerpted directly from article)
	smokers.						concentrations for menthol smokers compared with nonmenthol smokers among White smokers. Nicotine and carcinogen exposure as measured by NNAL and cotinine generally increases with CPD across race/ethnicity groups for U.S. smokers.
Rostron B.	Lung cancer mortality risk for U.S. menthol cigarette smokers.	2012	No funding source(s). Author affiliated with FDA	Nationally representative survey (NHIS-CCS)	Adult participants (age • 18) who were smokers identified with either menthol or nonmenthol preference (pack verified)	N=4832	The HR for lung cancer mortality for menthol smokers at ages 50 and over was 0.59 (95% CI = 0.37 – 0.95).
Sarkar M, Wang J, Liang Q	Metabolism of nicotine and 4-(methylnitrosami n o)-1-(3-pyridyl)-lbutanone (NNK) in menthol and non-menthol cigarette smokers	2013	No funding source(s). Authors affiliated with Altria Client Services	Multi-center, cross-sectional study (TES)	Adult participants (age •21) who reported smoking •1cpd for at least the past 12 months	N=1044 menthol; 2297 nonmenthol	Race, machine-smoked tar, age and menthol by age interaction term were statistically significant factors for the 3OHCOT glucuronide ratios. The biomarkers of exposure (NE, total NNAL, carboxyhemoglobin and serum cotinine) were not statistically significantly different (p>0.05).
Strasser AA, Ashare RL, Kaufman M, Tang KZ, Mesaros AC, Blair IA.	The effect of menthol on cigarette smoking behaviors, biomarkers and subjective	2013	NIH Grants	Human laboratory study	Adult smokers (age 21- 65); smoke •10 cpd, smoke menthol cigarettes at least 80% of the time	N=32	...the experimental group exhibited a marginal increase in total puff volume from period 1 (own brand) to period 2 (menthol; P = 0.06) and from period 2 (menthol) to period 3 (non-menthol; P = 0.06) and a significant increase between

Author Name(s)	Article Title	Year Pub.	Funded By	Type of Study	Subject Description (Including Special Population(s))	Sample Size (N)	Authors' Results/Conclusion(s) Related to Menthol* (excerpted directly from article)
	responses.						periods 1 and 3 (P = 0.02). There was a significant decrease in CO boost from period 1 (baseline) to period 2 (menthol; mean difference=1.6 ppm, SE=0.47, P=0.033), but there was no difference between period 2 and 3 (non-menthol; P = 0.32) for the experimental group... Cotinine values had a similar pattern as the nicotine values; there were no significant main effects or interaction effect.
Topp R, Winchester L, Mink AM, Kaufman JS, Jacks DE.	Comparison of the effects of ice and 3.5% menthol gel on blood flow and muscle strength of the lower arm.	2011	No funding(s) sources. Authors affiliated with the University of Louisville	Human laboratory study	Healthy adults (mean age 24.4)	N=17	...at 5 minutes after application of the menthol gel blood flow significantly declined in the radial artery by 42%.
Topp R, Winchester LJ, Schilero J, Jacks D.	Effect of topical menthol on ipsilateral and contralateral superficial blood flow following a bout of maximum voluntary muscle contraction.	2011	University of Louisville Foundation, Hygienic Research Fund	Human laboratory study	Healthy adults (average age 24.19±2.97)	N=16	...the application of either 3.5% menthol gel or 10% menthol wipe to the thigh decreases blood flow... The application of 3.5% menthol gel or a 10% menthol wipe reduced arterial popliteal diameter on the side receiving these treatments...
Valero ML, Mello de Queiroz F,	TRPM8 ion channels differentially	2012	Financed by the Max-Planck Society and grants SAF2010-14990	Nonclinical	Three human prostate cell lines (normal and cancerous)	N/A	We observed no consistent acceleration of growth after stimulation of the channel with menthol...

Reference Addendum (Continued)

Author Name(s)	Article Title	Year Pub.	Funded By	Type of Study	Subject Description (Including Special Population(s))	Sample Size (N)	Authors' Results/Conclusion(s) Related to Menthol* (excerpted directly from article)
Stühmer W, Viana F, Pardo LA.	modulate proliferation and cell cycle distribution of normal and cancer prostate cells.		and PROMETEO2010-046, and a predoctoral fellowship from the Spanish government.				
Villanti AC, Giovino GA, Barker DC, Mowery PD, Sevilimedu V, Abrams DB.	Menthol brand switching among adolescents and young adults in the National Youth Smoking Cessation Survey.	2012	Schroeder Institute for Tobacco Research and Policy Studies at Legacy	Longitudinal random-digit telephone survey	Smokers (age 16-24) who had ever smoked 20 lifetime cigarettes and had smoked within the past 30 days	N=1045	After 2 years, proportionately more baseline menthol smokers had switched to nonmenthol cigarettes (15.0%; 95% CI = 10.8%,19.2%) than baseline nonmenthol smokers had switched to menthol brands (6.9%; 95% CI = 4.9%,8.9%).
Vozoris NT.	Mentholated cigarettes and cardiovascular and pulmonary diseases: a population-based study.	2012	No funding source(s). Author affiliated with Kingston General Hospital; Queen's University	National representative survey (2001-2008 NHANES)	Current smokers (age 20) with ascertained menthol smoker status	N=5028	After also controlling for health professional– diagnosed, self-reported hypertension, diabetes mellitus, and dyslipidemia, the odds of stroke remained significantly increased among all (OR, 2.19; 95% CI, 1.05-4.58), women (OR, 3.54; 95% CI, 1.60- 7.84), and non–African American (OR, 3.02; 95% CI, 1.24- 7.34) mentholated cigarette smokers vs respective nonmentholated cigarette smokers.
Widome R, Brock B, Noble P, Forster JL.	The relationship of neighborhood demographic characteristics to	2013	Grant from the Robert Wood Johnson Foundation; Minnesota Department o fHealth	Cross-sectional study with US Census	Licensed tobacco vendors in St. Paul, MN	N=654 stores	...higher minority proportion (and lower income) areas were more likely to have greater amounts of ads for menthol tobacco products.

Author Name(s)	Article Title	Year Pub.	Funded By	Type of Study	Subject Description (Including Special Population(s))	Sample Size (N)	Authors' Results/Conclusion(s) Related to Menthol* (excerpted directly from article)
	point-of-sale tobacco advertising and marketing.						Stores in block groups that had greater proportions of African-Americans/ Blacks, Asians, people living in poverty, and/or under the age of 18 years tended to have more menthol advertising.
Willis DN, Liu B, Ha MA, Jordt SE, Morris JB.	Menthol attenuates respiratory irritation responses to multiple cigarette smoke irritants.	2011	NIH Grants and the American Asthma Foundation	Nonclinical	mice	N/A	...counterirritant effects of menthol in this mouse model are apparent at concentrations below or equal to those present in mentholated cigarette smoke.
Wilson N, Weerasekera D, Peace J, Edwards R.	Smokers have varying misperceptions about the harmfulness of menthol cigarettes: national survey data.	2011	Health Research Council of New Zealand	Cross-sectional analysis of ITC (International Tobacco Control Policy Evaluation Survey) data	Adult smokers from the 2008/2009 wave who participated in this telephone survey	N=923	...some groups of smokers (particularly menthol users and Pacific smokers) believed that smoking menthol cigarettes was less harmful than regular cigarettes.
Wise PM, Breslin PA, Dalton P.	Sweet taste and menthol increase cough reflex thresholds.	2012	NIH Grants and Kraft Foods	Human laboratory study	Healthy adults (age 23- 36); 12 nonsmokers, 1 light smoker	N=13	Inhalation of headspace above menthol solution decreased cough sensitivity, e.g., increased the concentration of capsaicin required to trigger cough, relative to inhalation of headspace above a solvent blank.
Wise PM, Preti G, Eades J, Wysocki CJ.	The effect of menthol vapor on nasal sensitivity to chemical	2011	Institutional funds from the Monell Chemical Senses Center	Human laboratory study	Healthy adults (age 21- 46	N=22	Pretreatment with menthol vapor decreased sensitivity to nasal irritation from acetic acid (participants required higher concentrations to lateralize) but

Author Name(s)	Article Title	Year Pub.	Funded By	Type of Study	Subject Description (Including Special Population(s))	Sample Size (N)	Authors' Results/Conclusion(s) Related to Menthol* (excerpted directly from article)
	irritation.						increased sensitivity to allyl isothiocyanate (lower concentrations were required).
Wu X, Desai KG,Mallery SR, Holpuch AS, Phelps MP, Schwendeman SP.	Mucoadhesive fenretinide patches for site-specific chemoprevention of oral cancer: enhancement of oral mucosal permeation of fenretinide by coincorporation of propylene glycol and menthol.	2012	Fanconi Anemia Research Fund and NIH grants	Nonclinical (porcine buccal preparation)	N/A	N/A	vitro and *in vivo* release of fenretinide from patch was not significantly increased by coincorporation of permeation enhancers, indicating that mass transfer across the tissue, and not the patch, largely determined the permeation rate control *in vivo*.
Yerger VB.	Menthol's potential effects on nicotine dependence: a tobacco industry perspective market.	2011	DHHS Contract	Documents research	N/A	N=309 documents	The tobacco industry knows that menthol overrides the harsh taste of tobacco and alleviates nicotine's irritating effects, synergistically interacts with nicotine, stimulates the trigeminal nerve to elicit a 'liking' response for a tobacco product, and makes low tar, low nicotine tobacco products more acceptable to smokers than non-mentholated low delivery products.
Brinkman MC, Chuang JC,	Exposure to and deposition of fine	2012	Contract from the Centers for Disease	Nonclinical and Laboratory	Smokers (age 18-30) who smoked at least 1	N=9	... there were no significant differences measured in daily MLE [mouth level

Author Name(s)	Article Title	Year Pub.	Funded By	Type of Study	Subject Description (Including Special Population(s))	Sample Size (N)	Authors' Results/Conclusion(s) Related to Menthol* (excerpted directly from article)
Gordon SM, Kim H, Kroeger RR, Polzin GM, Richter PA.	and ultrafine particles in smokers of menthol and nonmenthol cigarettes.		Control and Prevention (CDC)		pack/day for at least 6 months		exposure] and participant specific mainstream smoke when participants smoked the two test cigarettes. There were no significant differences in the level of urinary cotinine between the menthol and the nonmenthol cigarettes. Urinary 1-HOP levels were not significantly different between the two test cigarettes. The menthol test cigarette showed a significantly higher number (11%) and mass (33%) of ultrafine particles than the nonmenthol test cigarette. Participants smoked significantly fewer menthol cigarettes/day... as compared to nonmenthol test cigarettes. ...participants took longer puffs (0.24 s) and required a longer period of time (25 s) for each menthol cigarette, which resulted in a larger volume of smoke inhaled per menthol cigarette (73 ml/cigarette) as compared to nonmenthol.
Brody AL, Mukhin AG, La Charite J, Ta K, Farahi J, Sugar CA, Mamoun MS, Vellios E, Archie M,	Up-regulation of nicotinic acetylcholine receptors in menthol cigarette smokers.	2012	Tobacco-Related Disease Research Program, NIH grant, Veterans Affairs Type I Merit Review Award, endowment from the Richard Metzner Chair in Clinical	Clinical study	Healthy adult smokers (10-40 cpd)	N=22 menthol smokers, N=41 nonmenthol smokers	Menthol and non-menthol cigarette smokers did not differ on any demographic or rating scale measure, other than race/ethnicity... Follow-up tests revealed between-group differences for the brainstem, cerebellum and corpus callosum...

Reference Addendum (Continued)

Author Name(s)	Article Title	Year Pub.	Funded By	Type of Study	Subject Description (Including Special Population(s))	Sample Size (N)	Authors' Results/Conclusion(s) Related to Menthol* (excerpted directly from article)
Kozman M, Phuong J, Arlorio F, Mandelkern MA.			Neuropharmacology				
Buday T, Brozmanova M, Biringerova Z, Gavliakova S, Poliacek I, Calkovsky V, Shetthalli MV, Plevkova J.	Modulation of cough response by sensory inputs from the nose - role of trigeminal TRPA1 versus TRPM8 channels.	2012	VEGA no 1/0031/11 and Centre of Experimental and Clinical Respirology II (CEKR) co-financed from EU sources	Human laboratory study	Healthy non-smoking adults (average age 23)	N=18	Both menthol isomers after nasal administration significantly modulated urge to cough, cough threshold, and total cough response probably via the reduction of airway irritation induced during capsaicin challenge.
Caraballo RS, Holiday DB, Stellman SD, Mowery PD, Giovino GA, Muscat JE, Eriksen MP, Bernert JT, Richter PA, Kozlowski LT.	Comparison of serum cotinine concentration within and across smokers of menthol and nonmenthol cigarette brands among non-Hispanic black and non-Hispanic white U.S. adult smokers, 2001-2006.	2011	No funding source(s). Authors affiliated with the Centers for Disease Control and Prevention, RTI International, Georgia State University, Columbia University, State University of New York at Buffalo, Penn State College of Medicine	Cohort survey (NHANES 2001-2006)	Smokers (age •20) who had smoked on the day of or the day prior to the NHANES visit	N=1943	Smoking a menthol cigarette brand versus smoking a nonmenthol cigarette brand was not associated (P< 0.05) with mean serum cotinine concentration in either black or white smokers. ...only a minority (19.4%) of the sample of white smokers smoked menthol cigarettes, whereas the majority (73.9%) of black smokers smoked a menthol brand. Menthol cigarettes smoked by black smokers (1.24 mg) were on an average higher in FTC nicotine levels to the menthol cigarettes (0.94 mg) smoked by white smokers (P < 0.01).
Cheang WS,	Menthol relaxes	2013	National Basic Research	Nonclinical	Rat tissue, cell culture	N/A	The present study demonstrates that

Author Name(s)	Article Title	Year Pub.	Funded By	Type of Study	Subject Description (Including Special Population(s))	Sample Size (N)	Authors' Results/Conclusion(s) Related to Menthol* (excerpted directly from article)
Lam MY, Wong WT, Tian XY, Lau CW, Zhu Z, Yao X, Huang Y.	rat aortae, mesenteric and coronary arteries by inhibiting calcium influx		Program of China, a research grant from Research Grants Council of Hong Kong, and CUHK Focused Investment Scheme B.				menthol relaxes rat arteries through loweringCa2þ influx probably vianifedipine-sensitiveCa2þ channels in vascular smooth muscle. This effect appears independent of the reported TRPM8 activation.
Dauphinee AL,	Racial differences	2013	NIH grant	Longitudinal	6th-9th grade students	N=2589	On average, the proportion of cigarette ads that
Doxey JR, Schleicher NC, Fortmann SP, Henriksen L.	in cigarette brand recognition and impact on youth smoking.			study with some cross-sectional analyses	(age 11-15) in Vallejo, California		featured a menthol brand (menthol share of voice) was 36.9% (SD = 18.3), which was higher than the average for the state (25.7% (SD = 26.1)... ...provide the brand name: 52% for Camel, 36% for Marlboro, and 32% for Newport. The odds of smoking initiation increased by 49% for students who recognized the Newport brand at baseline.
Delnevo CD, Gundersen DA, Hrywna M, Echeverria SE, Steinberg MB.	Smoking-cessation prevalence among U.S. smokers of menthol versus non-menthol cigarettes.			Cross-sectional TUS-CPS	Black, White and Hispanic current smokers and those who have quit in the past 5 years	N=71,193 to 24,465 (depending on sample restrictions)	...there was a small but consistent relationship between menthol cigarettes and cessation, whereby smokers of menthol cigarettes were signif3/4cantly less likely to have quit smoking than smokers of non-menthol cigarettes.
D'Silva J, Boyle RG, Lien R, Rode P, Okuyemi KS.	Cessation outcomes among treatment-seeking menthol and nonmenthol	2012	No funding source(s). Authors were affiliated with ClearWay Minnesota; University of Minnesota;	Cross-sectional survey with single follow-up	Cigarette smokers who called the Minnesota Quitline and registered for services	N=1172 menthol smokers, N=5085 nonmenthol	...the odds of quitting for menthol smokers was not signif3/4cantly different from nonmenthol smokers (OR 1.29, 95% CI 0.77, 2.15) after controlling for the other covariates.

Reference Addendum (Continued)

Author Name(s)	Article Title	Year Pub.	Funded By	Type of Study	Subject Description (Including Special Population(s))	Sample Size (N)	Authors' Results/Conclusion(s) Related to Menthol* (excerpted directly from article)
	smokers.		Professional Data Analysts; Minnesota Department of Health			Smokers	
Faseru B, Choi WS, Krebill R, Mayo MS, Nollen NL, Okuyemi KS, Ahluwalia JS, Cox LS.	Factors associated with smoking menthol cigarettes among treatment-seeking African American light smokers.	2011	NIH Grant	Clinical trial	Treatment-seeking African-American light ("10 cpd) smokers	N=452 menthol, N=88 nonmenthol	Table 1 Baseline characteristics of AA menthol and non-menthol smokers in KIS III.
Faseru B, Nollen NL, Mayo MS, Krebill R, Choi WS, Benowitz NL, Tyndale RF, Okuyemi KS, Ahluwalia JS, Sanderson Cox L.	Predictors of cessation in African American light smokers enrolled in a bupropion clinical trial.	2013	NIH Grants; NRSA grant, American Cancer Society Institutional Research Grant	Clinical trial	Treatment-seeking African-American light ("10 cpd) smokers	N=540	Our current study has demonstrated a robust effect of menthol on smoking cessation. African American light smokers of menthol cigarettes were less likely to quit smoking compared to non-menthol cigarette smokers.
Fowler P, Smith K, Young J, Jeffrey L, Kirkland D, Pfuhler S, Carmichael P.	Reduction of misleading ("false") positive results in mammalian cell genotoxicity assays. I. Choice of cell type.	2012	European Cosmetic Industry Association, UK National Centre for the 3Rs (NC3Rs)	Nonclinical	6 *in vitro* cell lines	N/A	It was cytotoxic, inducing at least 50% reduction in RI at the top concentrations scored, but there were no increases in MN frequency. In other cases (e.g., d,l-menthol), testing was limited by cytotoxicity, and even though required levels of cytotoxicity were induced, MN were not.
Frasnelli J,	Perception of	2011	Postdoctoral fellowship	Human	Healthy adults with no	N=20	All stimuli clearly activated the

Author Name(s)	Article Title	Year Pub.	Funded By	Type of Study	Subject Description (Including Special Population(s))	Sample Size (N)	Authors' Results/Conclusion(s) Related to Menthol* (excerpted directly from article)
Albrecht J, Bryant B, Lundström JN.Frasnelli J, Albrecht J, Bryant B, Lundström JN.	specific trigeminal chemosensory agonists.		from the Canadian Institutes of Health Research	laboratory study	reductions in sense of smell		trigeminal system as demonstrated by the ease subjects had in lateralizing them. The scores for menthol and eucalyptol showed the highest correlation (r20 0.79; P< 0.001), Eucalyptol and menthol were described as predominantly cool (2.4 p and 2.3 p, respectively), fresh (both 1.4 p) and tickling (0.5 p and 0.7 p, respectively).
Gordon SM, Brinkman MC, Meng RQ, Anderson GM, Chuang JC, Kroeger RR, Reyes IL, Clark PI.	Effect of cigarette menthol content on mainstream smoke emissions.	2011	Battelle internal research and development funds	Nonclinical	N/A	N/A	Menthol in the TPM samples obtained from the cigarettes at each of the menthol levels investigated showed a linear increase with applied menthol concentration, but the amounts of nicotine, target TSNAs, PAHs, cotinine, and quinolone in the cigarettes remained essentially unchanged. Similarly, yields of the targeted VOCs in mainstream smoke from the MEN cigarettes that were measured in real-time on a puff-by-puff basis in whole smoke were largely unaffected by the levels of menthol present in the cigarettes.
Hans M, Wilhelm M, Swandulla D.	Menthol suppresses nicotinic acetylcholine receptor functioning in sensory neurons via allosteric	2012	Altria Client Services, Inc.	Nonclinical	Nicotinic acetylcholine receptors (native and recombinant)	N/A	...we show that nAChRs expressed in sensory neurons are reversibly inhibited by menthol with an IC50 of 111 lM. Single channel recordings from human a4b2 nAChR in HEK tsA201 cells revealed that menthol causes an increase in single channel amplitude, a shorting of channel open time and a prolongation of

Reference Addendum (Continued)

Author Name(s)	Article Title	Year Pub.	Funded By	Type of Study	Subject Description (Including Special Population(s))	Sample Size (N)	Authors' Results/Conclusion(s) Related to Menthol* (excerpted directly from article)
	modulation.						its close time. We conclude that the mechanism underlying the menthol-mediated inhibition of nAChR is due to an allosteric modulation of the nAChR by menthol.
Henriksen L, Schleicher NC, Dauphinee AL, Fortmann SP.	Targeted advertising, promotion, and price for menthol cigarettes in California high school neighborhoods.	2012	California's Tobacco-Related Disease Research Program grant	Cross-sectional study	Stores within walking distance of California high schools	N=407	For each 10 percentage point increase in the proportion of Black students, the proportion of menthol advertising increased by 5.9 percentage points... The menthol share of voice increased by 11.6 percentage points with each 10 percentage-point increase in the proportion of neighborhood residents ages 10–17 years. For each 10 percentage-point increase in the proportion of Black students, the odds of a store advertising a Newport promotion were 1.5 times greater
Hickman NJ 3rd, Delucchi KL, Prochaska JJ.	Menthol use among smokers with psychological distress: findings from the 2008 and 2009 National Survey on Drug Use and Health.	2012	NIH grants	Nationally representative cohort study (NSDUH)	Current smokers (age •18) who answered the item on menthol use	N=24157	The prevalence of menthol smoking among this national sample of current smokers was 33.3%. The prevalence of menthol use was higher among individuals with severe psychological distress, women, young adults, African Americans, Native Hawaiians/Pacific Islanders, persons with fewer years of education and lower income, the unmarried and uninsured.
Janssens A,	Ligand	2011	Grants from the Belgian	Nonclinical	TRPM8 ion channels	N/A	This indicates that TRPM8 can

Author Name(s)	Article Title	Year Pub.	Funded By	Type of Study	Subject Description (Including Special Population(s))	Sample Size (N)	Authors' Results/Conclusion(s) Related to Menthol* (excerpted directly from article)
Voets T.	stoichiometry of the cold- and menthol-activated channel TRPM8.		Federal Government, the Research Foundation-Flanders, and the Research Council of the KU Leuven		expressed in HEK293 cells		simultaneously bind up to four menthol molecules, resulting in a stepwise stabilization of the open state.
Jones MR, Apelberg BJ, Samet JM, Navas-Acien A.	Smoking, menthol cigarettes, and peripheral artery disease in U.S. adults.	2012	NIH Grants	Nationally representative survey from 1999-2004 (NHANES)	Adults (age • 40)	N=5973	Serum cotinine and blood cadmium concentrations were also higher in smokers of menthol cigarettes compared to smokers of nonmenthol cigarettes... We observed no significant difference in the association between smoking and peripheral artery disease for current smokers of nonmenthol and menthol cigarettes (p value for heterogeneity = 0.59).
Jones MR, Apelberg BJ, Tellez-Plaza M, Samet JM, Navas-Acien A.	Menthol cigarettes, race/ethnicity, and biomarkers of tobacco use in U.S. adults: the 1999-2010 National Health and Nutrition Examination Survey (NHANES).	2012	NIH grants	Cohort nationally representative survey from 1999-2010 (NHANES)	Adult current smokers (including White, African American and Mexican American smokers)	N=4603	In a representative sample of U.S. adult smokers, current menthol cigarette use was associated with increased concentration of blood cadmium, an established carcinogen and highly toxic metal, but not with other biomarkers. A total of 3,210 (74.3%) participants smoked nonmenthol cigarettes compared with 1,393 (25.7%) participants who smoked menthol cigarettes... After further adjustment for race/ethnicity, the corresponding ratios were markedly decreased and no longer statistically significant for serum cotinine (1.03; 95% CI, 0.9)

Reference Addendum (Continued)

Author Name(s)	Article Title	Year Pub.	Funded By	Type of Study	Subject Description (Including Special Population(s))	Sample Size (N)	Authors' Results/Conclusion(s) Related to Menthol* (excerpted directly from article)
Kabat GC, Shivappa N, HÃ©bert JR.	Mentholated cigarettes and smoking-related cancers revisited: an ecologic examination.	2012	NIH Grants	Multiple years of SEER data	Case and controls: lung. esophageal, oropharyngeal, laryngeal cancer	Not given/Not appropriate	Given the large differences in exposure to mentholated cigarettes by race and sex, if menthol had a discernible effect on the risk of smoking-related cancers, one might expect to see one or both of the following patterns: (1) higher incidence rates among Blacks of both sexes compared to their White counterparts; (2) differences in the temporal trends between Blacks and Whites of both sexes.
Kramlinger VM, von Weymarn LB, Murphy SE.	Inhibition and inactivation of cytochrome P450 2A6 and cytochrome P450 2A13 by menthofuran, Î2-nicotyrine and menthol.	2012	NIH Grants	Nonclinical	*In vitro*	N/A	Inhibition of CYP2A6 by menthol was 100 times less potent (Ki of 100mM). There was no indication that menthol inactivated CYP2A6 or CYP2A13.
Levy DT, Blackman K, Tauras J, Chaloupka FJ, Villanti AC, Niaura RS, Vallone DM, Abrams DB.	Quit attempts and quit rates among menthol and nonmenthol smokers in the United States.	2011	Legacy	Nationally representative cross-sectional TUC-CPS from 2003 and 2006/7	Adult smokers who had smoked at least 100 cigarettes and are either current or former smokers	Unknown	Table 1 presents the proportions of smokers and former smokers who quit within the past 5 years by cigarette type. In both 2003 and 2007, about 70% smoked nonmenthol, 26% smoked menthol, and 4% had no preference. Although they had a higher likelihood of a quit attempt, menthol smokers compared with nonmenthol smokers

Author Name(s)	Article Title	Year Pub.	Funded By	Type of Study	Subject Description (Including Special Population(s))	Sample Size (N)	Authors' Results/Conclusion(s) Related to Menthol* (excerpted directly from article)
							were 4% less likely to have quit successfully in the past year in 2003 and 12%less likely in 2007.
Lu S, Baad-Hansen L, List T, Zhang Z, Svensson P.	Somatosensory profiling of intra-oral capsaicin and menthol in healthy subjects	2013	NIH research grant	Human laboratory study	Healthy adults (mean age 31.5±7.5)	N=15	More than half (9/15) of the subjects reported mild levels of pain during menthol application. Our study showed that topical application of menthol on the gingiva elicited cold and warmth hyperesthesia...
Millqvist E, Ternesten-Hasséus E, Bende M.	Inhalation of menthol reduces capsaicin cough sensitivity and influences inspiratory flows in chronic cough.	2013	Grants from the Regional Health Care Authority of West Sweden, the Swedish Asthma and Allergy Association and the Swedish Heart and Lung Foundation	Human laboratory study	Patients: non-smokers with histories of cough and other airway symptoms induced by environmental irritants (average age 51). Controls: healthy nonsmokers (average age 52).	N=14 (patients) N=15 (controls)	We conclude that in patients with chronic cough that is not caused by asthma, COPD or infections, pre-inhalation of menthol reduces cough sensitivity to inhaled capsaicin and influences inspiratory flows.
Muscat JE, Liu HP, Stellman SD, Richie JP Jr.	Menthol smoking in relation to time to first cigarette and cotinine: results from a community-based study.	2012	NIH Grants; contracts from DHHS; Pennsylvania Department of Health	Human laboratory study	Daily smokers (•5 cpd for one or more years)	N=495	. Overall there was a trend between menthol smoking and a shorter TTFC ($P < 0.02$). When analyzed by race, the trend was significant in black subjects ($P < 0.04$). The time to first cigarette ($P < 0.01$) but not menthol ($P = 0.66$) was significantly associated with cotinine levels.
Naziro÷lu M, Ozgül C.	Effects of antagonists and heat on TRPM8 channel currents	2012	No funding source(s). Authors affiliated with University of Suleyman Demirel, Turkey	Nonclinical	Rat dorsal root ganglia	N/A	In the current study, TRPM8 channels were activated by menthol.

Reference Addendum (Continued)

Author Name(s)	Article Title	Year Pub.	Funded By	Type of Study	Subject Description (Including Special Population(s))	Sample Size (N)	Authors' Results/Conclusion(s) Related to Menthol* (excerpted directly from article)
	in dorsal root ganglion neuron activated by nociceptive cold stress and menthol.						
Nelson PR, Chen P, Dixon M, Steichen T.	A survey of mouth level exposure to cigarette smoke in the United States.	2011	No funding source(s). Authors affiliated with R.J. Reynolds Tobacco Company	Human study	Healthy smokers (•7 cpd) who smoked one of the selected brand styles as their usual brand style	N= 1330	The regression lines for the menthol cigarettes fell slightly below those for the non-menthol cigarettes suggesting a trend towards slightly lower MLEs per cigarette for the menthol brand-styles. However, differences in the slopes and intercepts of the regression lines were not statistically significant.
Nonnemaker J, Hersey J, Homsi G, Busey A, Allen J, Vallone D.	Initiation with menthol cigarettes and youth smoking uptake.	2012	DHHS contract	Cross-sectional survey	Middle and high school students from 83 schools in seven communities and five states	N=638 (progression analysis) or N=399 (dependence analysis)	The models reveal a positive and statistically significant association between menthol at initiation [odds ratio (OR) = 1.8, confidence interval (CI): 1.02–3.16) and escalation to established smoking. As shown, initiation with menthol is associated positively and significantly with nicotine dependence (b = 1.25, CI: 0.1–2.4).
Pereira EJ, Sim L, Driver H, Parker C, Fitzpatrick M.	The effect of inhaled menthol on upper airway resistance in humans: A	2013	Research grants from the Ontario Thoracic Society, William M. Spear Foundation, Queen's University and	Human laboratory study	Healthy adults (age 21±0.5 years)	N=10	...90% of participants reported that they could breathe easier on the menthol test day. The present study demonstrated that cold receptor stimulation of the upper airway

Author Name(s)	Article Title	Year Pub.	Funded By	Type of Study	Subject Description (Including Special Population(s))	Sample Size (N)	Authors' Results/Conclusion(s) Related to Menthol* (excerpted directly from article)
	randomized controlled crossover study.		Clinical Teachers Association at Queen's University				with inhaled menthol does not alter UAR [upper airway respiration] in conscious resting human subjects.
Reitzel LR, Li Y, Stewart DW, Cao Y, Wetter DW, Waters AJ, Vidrine JI.	Race moderates the effect of menthol cigarette use on short-term smoking abstinence.	2013	NIH Grant; CDC grant, The University of Texas MD Anderson Cancer Center	Cohort study	Current smokers (age 18-65), smoking •5 cpd for at least a year, willingness to quit	N=183	The main effects of menthol use status on continuous short-term smoking abstinence were not significant... Menthol use was significantly associated with short-term continuous smoking abstinence among White participants... White menthol users were about 5 times less likely to maintain continuous smoking abstinence than White nonmenthol users (odds ratio = 0.21, 95% CI = 0.05–0.98).
Reitzel LR, Nguyen N, Cao Y, Vidrine JI, Daza P, Mullen PD, Velasquez MM, Li Y, Cinciripini PM, Cofta-Woerpel L, Wetter DW.	Race/ethnicity moderates the effect of prepartum menthol cigarette use on postpartum smoking abstinence.	2011	NIH Grants	Clinical trial	Women who smoked prior to pregnancy and quit either during pregnancy or within 2 months of becoming pregnant	N= 123 menthol smokers, 121 nonmenthol smokers	White menthol users were less likely to maintain continuous abstinence than White non-menthol users.
Rosenbloom J, Rees VW, Reid K, Wong J, Kinnunen T.	A cross-sectional study on tobacco use and dependence among women: Does menthol matter?	2012	NIH Grant, the Harvard School Office for Enrichment Programs and the Harvard School of Dental Medicine	Cross-sectional study	Women smokers	N=198 African American, N=730 White	A greater proportion of menthol smokers smoked their first cigarette within five minutes of waking ($p < 0.01$)... The ANOVAs conducted showed no significant menthol preference main effects on cigarettes per day, age of smoking initiation...
Rostron B.	NNAL exposure	2012	No funding source(s).	Nationally	NHANES smoker	N=1614	Menthol cigarette use was associated

Reference Addendum (Continued)

Author Name(s)	Article Title	Year Pub.	Funded By	Type of Study	Subject Description (Including Special Population(s))	Sample Size (N)	Authors' Results/Conclusion(s) Related to Menthol* (excerpted directly from article)
	by race and menthol cigarette use among US smokers.	(epub)	Author affiliated with FDA	representative survey (NHANES)	participants from 2007- 2010 (age •20)		with lower NNAL concentrations among smokers overall. This difference was principally due to lower NNAL concentrations for menthol smokers compared with nonmenthol smokers among White smokers. Nicotine and carcinogen exposure as measured by NNAL and cotinine generally increases with CPD across race/ethnicity groups for U.S. smokers.
Rostron B.	Lung cancer mortality risk for U.S. menthol cigarette smokers.	2012	No funding source(s). Author affiliated with FDA	Nationally representative survey (NHIS-CCS)	Adult participants (age • 18) who were smokers identified with either menthol or nonmenthol preference (pack verified)	N=4832	The HR for lung cancer mortality for menthol smokers at ages 50 and over was 0.59 (95% CI = 0.37 – 0.95).
Sarkar M, Wang J, Liang Q	Metabolism of nicotine and 4-(methylnitrosami n o)-1-(3-pyridyl)-lbutanone (NNK) in menthol and non-menthol cigarette smokers	2013	No funding source(s). Authors affiliated with Altria Client Services	Multi-center, cross-sectional study (TES)	Adult participants (age •21) who reported smoking •1cpd for at least the past 12 months	N=1044 menthol; 2297 nonmenthol	Race, machine-smoked tar, age and menthol by age interaction term were statistically significant factors for the 3OHCOT glucuronide ratios. The biomarkers of exposure (NE, total NNAL, carboxyhemoglobin and serum cotinine) were not statistically significantly different ($p>0.05$).
Strasser AA, Ashare RL, Kaufman M,	The effect of menthol on cigarette smoking	2013	NIH Grants	Human laboratory study	Adult smokers (age 21- 65); smoke •10 cpd, smoke menthol	N=32	...the experimental group exhibited a marginal increase in total puff volume from period 1 (own brand) to period 2

Author Name(s)	Article Title	Year Pub.	Funded By	Type of Study	Subject Description (Including Special Population(s))	Sample Size (N)	Authors' Results/Conclusion(s) Related to Menthol* (excerpted directly from article)
Tang KZ, Mesaros AC, Blair IA.	behaviors, biomarkers and subjective responses.				cigarettes at least 80% of the time		(menthol; P = 0.06) and from period 2 (menthol) to period 3 (non-menthol; P = 0.06) and a significant increase between periods 1 and 3 (P = 0.02). There was a significant decrease in CO boost from period 1 (baseline) to period 2 (menthol; mean difference=1.6 ppm, SE=0.47, P=0.033), but there was no difference between period 2 and 3 (non-menthol; P = 0.32) for the experimental group... Cotinine values had a similar pattern as the nicotine values; there were no significant main effects or interaction effect.
Topp R, Winchester L, Mink AM, Kaufman JS, Jacks DE.	Comparison of the effects of ice and 3.5% menthol gel on blood flow and muscle strength of the lower arm.	2011	No funding(s) sources. Authors affiliated with the University of Louisville	Human laboratory study	Healthy adults (mean age 24.4)	N=17	...at 5 minutes after application of the menthol gel blood flow significantly declined in the radial artery by 42%.
Topp R, Winchester LJ, Schilero J, Jacks D.	Effect of topical menthol on ipsilateral and contralateral superficial blood flow following a bout of maximum voluntary muscle contraction.	2011	University of Louisville Foundation, Hygienic Research Fund	Human laboratory study	Healthy adults (average age 24.19±2.97)	N=16	...the application of either 3.5% menthol gel or 10% menthol wipe to the thigh decreases blood flow... The application of 3.5% menthol gel or a 10% menthol wipe reduced arterial popliteal diameter on the side receiving these treatments...

Reference Addendum (Continued)

Author Name(s)	Article Title	Year Pub.	Funded By	Type of Study	Subject Description (Including Special Population(s))	Sample Size (N)	Authors' Results/Conclusion(s) Related to Menthol* (excerpted directly from article)
Valero ML, Mello de Queiroz F, Stühmer W, Viana F, Pardo LA.	TRPM8 ion channels differentially modulate proliferation and cell cycle distribution of normal and cancer prostate cells.	2012	Financed by the Max-Planck Society and grants SAF2010-14990 and PROMETEO2010-046, and a predoctoral fellowship from the Spanish government.	Nonclinical	Three human prostate cell lines (normal and cancerous)	N/A	We observed no consistent acceleration of growth after stimulation of the channel with menthol...
Villanti AC, Giovino GA, Barker DC, Mowery PD, Sevilimedu V, Abrams DB.	Menthol brand switching among adolescents and young adults in the National Youth Smoking Cessation Survey.	2012	Schroeder Institute for Tobacco Research and Policy Studies at Legacy	Longitudinal random-digit telephone survey	Smokers (age 16-24) who had ever smoked 20 lifetime cigarettes and had smoked within the past 30 days	N=1045	After 2 years, proportionately more baseline menthol smokers had switched to nonmenthol cigarettes (15.0%; 95% CI = 10.8%,19.2%) than baseline nonmenthol smokers had switched to menthol brands (6.9%; 95% CI = 4.9%,8.9%).
Vozoris NT.	Mentholated cigarettes and cardiovascular and pulmonary diseases: a population-based study.	2012	No funding source(s). Author affiliated with Kingston General Hospital; Queen's University	National representative survey (2001-2008 NHANES)	Current smokers (age •20) with ascertained menthol smoker status	N=5028	After also controlling for health professional– diagnosed, self-reported hypertension, diabetes mellitus, and dyslipidemia, the odds of stroke remained significantly increased among all (OR, 2.19; 95% CI, 1.05-4.58), women (OR, 3.54; 95% CI, 1.60- 7.84), and non–African American (OR, 3.02; 95% CI, 1.24- 7.34) mentholated cigarette smokers vs respective nonmentholated cigarette smokers.
Widome R,	The relationship	2013	Grant from the Robert	Cross-sectional	Licensed tobacco	N=654 stores	...higher minority proportion (and lower

Author Name(s)	Article Title	Year Pub.	Funded By	Type of Study	Subject Description (Including Special Population(s))	Sample Size (N)	Authors' Results/Conclusion(s) Related to Menthol* (excerpted directly from article)
Brock B, Noble P, Forster JL.	of neighborhood demographic characteristics to point-of-sale tobacco advertising and marketing.		Wood Johnson Foundation; Minnesota Department o fHealth	study with US Census	vendors in St. Paul, MN		income) areas were more likely to have greater amounts of ads for menthol tobacco products. Stores in block groups that had greater proportions of African-Americans/ Blacks, Asians, people living in poverty, and/or under the age of 18 years tended to have more menthol advertising.
Willis DN, Liu B, Ha MA, Jordt SE, Morris JB.	Menthol attenuates respiratory irritation responses to multiple cigarette smoke irritants.	2011	NIH Grants and the American Asthma Foundation	Nonclinical	mice	N/A	...counterirritant effects of menthol in this mouse model are apparent at concentrations below or equal to those present in mentholated cigarette smoke.
Wilson N, Weerasekera D, Peace J, Edwards R.	Smokers have varying misperceptions about the harmfulness of menthol cigarettes: national survey data.	2011	Health Research Council of New Zealand	Cross-sectional analysis of ITC (International Tobacco Control Policy Evaluation Survey) data	Adult smokers from the 2008/2009 wave who participated in this telephone survey	N=923	...some groups of smokers (particularly menthol users and Pacific smokers) believed that smoking menthol cigarettes was less harmful than regular cigarettes.
Wise PM, Breslin PA, Dalton P.	Sweet taste and menthol increase cough reflex thresholds.	2012	NIH Grants and Kraft Foods	Human laboratory study	Healthy adults (age 23- 36); 12 nonsmokers, 1 light smoker	N=13	Inhalation of headspace above menthol solution decreased cough sensitivity, e.g., increased the concentration of capsaicin required to trigger cough, relative to inhalation of headspace above a solvent blank.

Reference Addendum (Continued)

Author Name(s)	Article Title	Year Pub.	Funded By	Type of Study	Subject Description (Including Special Population(s))	Sample Size (N)	Authors' Results/Conclusion(s) Related to Menthol* (excerpted directly from article)
Wise PM, Preti G, Eades J, Wysocki CJ.	The effect of menthol vapor on nasal sensitivity to chemical irritation.	2011	Institutional funds from the Monell Chemical Senses Center	Human laboratory study	Healthy adults (age 21-46	N=22	Pretreatment with menthol vapor decreased sensitivity to nasal irritation from acetic acid (participants required higher concentrations to lateralize) but increased sensitivity to allyl isothiocyanate (lower concentrations were required).
Wu X, Desai KG,Mallery SR, Holpuch AS, Phelps MP, Schwendeman SP.	Mucoadhesive fenretinide patches for site- specific chemoprevention of oral cancer: enhancement of oral mucosal permeation of fenretinide by coincorporation of propylene glycol and menthol.	2012	Fanconi Anemia Research Fund and NIH grants	Nonclinical (porcine buccal preparation)	N/A	N/A	vitro and *in vivo* release of fenretinide from patch was not significantly increased by coincorporation of permeation enhancers, indicating that mass transfer across the tissue, and not the patch, largely determined the permeation rate control *in vivo*.
Yerger VB.	Menthol's potential effects on nicotine dependence: a tobacco industry perspective.	2011	DHHS Contract	Documents research	N/A	N=309 documents	The tobacco industry knows that menthol overrides the harsh taste of tobacco and alleviates nicotine's irritating effects, synergistically interacts with nicotine, stimulates the trigeminal nerve to elicit a 'liking' response for a tobacco product, and makes low tar, low nicotine tobacco products more acceptable to smokers than non-mentholated low delivery products.

* Note: these statements are taken directly from articles and may not include all relevant results/conclusions.

References

Abobo, C. V., Ma, J., & Liang, D. (2012). Effect of menthol on nicotine pharmacokinetics in rats after cigarette smoke inhalation. *Nicotine Tob.Res., 14,* 801-808. ntr287;10.1093/ntr/ntr287.

Anderson, S. J. (2011). Menthol cigarettes and smoking cessation behaviour: a review of tobacco industry documents. *Tobacco control, 20 Suppl 2,* ii49-ii56. 20/Suppl_2/ii49;10.1136/tc.2010.041947.

Ashley, M., Dixon, M., Sisodiya, A., & Prasad, K. (2012). Lack of effect of menthol level and type on smokers' estimated mouth level exposures to tar and nicotine and perceived sensory characteristics of cigarette smoke. *Regulatory toxicology and pharmacology : RTP, 63,* 381-390. S0273-2300(12)00089- X;10.1016/j.yrtph.2012.04.010.

Benowitz, N. L., Dains, K. M., Dempsey, D., Wilson, M., & Jacob, P. (2011). Racial differences in the relationship between number of cigarettes smoked and nicotine and carcinogen exposure. *Nicotine & tobacco research : official journal of the Society for Research on Nicotine and Tobacco, 13,* 772-783. ntr072;10.1093/ntr/ntr072.

Bodnar, J. A., Morgan, W. T., Murphy, P. A., & Ogden, M. W. (2012). Mainstream smoke chemistry analysis of samples from the 2009 US cigarette market. *Regulatory toxicology and pharmacology : RTP, 64,* 35-42. S0273-2300(12)00093-1;10.1016/j. yrtph.2012.05.011.

Brinkman, M. C., Chuang, J. C., Gordon, S. M., Kim, H., Kroeger, R. R., Polzin, G. M. et al. (2012). Exposure to and deposition of fine and ultrafine particles in smokers of menthol and nonmenthol cigarettes. *Inhalation Toxicology, 24,* 255-269. 10.3109/08958378.2012.667218.

Brody, A. L., Mukhin, A. G., La, C. J., Ta, K., Farahi, J., Sugar, C. A. et al. (2012). Up-regulation of nicotinic acetylcholine receptors in menthol cigarette smokers. *The international journal of* neuropsychopharmacology / official scientific journal of the Collegium Internationale Neuropsychopharmacologicum (CINP), 1-10. S1461145712001022;10.1017/S1461145712001022.

Buday, T., Brozmanova, M., Biringerova, Z., Gavliakova, S., Poliacek, I., Calkovsky, V. et al. (2012). Modulation of cough response by sensory inputs from the nose - role of trigeminal TRPA1 versus TRPM8 channels. Cough (London, England), 8, 11. 1745-9974-8-11;10.1186/1745-9974-8-11.

Caraballo, R. S., Holiday, D. B., Stellman, S. D., Mowery, P. D., Giovino, G. A., Muscat, J. E. et al. (2011). Comparison of serum cotinine concentration within and across smokers of menthol and nonmenthol cigarette brands among non-Hispanic black and non-Hispanic white U.S. adult smokers, 2001-2006. Cancer Epidemiol Biomarkers Prev, 20, 1329-1340. 1055-9965.EPI-10-1330;10.1158/1055- 9965.EPI-10-1330.

Cheang, W. S., Lam, M. Y., Wong, W. T., Tian, X. Y., Lau, C. W., Zhu, Z. et al. (2013). Menthol relaxes rat aortae, mesenteric and coronary arteries by inhibiting calcium influx. European journal of pharmacology, 702, 79-84. S0014-2999(13)00043-5;10.1016/j.ejphar.2013.01.028.

D'Silva, J., Boyle, R. G., Lien, R., Rode, P., & Okuyemi, K. S. (2012). Cessation outcomes among treatment-seeking menthol and nonmenthol smokers. Am J Prev.Med., 43, S242-S248. S0749- 3797(12)00539-9;10.1016/j.amepre.2012.07.033.

Dauphinee, A. L., Doxey, J. R., Schleicher, N. C., Fortmann, S. P., & Henriksen, L. (2013). Racial differences in cigarette brand recognition and impact on youth smoking. Bmc Public Health, 13, 170. 1471-2458-13-170;10.1186/1471-2458-13-170.

Delnevo, C. D., Gundersen, D. A., Hrywna, M., Echeverria, S. E., & Steinberg, M. B. (2011). Smoking-Cessation Prevalence Among US Smokers of Menthol Versus Non-Menthol Cigarettes. *American journal of preventive medicine, 41,* 357-365.

Faseru, B., Nollen, N. L., Mayo, M. S., Krebill, R., Choi, W. S., Benowitz, N. L. et al. (2013). Predictors of cessation in African American light smokers enrolled in a bupropion clinical trial. *Addictive behaviors, 38,* 1796-1803. S0306-4603(12)00383-8;10.1016/j.addbeh.2012.11.010.

Fowler, P., Smith, K., Young, J., Jeffrey, L., Kirkland, D., Pfuhler, S. et al. (2012). Reduction of misleading ("false") positive results in mammalian cell genotoxicity assays. I. Choice of cell type. *Mutation research, 742,* 11-25. S1383-5718(11)00342-1;10.1016/j.mrgentox.2011.10.014.

Frasnelli, J., Albrecht, J., Bryant, B., & Lundstrom, J. N. (2011). Perception of specific trigeminal chemosensory agonists. *Neuroscience, 189,* 377-383. S0306-4522(11)00527-6;10.1016/j.neuroscience.2011.04.065.

Gordon, S. M., Brinkman, M. C., Meng, R. Q., Anderson, G. M., Chuang, J. C., Kroeger, R. R. et al. (2011). Effect of cigarette menthol content on mainstream smoke emissions. *Chemical Research in Toxicology, 24,* 1744-1753. 10.1021/tx200285s.

Hans, M., Wilhelm, M., & Swandulla, D. (2012). Menthol suppresses nicotinic acetylcholine receptor functioning in sensory neurons via allosteric modulation. *Chemical senses, 37,* 463-469. bjr128;10.1093/chemse/bjr128.

Henriksen, L., Schleicher, N. C., Dauphinee, A. L., & Fortmann, S. P. (2012). Targeted advertising, promotion, and price for menthol cigarettes in California high school neighborhoods. *Nicotine Tob. Res., 14,* 116-121. ntr122;10.1093/ntr/ntr122.

Hickman, N. J., III, Delucchi, K. L., & Prochaska, J. J. (2012). Menthol use among smokers with psychological distress: findings from the 2008 and 2009 National Survey on Drug Use and Health. *Tobacco control,* tobaccocontrol-2012-050479;10.1136/tobaccocontrol-2012-050479.

Janssens, A. & Voets, T. (2011). Ligand stoichiometry of the cold- and menthol-activated channel TRPM8. *The Journal of physiology, 589,* 4827-4835. jphysiol.2011.216523;10.1113/jphysiol.2011.216523.

Jones, M. R., Apelberg, B. J., Samet, J. M., & Navas-Acien, A. (2012). Smoking, Menthol Cigarettes, and Peripheral Artery Disease in U.S. Adults. *Nicotine Tob. Res.,* nts253;10.1093/ntr/nts253.

Jones, M. R., Apelberg, B. J., Tellez-Plaza, M., Samet, J. M., & Navas-Acien, A. (2013). Menthol cigarettes, race/ethnicity, and biomarkers of tobacco use in U.S. adults: the 1999-2010 National Health and Nutrition Examination Survey (NHANES). *Cancer epidemiology, biomarkers & prevention : a publication of the American Association for Cancer Research, cosponsored by the American Society of Preventive Oncology, 22,* 224-232. 1055-9965.EPI-12-0912;10.1158/1055-9965.EPI-12-0912.

Kabat, G. C., Shivappa, N., & Hebert, J. R. (2012). Mentholated cigarettes and smoking-related cancers revisited: an ecologic examination. *Regulatory toxicology and pharmacology : RTP, 63,* 132-139. S0273-2300(12)00042-6;10.1016/j.yrtph.2012.03.002.

Kramlinger, V. M., von Weymarn, L. B., & Murphy, S. E. (2012). Inhibition and inactivation of cytochrome P450 2A6 and cytochrome P450 2A13 by menthofuran, beta-nicotyrine and menthol. *Chemico biological interactions, 197,* 87-92. S0009-2797(12)00061-0;10.1016/j.cbi.2012.03.009.

Levy, D. T., Blackman, K., Tauras, J., Chaloupka, F. J., Villanti, A. C., Niaura, R. S. et al. (2011). Quit Attempts and Quit Rates Among Menthol and Nonmenthol Smokers in the United States. *American journal of public health, 101,* 1241-1247.

Lu, S., Baad-Hansen, L., List, T., Zhang, Z., & Svensson, P. (2013). Somatosensory profiling of intra-oral capsaicin and menthol in healthy subjects. *European journal of oral sciences, 121,* 29-35. 10.1111/eos.12014.

Millqvist, E., Ternesten-Hasseus, E., & Bende, M. (2013). Inhalation of menthol reduces capsaicin cough sensitivity and influences inspiratory flows in chronic cough. *Respiratory medicine, 107,* 433-438. S0954-6111(12)00428-3;10.1016/j.rmed. 2012.11. 017.

Muscat, J. E., Liu, H. P., Stellman, S. D., & Richie, J. P., Jr. (2012). Menthol smoking in relation to time to first cigarette and cotinine: results from a community-based study. *Regulatory toxicology and pharmacology : RTP, 63,* 166-170. S0273-2300(12)00059-1;10.1016/j.yrtph.2012.03.012.

Naziroglu, M. & Ozgul, C. (2012). Effects of antagonists and heat on TRPM8 channel currents in dorsal root ganglion neuron activated by nociceptive cold stress and menthol. *Neurochemical research, 37,* 314-320. 10.1007/s11064-011-0614-z.

Nelson, P. R., Chen, P., Dixon, M., & Steichen, T. (2011). A survey of mouth level exposure to cigarette smoke in the United States. *Regulatory toxicology and pharmacology : RTP, 61,* S25-S38. S0273-2300(10)00180-7;10.1016/j.yrtph.2010.10.001.

Nonnemaker, J., Hersey, J., Homsi, G., Busey, A., Allen, J., & Vallone, D. (2013). Initiation with menthol cigarettes and youth smoking uptake. *Addiction (Abingdon, England), 108,* 171-178. 10.1111/j.1360-0443.2012.04045.x.

Pereira, E. J., Sim, L., Driver, H., Parker, C., & Fitzpatrick, M. (2013). The effect of inhaled menthol on upper airway resistance in humans: A randomized controlled crossover study. *Canadian respiratory journal : journal of the Canadian Thoracic Society, 20,* e1-e4.

Reitzel, L. R., Li, Y., Stewart, D. W., Cao, Y., Wetter, D. W., Waters, A. J. et al. (2013). Race Moderates the Effect of Menthol Cigarette Use on Short-Term Smoking Abstinence. *Nicotine Tob.Res.,* nts335;10.1093/ntr/nts335.

Reitzel, L. R., Nguyen, N., Cao, Y., Vidrine, J. I., Daza, P., Mullen, P. D. et al. (2011). Race/ethnicity moderates the effect of prepartum menthol cigarette use on postpartum smoking abstinence. *Nicotine Tob.Res., 13,* 1305-1310. ntr095;10.1093/ntr/ntr095.

Rosenbloom, J., Rees, V. W., Reid, K., Wong, J., & Kinnunen, T. (2012). A cross-sectional study on tobacco use and dependence among women: Does menthol matter? *Tobacco induced diseases, 10,* 19. 1617-9625-10-19;10.1186/1617-9625-10-19.

Rostron, B. (2012a). Lung cancer mortality risk for U.S. menthol cigarette smokers. *Nicotine Tob.Res., 14,* 1140-1144. nts014;10.1093/ntr/nts014.

Rostron, B. (2012b). NNAL Exposure by Race and Menthol Cigarette Use among US Smokers. *Nicotine Tob.Res.,* nts223;10.1093/ntr/nts223.

Rostron, B. (2013). Methodology, Menthol, and Mortality. *Nicotine & Tobacco Research, 15,* 619.

Sarkar, M., Wang, J., & Liang, Q. (2012). Metabolism of nicotine and 4-(methylnitrosamino)-1-(3- pyridyl)-1-butanone (NNK) in menthol and non-menthol cigarette smokers. *Drug metabolism letters,* DML-EPUB-20121105-3.

Strasser, A. A., Ashare, R. L., Kaufman, M., Tang, K. Z., Mesaros, A. C., & Blair, I. A. (2013). The effect of menthol on cigarette smoking behaviors, biomarkers and subjective responses. *Cancer epidemiology, biomarkers & prevention : a publication of the American Association for Cancer Research,* cosponsored by the American Society of Preventive Oncology, 22, 382-389. 1055-9965.EPI-12- 1097;10.1158/1055-9965.EPI-12-1097.

Valero, M. L., Mello de, Q. F., Stuhmer, W., Viana, F., & Pardo, L. A. (2012). TRPM8 ion channels differentially modulate proliferation and cell cycle distribution of normal and cancer prostate cells. Plos One, 7, e51825. 10.1371/journal.pone.0051825;PONE-D-12-19488.

Villanti, A. C., Giovino, G. A., Barker, D. C., Mowery, P. D., Sevilimedu, V., & Abrams, D. B. (2012). Menthol brand switching among adolescents and young adults in the National Youth Smoking Cessation Survey. Am J Public Health, 102, 1310-1312. 10.2105/AJPH.2011.300632.

Villanti, A. C., Giovino, G. A., Burns, D. M., & Abrams, D. B. (2013). Menthol cigarettes and mortality: keeping focus on the public health standard. Nicotine Tob.Res., 15, 617-618. nts176;10.1093/ntr/nts176.

Vozoris, N. T. (2012). Mentholated cigarettes and cardiovascular and pulmonary diseases: a population-based study. Arch.Intern.Med., 172, 590-591. 172/7/590;10.1001/archinternmed.2012.320.

Widome, R., Brock, B., Noble, P., & Forster, J. L. (2012). The relationship of neighborhood demographic characteristics to point-of-sale tobacco advertising and marketing. Ethnicity & health, 10.1080/13557858.2012.701273.

Willis, D. N., Liu, B., Ha, M. A., Jordt, S. E., & Morris, J. B. (2011). Menthol attenuates respiratory irritation responses to multiple cigarette smoke irritants. FASEB journal : official publication of the Federation of American Societies for Experimental Biology, 25, 4434-4444. fj.11-188383;10.1096/fj.11- 188383.

Wilson, N., Weerasekera, D., Peace, J., & Edwards, R. (2011). Smokers have varying misperceptions about the harmfulness of menthol cigarettes: national survey data. *Australian and New Zealand Journal of Public Health, 35,* 364-367.

Wise, P. M., Breslin, P. A., & Dalton, P. (2012). Sweet taste and menthol increase cough reflex thresholds. *Pulmonary pharmacology & therapeutics, 25,* 236-241. S1094-5539(12)00047- 8;10.1016/j.pupt.2012.03.005.

Wise, P. M., Preti, G., Eades, J., & Wysocki, C. J. (2011). The effect of menthol vapor on nasal sensitivity to chemical irritation. *Nicotine Tob.Res., 13,* 989-997. ntr107;10.1093/ntr/ntr107.

Wu, X., Desai, K. G., Mallery, S. R., Holpuch, A. S., Phelps, M. P., & Schwendeman, S. P. (2012). Mucoadhesive fenretinide patches for site-specific chemoprevention of oral cancer: enhancement of oral mucosal permeation of fenretinide by coincorporation of propylene glycol and menthol. *Molecular pharmaceutics, 9,* 937-945. 10.1021/mp200655k.

Yerger, V. B. (2011). Menthol's potential effects on nicotine dependence: a tobacco industry perspective. *Tobacco control, 20 Suppl 2,* ii29-ii36. 20/Suppl_2/ii29;10.1136/ tc.2010.041970.

Index

A

accounting, 38
acculturation, 104, 124
acetic acid, 168, 170, 203, 220
acetylcholine, 170, 189, 193, 205, 209, 221, 222
acid, 6, 8, 15, 19, 39, 48, 168, 169
action potential, 20
additives, 7, 10, 14, 17, 18
adenocarcinoma, 152
adjustment, 23, 38, 40, 41, 115, 116, 117, 152, 177, 195, 211
adolescents, 3, 38, 60, 68, 69, 71, 72, 74, 76, 77, 78, 80, 81, 83, 85, 88, 90, 92, 94, 97, 101, 103, 107, 112, 114, 116, 120, 123, 138, 140, 154, 178, 202, 218, 224
adulthood, vii, 1, 4, 66, 96
adults, 54, 58, 60, 62, 64, 66, 69, 70, 73, 77, 83, 89, 90, 91, 94, 95, 96, 97, 98, 102, 103, 105, 114, 116, 117, 120, 123, 125, 134, 140, 143, 147, 168, 184, 190, 192, 195, 197, 198, 201, 203, 206, 208, 211, 213, 214, 217, 219, 220, 222
adverse effects, 88
advertisements, 70, 71, 72, 74, 75, 76, 84, 88, 91, 93, 95, 176, 177
African American women, 37, 38
African American(s), vii, 1, 3, 25, 31, 37, 38, 39, 42, 50, 60, 66, 69, 70, 71, 72, 73, 74, 75, 76, 80, 84, 87, 91, 93, 99, 100, 101, 103, 108, 112, 115, 117, 119, 123, 128, 129, 132, 133, 134, 135, 136, 137, 138, 140, 145, 146, 147, 148, 150, 151, 153, 154, 155, 156, 166, 175, 176, 177, 183, 184, 192, 194, 202, 208, 210, 218
agonist, 20, 169
Alaska, 54, 55, 58, 98, 138
Alaska Natives, 54, 55, 98, 138
alcohol consumption, 151
alcohol use, 37
aldehydes, 7
American Heart Association, 43, 52, 83, 94
amplitude, 193, 209
analgesic, 21, 22, 26, 34
androgen, 16, 19
antigen, 40
antitumor, 21
aromatic hydrocarbons, 166
arteries, 170, 190, 206
artery, 173, 184, 195, 201, 211, 217
Asian Americans, 55, 56, 60, 80, 97, 98, 103, 138
assessment, 2, 5, 12, 17, 19, 55, 96, 113, 118, 122, 130, 133, 134, 177
asthma, 153, 168, 197, 213
atherosclerosis, 109, 113, 129, 132, 146, 147, 160, 163
attachment, 170
attitudes, 71, 72, 73, 88, 93
awareness, 88

B

ban, viii, 2
behaviors, 14, 54, 55, 59, 60, 61, 62, 71, 72, 104, 105, 112, 121, 125, 200, 216, 222, 224
benefits, 69, 74, 83
bias, 2, 38, 59, 101, 120, 138, 148, 149, 154
bilirubin, 40
bioassay, 11, 17
biomarkers, vii, 3, 23, 27, 34, 36, 39, 40, 41, 44, 47, 52, 53, 171, 173, 175, 195, 200, 211, 216, 222, 224
Black students, 194, 210
black women, 48
Blacks, 43, 75, 83, 84, 91, 147, 196, 202, 212, 218
bladder cancer, 13, 18
blood, 3, 22, 28, 29, 36, 39, 40, 156, 184, 195, 201, 211, 217

blood flow, 201, 217
blood pressure, 184
blood transfusion, 156
body composition, 37
body mass index (BMI), 4, 6, 38, 39, 115, 148, 149, 150, 151, 152, 153, 173
body weight, 38, 46
bowel, 15, 19
brain, 7
brain activity, 7
brainstem, 170, 189, 205
brand loyalty, 69
breast cancer, 148, 151
breathing, 20, 168
bronchoconstriction, 32
burn, 8, 11, 13, 17, 18
businesses, 87

C

Ca^{2+}, 8, 13, 16, 18, 19, 20, 21, 28, 31, 35, 170
cadmium, 195, 211
calcification, 134, 153
calcium, 8, 21, 170, 190, 206, 221
campaigns, 71, 79
cancer, 4, 8, 12, 13, 15, 16, 21, 22, 28, 29, 35, 48, 62, 64, 139, 140, 148, 149, 150, 151, 152, 154, 155, 157, 158, 159, 160, 161, 163, 183, 200, 202, 204, 216, 218, 220, 223, 224
cancer cells, 12, 21, 28
carbon, 3, 22, 28, 29, 31, 34, 36, 44, 45, 50, 52, 53, 135, 171
carbon monoxide, 3, 22, 28, 29, 31, 34, 36, 44, 45, 50, 52, 53, 135, 171
carcinogen, 47, 52, 53, 174, 187, 195, 200, 211, 216, 221
carcinogenesis, 9, 14, 19
carcinogenicity, 7, 10, 17
carcinoma, 148
cardiovascular disease, 4, 148, 150, 153
career development, 142, 147
case studies, 148
cation, 20
Caucasians, 70, 155
causality, 2, 12
CDC, 6, 69, 70, 188, 199, 204, 215
cell culture, 190, 206
cell cycle, 202, 218, 224
cell death, 8, 12, 13, 18
cell line(s), 8, 13, 15, 16, 18, 19, 167, 170, 201, 218
cell size, 100
Census, 75, 202, 218
cerebellum, 170, 189, 205
cervical cancer, 152
challenges, 168
channel blocker, 169
chemical(s), 7, 10, 12, 14, 15, 17, 18, 21, 22, 26, 36, 40, 168, 170, 203, 220, 224
chemoprevention, 204, 220, 224
chicken, 10
children, vii, 1, 69, 97
China, 13, 18, 28, 35, 190, 206
cholesterol, 40
chromosome, 14, 18
chronic obstructive pulmonary disease, 144, 160, 168
cigarette smoke, 5, 9, 11, 12, 14, 15, 17, 23, 24, 25, 30, 36, 37, 41, 42, 43, 44, 46, 50, 52, 53, 55, 59, 65, 70, 73, 88, 89, 106, 109, 119, 120, 121, 122, 124, 126, 129, 137, 143, 146, 160, 161, 170, 172, 173, 179, 184, 185, 186, 187, 188, 189, 192, 198, 200, 202, 203,205, 208, 214, 216, 218, 219, 221, 223, 224
cigarette smokers, 5, 23, 24, 25, 30, 41, 42, 43, 44, 46, 50, 52, 53, 55, 59, 65, 70, 89, 106, 109, 119, 120, 121, 122, 124, 126, 143, 161, 173, 184, 187, 189, 192, 200, 202, 205, 208, 216, 218, 221, 223, 224
cigarette smoking, vii, 1, 4, 5, 23, 24, 25, 30, 34, 37, 40, 41, 42, 54, 55, 64, 65, 66, 68, 75, 80, 83, 93, 94, 96, 98, 101, 102, 108, 110, 113, 116, 127, 130, 133, 134, 135, 136, 146, 147, 148, 149, 150, 152, 154, 155, 158, 163, 200, 216, 224
city(ies), 28, 35, 92, 96, 148, 151, 152, 158
classification, 154, 166
clean air, 168
clinical trials, 122
colon, 10, 17, 148, 149, 151
colon cancer, 10, 17, 149, 151
combustion, 7
commercial, 22
community(ies), 4, 38, 69, 70, 71, 74, 77, 79, 82, 83, 90, 91, 93, 94, 96, 99, 114, 115, 116, 118, 133, 150, 156, 176, 178, 180, 197, 198, 213, 214, 223
complex interactions, 87
composition, 148
compounds, 170
computation, 134
conference, 151
congestive heart failure, 184
conjugation, 22, 37
constituents, 3, 7, 10, 15, 19, 21, 23, 31, 36, 38, 41, 48, 50, 166, 175
consumer choice, 69
consumer goods, 74
consumers, 70, 74, 76

consumption, viii, 2, 27, 44, 46, 55, 119, 162
content analysis, 76
contextualization, 69
contraband, viii, 2
control group, 168, 171
controlled studies, 41
convergence, 12
cooling, 3, 5, 12, 19, 20, 22, 23, 26, 29, 34, 35, 102, 168, 169, 181, 182, 185, 186, 188
COPD, 6, 44, 52, 153, 184, 197, 213
coronary arteries, 170, 190, 206, 221
coronary artery disease, 116, 134, 153
coronary heart disease, 150, 153
corpus callosum, 170, 189, 205
correlation(s), 4, 37, 192, 208
cosmetic, 19
cotinine, 3, 21, 22, 23, 24, 29, 36, 37, 38, 39, 40, 41, 42, 43, 44, 45, 46, 48, 49, 50, 52, 53, 134, 166, 172, 173, 174, 175, 176, 182, 184, 185, 187, 188, 190, 193, 195, 197, 200, 204, 206, 209, 211, 213, 216, 221, 223
cough, 7, 12, 21, 28, 168, 182, 185, 188, 190, 197, 203, 206, 213, 219, 221, 223, 224
cough reflex, 203, 219, 224
cough suppressant, 21
coughing, 21, 168
counseling, 122
counterirritant, 203, 219
craving, 4, 113, 117, 121, 180
creatinine, 39, 40, 174
cross-sectional study, 36, 38, 55, 97, 115, 118, 137, 143, 150, 172, 173, 175, 178, 180, 182, 199, 200, 215, 216, 223
CSCs, 11
CT, 85, 122, 127, 132
cultural norms, 71
culture, 21
customers, 149
CV, 185, 187
cycles, 172
cytochrome, 196, 212, 223
cytotoxicity, 8, 14, 18, 21, 28, 167, 192, 208

D

data analysis, 100, 118, 120
data collection, 100
data set, 100, 117
database, viii, 7, 165
deaths, 5
decongestant, 7
deficiencies, 126
demographic characteristics, 40, 58, 114, 118, 119, 202, 218, 224
demographic data, 53, 177, 180
demographic factors, 38, 135, 149, 151, 152, 154, 174, 181, 184
Department of Defense, 25, 34
Department of Health and Human Services, vii, 1, 5, 32, 36, 53, 66, 68, 76, 89, 90, 93, 95, 96, 110, 113
depolarization, 13, 21
deposition, 188, 204, 221
depression, 20
depth, 22
derivatives, 20, 28, 34
desensitization, 3, 19, 20, 21, 26, 28, 34
detoxification, 39, 47, 48
diabetes, 184, 202, 218
diet, 48, 161
dilation, 170
direct action, 32, 36
direct measure, 102
discordance, 169
diseases, 4, 10, 27, 141, 149, 184, 223
distress, 175
distribution, 5, 53, 99, 100, 116, 118, 202, 218, 224
District of Columbia, 94, 137
DNA, 7, 28, 35
doctors, 139, 141
dogs, 20, 30, 35
dosage, 45
down-regulation, 19
drawing, viii, 2, 74
drug treatment, 182
drugs, 16, 42
duodenum, 9
dyslipidemia, 184, 202, 218

E

economic status, 6
education, 39, 55, 57, 58, 61, 62, 73, 100, 104, 108, 114, 128, 136, 148, 149, 150, 175, 194, 210
educational attainment, 150, 152, 153
emergency, 4, 153
employees, 54
endocrine, 42
endorsements, 70
England, 221, 223
enrollment, 109, 129, 136, 146, 160
environment, 82, 177
environmental tobacco, 14, 38
enzymes, 128
epidemiologic, 114, 122, 148, 150
epidemiology, 122, 222, 224

epithelial cells, 8, 14, 16
esophageal cancer, 4, 151, 152, 158, 163
esophagus, 152
ethanol, 21, 25, 34
ethnic background, 101, 102, 103
ethnic groups, 53, 65, 68, 79, 80, 92, 96, 97, 102, 110, 113, 115, 116
ethnic minority, 62, 66, 80, 93, 105, 142
ethnicity, 37, 38, 39, 40, 55, 59, 61, 63, 69, 72, 84, 97, 99, 100, 104, 107, 112, 114, 116, 117, 118, 119, 122, 126, 127, 133, 143, 144, 147, 173, 174, 182, 189, 195, 199, 200, 205, 211, 215, 216, 222, 223
EU, 190, 206
evidence, vii, viii, 1, 2, 3, 4, 5, 7, 8, 9, 16, 19, 23, 32, 36, 37, 41, 59, 65, 68, 70, 71, 74, 80, 81, 84, 101, 102, 110, 113, 120, 130, 133, 138, 139, 142, 144, 146, 147, 154, 159, 160, 163, 167, 170, 171, 175, 176, 178, 179, 181, 183, 184
exclusion, 156
excretion, 38
exercise, 73
expenditures, 70, 74
experimental design, 11
exposure, 3, 7, 9, 20, 21, 22, 23, 24, 25, 26, 27, 31, 36, 38, 39, 41, 42, 43, 44, 46, 47, 48, 50, 52, 53, 72, 74, 76, 83, 84, 88, 93, 94, 121, 122, 128, 132, 149, 152, 153, 168, 169, 170, 171, 173, 174, 175, 178, 185, 187, 188, 195, 198, 199, 200, 204, 212, 214, 215, 216, 221, 223
extension strategies, 71

F

false positive, 167
family history, 148, 150
family income, 55, 60, 103, 123, 140
fantasy, 76
Federal Government, 194, 210
feelings, 133
female prisoners, 139, 141
female rat, 11
fibers, 20, 34
fibrinogen, 40
flavor, vii, viii, 1, 2, 11, 13, 17, 19, 108, 166
flavour, 87, 144
flaws, 137, 138
FMC, 82
focus groups, 73, 90
food, 12, 17, 69
food additives, 12, 17
Food and Drug Administration(FDA), vii, viii, 1, 2, 3, 4, 5, 6, 7, 16, 39, 40, 58, 59, 69, 92, 111, 114, 118, 120, 122, 131, 138, 146, 148, 150, 154, 155, 165, 199, 200, 216
force, 118
formation, 7, 21, 25, 34
fruits, 15, 19
funds, 30, 35, 50, 52, 53, 80, 185, 187, 193, 203, 209, 220

G

ganglion, 169, 197, 214, 223
gel, 201, 217
gender differences, 73
gene expression, 21, 28
generalizability, 98, 99, 114, 115, 116, 118, 120, 134, 136, 138, 149, 153, 179
genetic marker, 149
genotype, 49
geography, 92, 96
Georgia, 82, 84, 90, 94, 95, 190, 206
Germany, 151
glossopharyngeal nerve, 27
glycol, 204, 220, 224
grades, 56, 66, 76, 79, 97, 106, 118, 119
grants, 17, 31, 35, 46, 50, 52, 53, 85, 87, 95, 106, 112, 113, 128, 132, 144, 145, 147, 154, 156, 161, 164, 194, 195, 198, 201, 204, 210, 211, 214, 218, 220
growth, 8, 9, 10, 13, 14, 15, 19, 21, 31, 82, 167, 201, 218
Guinea, 28, 29, 30, 32

H

half-life, 37, 41, 42, 44, 172, 185, 188
Hawaii, 71, 84, 94
hazards, 144, 160, 183
HCC, 25, 34
health, vii, 1, 2, 4, 5, 31, 37, 40, 50, 53, 64, 70, 74, 76, 83, 87, 90, 92, 96, 108, 113, 116, 117, 122, 128, 129, 134, 136, 144, 145, 147, 150, 152, 153, 159, 160, 161, 163, 177, 184, 185, 188, 202, 218, 224
Health and Human Services, vii, 1, 6, 66
health condition, 4
health effects, 128, 145, 150
health insurance, 122, 150, 152
health risks, vii, 1, 37, 144, 147, 153, 160, 163
healthfulness, 178
heart attack, 88
hemoglobin, 39
heterogeneity, 195, 211

HHS, vii, 1, 6
high density lipoprotein, 40
high school, 54, 55, 56, 57, 60, 62, 63, 66, 79, 81, 84, 93, 94, 97, 100, 103, 107, 118, 119, 124, 126, 140, 177, 179, 194, 198, 210, 214, 222
high school diploma, 54
Hispanics, vii, 1, 3, 55, 56, 66, 69, 73, 75, 80, 97, 98, 100, 137, 138
history, 27, 28, 37, 44, 133, 149, 155, 173, 178
homeostasis, 16
Hong Kong, 190, 206
host, 161
household income, 71, 150
human, 3, 8, 12, 13, 14, 15, 16, 18, 19, 20, 21, 29, 31, 35, 167, 193, 198, 201, 209, 214, 218
human leukemia cells, 8
human skin, 20
human subjects, 198, 214
hybridization, 16
hydrocarbons, 7
hyperesthesia, 197, 213
hypersensitivity, 168
hypertension, 184, 202, 218
hypothesis, 22, 40, 72, 74, 155

I

image(s), 73, 76
imitation, 69
immigrants, 91
in vitro, 3, 8, 9, 10, 12, 13, 14, 18, 19, 20, 21, 23, 31, 32, 170, 192, 208
in vivo, 3, 9, 13, 18, 19, 20, 21, 23, 32, 204, 220
incidence, 11, 150, 155, 183, 196, 212
income, 39, 54, 57, 61, 91, 92, 100, 104, 114, 175, 194, 202, 210, 218
India, 14, 18
individuals, 61, 88, 98, 104, 108, 115, 117, 124, 129, 138, 140, 142, 153, 194, 210
induction, 13, 28, 167
industry, vii, viii, 1, 2, 5, 7, 9, 14, 22, 32, 36, 40, 69, 70, 71, 72, 74, 76, 82, 85, 86, 91, 92, 93, 95, 96, 101, 102, 107, 108, 112, 151, 181, 182, 185, 188, 204, 220, 221, 224
infection, 168
inferences, 29
ingredients, 8, 10, 11, 14, 17, 18
inhibition, 8, 10, 14, 15, 18, 19, 20, 21, 29, 32, 128, 170, 194, 210
inhibitor, 170
initiation, vii, 1, 4, 5, 14, 54, 61, 62, 68, 72, 79, 81, 86, 93, 95, 96, 98, 100, 101, 102, 103, 104, 105, 106, 107, 112, 119, 178, 179, 191, 198, 199, 207, 214, 215
initiation rates, vii, 1, 96
institutionalized individuals, 62, 105
interaction effect, 200, 216
internal consistency, 129
intervention, 133, 136, 142
intravesical chemotherapy, 13
ion channels, 30, 35, 194, 201, 210, 218, 224
Iowa, 31, 36
ipsilateral, 201, 217
isomers, 190, 206
Israel, 102, 103
issues, 5, 116
Italy, 26, 34

J

Japan, 12, 15, 16, 17, 19, 27, 34, 71, 81, 93, 169
Jews, 103

K

K^+, 20
kidney, 20
Korea, 12, 18

L

large intestine, 9
laryngeal cancer, 183, 196, 212
larynx, 20, 29, 152
Latin America, 87, 95
Latinos, 66, 106, 126, 135, 143
LDL, 6, 40
lead, 7, 21, 53, 137, 143, 148
lean body mass, 37
lesions, 8
leukemia, 9, 10, 13, 15, 17, 18, 19
lifetime, 55, 56, 137, 142, 147, 152, 176, 202, 218
ligand, 170
light, 46, 64, 73, 75, 89, 99, 109, 113, 114, 116, 177, 179, 182, 192, 203, 208, 219, 222
liver, 8, 10, 14, 18, 21, 29, 35, 42, 167
local anesthesia, 7
longitudinal study, 116, 133, 136, 180
long-term customer, 92
lovastatin, 14
low-density lipoprotein, 6
lower prices, 84
loyalty, 69
lumen, 20, 29

lung cancer, 4, 39, 128, 134, 140, 148, 149, 150, 151, 152, 153, 154, 155, 156, 158, 159, 161, 163, 183, 200, 216
lung function, 16, 153
lymphocytes, 14, 167

M

macrophages, 9
magazines, 70, 71, 82, 86, 88, 95
magnitude, 21
mainstream smoke, 11, 17, 161, 166, 172, 188, 193, 204, 209, 222
majority, vii, 1, 3, 31, 50, 59, 66, 69, 90, 99, 114, 116, 117, 118, 190, 206
malignant melanoma, 16
management, 16, 122
manufacturing, 14
marital status, 57, 65, 99, 110, 117, 130
market share, 69, 78, 85, 89, 95, 183
marketing, vii, 3, 69, 70, 71, 72, 74, 76, 79, 80, 81, 82, 83, 84, 85, 86, 87, 90, 91, 92, 93, 94, 95, 96, 102, 176, 178, 202, 218, 224
marketing mix, 3, 70, 74, 82, 94
marketing strategy, 70, 71
marketplace, vii, 2
mass, 4, 166, 188, 204, 220
materials, viii, 2
matter, 7, 166, 199, 215, 223
MB, 11, 17, 87, 88, 95, 106, 112, 121, 122, 125, 126, 132, 139, 141, 143, 147, 191, 207
measurement(s), 39, 40, 166, 170, 171
media, 80, 90, 91, 93, 95
median, 22, 40, 115
medical, vii, 1, 74, 122
medication, 45, 134, 135
medicine, 222, 223
melanoma, 10, 15, 16, 17, 19, 155
mellitus, 184
membership, 142
membranes, 8, 10
messages, 74, 91, 96
meta-analysis, 151
Metabolic, 21, 47
metabolism, 3, 21, 22, 23, 25, 29, 34, 37, 38, 41, 42, 44, 45, 46, 47, 48, 52, 170, 172, 175, 224
metabolites, 3, 36, 38, 47, 52
methodology, viii, 165
metropolitan areas, 54
Miami, 139, 142
mice, 9, 11, 12, 17, 21, 203, 219
micrograms, 28
micronucleus, 167
microscopy, 25
Ministry of Education, 12, 15, 16, 18, 19, 27, 34
Minneapolis, 142
minorities, vii, 1, 100
minority groups, 3, 54, 59
Missouri, 76, 93, 129, 132
mitochondria, 8, 10
model system, 10
models, 3, 19, 40, 71, 88, 95, 114, 118, 198, 214
moderates, 199, 215, 223
molecules, 170, 194, 210
monoterpenoids, 14, 19
morbidity, 53
mortality, 53, 136, 141, 150, 153, 155, 183, 200, 216, 223, 224
mortality risk, 200, 216, 223
MR, 28, 29, 34, 35, 45, 90, 154, 156, 195, 211
mucosa, 21, 25, 31, 36, 167, 168
multidimensional, 129, 130, 133
multivariate analysis, 150
muscle contraction, 201, 217
muscle strength, 201, 217
music, 82
mustard oil, 169
mutant, 28
myocardial infarction, 184

N

National Health and Nutrition Examination Survey (NHANES), 6, 38, 40, 43, 44, 52, 58, 59, 61, 104, 111, 113, 124, 131, 133, 140, 157, 162, 164, 166, 173, 174, 176, 184, 190, 195, 199, 202, 206, 211, 215, 216, 218, 222
National Institute of Mental Health, 14, 18
National Institutes of Health, 15, 19, 25, 27, 30, 31, 34, 35, 41, 42, 47, 49, 52, 53, 85, 108, 109, 113, 121, 122, 129, 132, 144, 147, 154, 155, 160, 163
national strategy, 70
National Survey, 6, 58, 64, 65, 70, 89, 108, 110, 113, 175, 194, 210, 222
NDI, 6
nerve, 20, 27
neuroblastoma, 21, 31, 35
neurokinin, 32, 36
neurons, 27, 169, 193, 209, 222
neuropathic pain, 30
neuropsychopharmacology, 221
neuroscience, 222
New England, 90
New Zealand, 177, 178, 203, 219, 224
nicotine, 3, 4, 5, 7, 14, 19, 21, 22, 23, 24, 25, 26, 29, 30, 31, 34, 35, 36, 37, 38, 39, 40, 41, 42, 43, 44,

45, 46, 49, 50, 52, 53, 54, 55, 63, 87, 88, 98, 106, 107, 111, 113, 114, 116, 117, 118, 119, 120, 121, 122, 126, 127, 128, 130, 131, 132, 133, 139, 142, 144, 147, 162, 164, 166, 169, 170, 172, 173, 174, 180, 181, 185, 186, 187, 188, 190, 193, 198, 200, 204, 206, 209, 214, 216, 220, 221, 224
nitrosamines, 3, 19, 166
nonsmokers, 14, 43, 73, 88, 91, 150, 168, 197, 203, 213, 219

O

OAS, 70
obstruction, 136, 150, 153
oesophageal, 158, 163
oil, 169
old age, 97, 100
oral cavity, 152
outpatient, 106, 125, 126, 141, 143
oxidation, 21, 29, 35

P

Pacific, 54, 55, 59, 60, 66, 91, 92, 97, 102, 103, 175, 177, 194, 203, 210, 219
Pacific Islanders, 54, 55, 66, 175, 194, 210
pain, 12, 168, 182, 185, 188, 197, 213
pairing, 99
Pakistan, 35
palliative, 101
pancreatic cancer, 152
parallel, 31
parents, 102, 177
participants, 20, 22, 23, 37, 38, 39, 41, 44, 46, 48, 58, 71, 73, 74, 90, 97, 98, 99, 114, 134, 137, 140, 148, 150, 153, 157, 168, 169, 170, 174, 175, 178, 179, 180, 188, 195, 198, 199, 200, 203, 204, 211, 214, 215, 216, 220
peripheral blood, 14, 167
permeability, 8, 167
permeation, 25, 204, 220, 224
PET scan, 170, 180
pharmaceutics, 224
pharmacokinetics, 43, 172, 185, 187, 221
pharmacology, 23, 24, 221, 222, 223, 224
pharmacotherapy, 182
pharynx, 151
phenotypes, 47
Philadelphia, 154
photographs, 86
physicians, 70, 156
physiology, vii, 222
pigs, 20, 21, 27, 28, 32, 35
placebo, 99, 114, 134, 135, 143, 182
plasma levels, 172
plasma membrane, 14, 18
platform, 70
platinum, 10
Poland, 169
policy, 19, 53, 90
policy makers, 53
population, 2, 3, 4, 10, 12, 14, 16, 24, 26, 28, 30, 32, 42, 44, 46, 48, 50, 54, 55, 57, 58, 60, 62, 64, 65, 66, 68, 71, 73, 75, 76, 78, 80, 81, 82, 84, 86, 88, 89, 90, 92, 97, 102, 103, 104, 106, 108, 110, 113, 114, 115, 116, 118, 122, 124, 126, 128, 130, 133, 134,136, 137, 140, 142, 144, 146, 147, 148, 149, 152, 153, 155, 156, 157, 158, 160, 161, 162, 179, 180, 202, 218, 224
population group, 103
positive correlation, 37
poverty, 38, 177, 202, 218
poverty line, 177
predictive validity, 114, 122
prefrontal cortex, 170
pregnancy, 182, 199, 215
preparation, 12, 167, 204, 220
President, 66, 68
prevention, 66, 91, 144, 150, 160, 222, 224
prisoners, 138
private schools, 55, 56, 97, 118, 119
probability, 162
probe, 30
product design, 86
professionals, 53
project, 12, 18, 177
proliferation, 8, 15, 19, 167, 202, 218, 224
propane, 10
propylene, 204, 220, 224
prostate cancer, 12, 16, 18, 19, 30
psychological distress, 175, 194, 210, 222
psychotropic medications, 175
public assistance, 177
public health, vii, viii, 1, 2, 5, 19, 53, 96, 133, 165, 223, 224
pulmonary diseases, 202, 218, 224
pulmonary function test, 134, 153
pyrolysis, 7, 10, 15, 19

Q

questionnaire, 48, 157

R

race, 7, 36, 37, 38, 39, 40, 43, 46, 50, 52, 55, 57, 59, 61, 63, 65, 69, 72, 73, 84, 86, 97, 99, 100, 104, 107, 110, 112, 114, 115, 116, 117, 118, 119, 122, 126, 127, 130, 133, 136, 142, 143, 144, 147, 148, 149, 150, 152, 153, 167, 173, 174, 178, 180, 181, 182, 183, 189, 195, 197, 199, 200, 205, 211, 212, 213, 216, 222
racial differences, 29, 36, 39, 48
radio, 69
radiotherapy, 156
rating scale, 189, 205
reactivity, 7
readership, 70
reality, 74
recall, 101, 120
receptors, 3, 8, 15, 19, 20, 21, 29, 30, 35, 167, 169, 170, 189, 193, 205, 209, 221
recognition, 177, 178, 191, 207, 222
recommendations, vii, 2
recovery, 26
recruiting, 85
regression, 37, 39, 40, 50, 63, 107, 119, 126, 135, 158, 198, 214
regression analysis, 40
regression line, 198, 214
regression model, 37, 39, 50, 63, 107, 126
relaxation, 20
relevance, viii, 2, 9
reliability, 54, 56
relief, 7, 12, 185, 188
requirements, 182
researchers, vii, 1, 9, 19, 59, 72, 74, 100, 119, 120, 135, 136, 148, 149, 152, 153, 166, 168, 170, 173, 180
resistance, 168, 198, 214, 223
respiration, 198, 214
response, 20, 21, 29, 53, 55, 58, 60, 80, 97, 103, 114, 118, 119, 137, 149, 167, 168, 169, 170, 182, 190, 204, 206, 220, 221
responsiveness, 20, 21
restrictions, vii, 1, 5, 55, 116, 117, 175, 191, 207
retail, 71, 82, 84, 176
risk(s), vii, viii, 2, 3, 4, 5, 12, 21, 31, 39, 46, 48, 50, 62, 69, 73, 74, 80, 88, 90, 91, 95, 116, 120, 128, 130, 133, 134, 139, 140, 144, 145, 148, 149, 150, 151, 152, 153, 154, 155, 156, 158, 159, 161, 163, 176, 180, 183, 184, 196, 212
risk factors, 116, 134, 150, 152, 153, 184
risk perception, 74, 90, 95, 180
rodents, 26
room temperature, 20
root, 169, 197, 213, 214, 223
rules, 116

S

saliva, 3, 36
sample design, 63, 106, 119
sample survey, 162
schizophrenia, 36, 37, 50, 53
school, 55, 56, 60, 63, 76, 79, 80, 83, 84, 85, 91, 97, 100, 103, 105, 107, 116, 118, 119, 124, 126, 140, 179, 198, 214
school performance, 83
science, vii, viii, 2, 133, 184
scientific papers, 7
secondary data, 40, 100, 101, 102, 113, 115, 117, 118, 119, 120, 150, 152, 153
secondary schools, 85
Section 907, vii, 1
selectivity, 30
self-reports, 60, 103, 123, 140
sensation(s), 19, 21, 23, 73, 108, 168, 169
senses, 222
sensitivity, 10, 14, 21, 74, 89, 116, 117, 168, 170, 197, 203, 204, 213, 219, 220, 223, 224
sensory experience, 101
serum, 23, 36, 37, 38, 39, 40, 41, 43, 44, 48, 49, 50, 52, 53, 134, 173, 174, 175, 184, 190, 195, 200, 206, 211, 216, 221
services, 179, 191, 207
SES, 3, 6, 114, 118
sex, 11, 38, 40, 65, 110, 115, 130, 135, 136, 148, 149, 150, 152, 153, 183, 195, 212
showing, 7, 40
sidestream smoke, 8, 11, 17
signs, 5, 153
sister chromatid exchange, 7, 12, 14, 18
skin, 9, 11, 17, 155
smoke exposure, 11, 23, 24, 27, 34, 36, 41, 42, 44, 52
smoking cessation, 4, 45, 54, 68, 98, 99, 106, 109, 112, 113, 114, 115, 116, 122, 126, 127, 128, 130, 132, 133, 134, 135, 136, 138, 139, 141, 143, 144, 145, 146, 147, 150, 153, 160, 163, 175, 179, 181, 182, 183, 185, 188, 192, 208, 221
smooth muscle, 20, 27, 32, 34, 36, 170, 190, 206
social change, 81
socioeconomic status, 3, 53, 101, 118, 151
solution, 21, 203, 219
special education, 55
spleen, 9, 13
SS, 13, 18, 129, 132, 139, 140, 142, 147, 154, 155
stabilization, 170, 194, 210

state(s), 30, 31, 50, 76, 85, 168, 170, 176, 185, 187, 191, 194, 198, 207, 210, 214
stimulant, 20, 30
stimulation, 20, 167, 168, 169, 198, 201, 214, 218
stimulus, 21, 30
stoichiometry, 170, 194, 210, 222
stress, 198, 214, 223
stroke, 184, 202, 218
structure, 17, 129
style, 172, 198, 214
subgroups, 106, 126, 133, 143, 151, 152, 182
subscribers, 157
substance abuse, 45
success rate, 139, 141
survival, 16, 19, 167
survivors, 149
susceptibility, 83, 94
Sweden, 126, 132, 197, 213
symptoms, 14, 62, 119, 122, 197, 213
syndrome, 130, 133
synthesis, 8

T

Taiwan, 13, 18, 28, 35
tar, 22, 32, 39, 87, 114, 118, 169, 172, 177, 181, 186, 187, 188, 200, 204, 216, 220, 221
target, 11, 16, 70, 71, 75, 91, 122, 166, 169, 177, 186, 188, 193, 209
teens, 56, 69, 72
telephone, 54, 91, 99, 114, 116, 117, 124, 133, 202, 203, 218, 219
television commercial, 69
temperature, 20
terpenes, 8, 14
territory, 55, 64, 108, 127
testing, 13, 18, 21, 107, 167, 192, 208
thalamus, 170
therapeutic benefits, 12
therapeutics, 224
therapy, 30, 46, 142, 147
threats, 2
threshold level, 30
tissue, 21, 25, 31, 34, 167, 190, 204, 206, 220
tobacco smoke, 3, 19, 23, 38, 40, 46, 48, 128, 132, 167, 168, 171
tobacco smoking, 92
total cholesterol, 40
toxicity, 3, 9, 10, 11, 12, 17, 166, 167
toxicology, vii, 7, 9, 11, 17, 221, 222, 223
toxicology studies, 11, 17
toys, 84
trachea, 10
tracks, 102
trade, 82
training, 14, 18
trajectory, 70
transformation, 138
transport, 12
treatment, 30, 38, 46, 99, 106, 112, 114, 116, 117, 120, 121, 122, 124, 125, 126, 127, 128, 132, 134, 135, 136, 139, 141, 143, 145, 147, 170, 178, 182, 191, 192, 207, 208, 221
trial, 4, 12, 36, 38, 46, 99, 115, 116, 117, 122, 128, 133, 134, 135, 136, 139, 141, 143, 144, 145, 147, 160, 182, 192, 199, 208, 215, 222
trigeminal nerve, 169, 181, 204, 220
triglycerides, 40
Trinidad, 54, 58, 66, 68, 92, 96
tumor(s), 8, 9, 14, 16, 18
tumor cells, 14, 18
tumor progression, 16
Turkey, 197, 213

U

uninsured, 175, 194, 210
United Kingdom (UK), 28, 35, 115, 139, 141, 153, 192, 208
United States (USA), vii, viii, 1, 2, 5, 15, 16, 19, 31, 53, 59, 60, 62, 64, 65, 68, 72, 77, 78, 80, 82, 84, 89, 91, 93, 94, 96, 99, 100, 102, 103, 104, 105, 108, 110, 112, 113, 115, 117, 121, 122, 123, 124, 127, 130, 132, 139, 140, 144, 147, 149, 153, 157, 163, 196, 198, 212, 214, 223
universities, 10, 17
urban, 4, 71, 74, 82, 114, 116
urinary tract, 152
urine, 3, 36, 39, 40, 172, 173, 174
US Department of Health and Human Services, 113

V

validation, 57, 93, 154, 156
vapor, 168, 203, 220, 224
variables, 39, 40, 46, 49, 99, 115, 117, 134, 135, 136, 137
variations, 72
varieties, 62, 64, 89
vegetables, 15, 19
ventilation, 20, 29, 30, 35, 154
volatile organic compounds, 166
voting, viii, 2

W

waking, 4, 6, 62, 105, 113, 114, 115, 120, 122, 125, 135, 179, 180, 199, 215
walking, 177, 194, 210
weakness, 148
wellness, 4
white blood cells, 40
Wisconsin, 114, 129, 132
withdrawal, 122
workers, 54

Y

yield, 22, 27, 44, 73, 161, 172, 186, 188
young adults, 4, 5, 58, 66, 68, 73, 79, 91, 92, 96, 107, 110, 112, 113, 175, 194, 202, 210, 218, 224
young women, 81